AF771834

Enhancing Behavioral Health in Latino Populations

Lorraine T. Benuto • William O'Donohue
Editors

Enhancing Behavioral Health in Latino Populations

Reducing Disparities Through Integrated Behavioral and Primary Care

Springer

Editors
Lorraine T. Benuto
Department of Psychology
University of Nevada
Reno, NV, USA

William O'Donohue
Department of Psychology
University of Nevada
Reno, NV, USA

ISBN 978-3-319-42531-3 ISBN 978-3-319-42533-7 (eBook)
DOI 10.1007/978-3-319-42533-7

Library of Congress Control Number: 2016953115

© Springer International Publishing Switzerland 2016
This work is subject to copyright. All rights are reserved by the Publisher, whether the whole or part of the material is concerned, specifically the rights of translation, reprinting, reuse of illustrations, recitation, broadcasting, reproduction on microfilms or in any other physical way, and transmission or information storage and retrieval, electronic adaptation, computer software, or by similar or dissimilar methodology now known or hereafter developed.
The use of general descriptive names, registered names, trademarks, service marks, etc. in this publication does not imply, even in the absence of a specific statement, that such names are exempt from the relevant protective laws and regulations and therefore free for general use.
The publisher, the authors and the editors are safe to assume that the advice and information in this book are believed to be true and accurate at the date of publication. Neither the publisher nor the authors or the editors give a warranty, express or implied, with respect to the material contained herein or for any errors or omissions that may have been made.

Printed on acid-free paper

This Springer imprint is published by Springer Nature
The registered company is Springer International Publishing AG
The registered company address is: Gewerbestrasse 11, 6330 Cham, Switzerland

Para William O'Donohue y Jane Fisher, por ser excelentes mentores. ¡Mil gracias!

-L.T.B.

To George Will, Thomas Sowell, Milton Friedman, and Karl Popper who helped me think for clearly about important social issues

-W.T.O.

Contents

Chapter 1
Integrated Care: A Potential Solution to Behavioral Health Disparities Among Latinos

Lorraine T. Benuto and William O'Donohue

Introduction: A Potential Solution to Behavioral Health Disparities Among Latinos

Latinos in the United States

Latinos constitute the largest minority group in the United States making up approximately 16 % of the total US population (U.S. Census Bureau, 2010). The Center for Disease Control defines Latinos and Hispanics as peoples of "Cuban, Mexican, Puerto Rican, South or Central American, or other Spanish culture or origin, regardless of race." In addition to nationality, there is substantial heterogeneity among Latinos with regard to immigrant status, English-language fluency, and acculturation, socioeconomic level, among other factors.

In the United States, persons of Mexican origin comprise the largest proportion of Latinos (almost two-thirds), with the remaining third distributed primarily among persons of Puerto Rican, Cuban, and Central American origin (U.S. Census Bureau, 2010). With regard to immigrant status, of the 55 million people in 2014 who identified themselves as of Hispanic or Latino origin, 35 % (19.4 million) were recent immigrants (U.S. Census Bureau, 2010). This constitutes about 6 % of the total US population. The other two-thirds of Latinos (64 %) living in the United Sates were born in the U.S. (Zong & Batalova, 2016). Given the high number of Latino immigrants in the United States, it is not surprising that a large portion of Latinos aren't fluent in English. Approximately 78 % of Latinos aged 5 and older speak Spanish as their primary language in the home (Weil, 2010), and less than half of Latino

L.T. Benuto, Ph.D. (✉) • W. O'Donohue, Ph.D.
Department of Psychology, University of Nevada, Reno, NV 89557, USA
e-mail: dr.benuto@gmail.com

© Springer International Publishing Switzerland 2016

L.T. Benuto, W. O'Donohue (eds.), *Enhancing Behavioral Health in Latino Populations*, DOI 10.1007/978-3-319-42533-7_1

immigrants residing in the United States have *even* limited English-language proficiency (Patten, 2012). In addition to the above, acculturation level is also a relevant factor that contributes to the heterogeneity of the Latino population in the United States.

Contemporary Issues in the Latino Community

Benuto (2017) summarized the contemporary issues that Latinos face. These include issues related to cultural self-identification, acculturation level, immigration status, discrimination, English-language proficiency, and poverty. With regard to cultural self-identification and acculturation, ethnic identity can be a key component of psychosocial development and it may serve as a resource for people who experience discrimination or inequitable treatment (Brittian, Umaña-Taylor, & Derlan, 2013) and self-identity is relevant to acculturation. Acculturation is characterized by adaptation to the host culture, maintenance of the cultural practices and values of coulter or origin, or a combination of both (Berry, 2005). Latinos and other ethnic minority groups may experience a phenomenon known as acculturative stress, which is a stress reaction to the life events that are related to the acculturation process (Berry, 2005). Prevalence of mental health conditions also have been noted to be related to acculturation level. Specifically Latinos who were born in the United States have higher rates of mental health disorders (Alegría et al., 2008) and because acculturation may result in added stressors or maladaptive coping and a loss of indigenous protective factors (Alamilla, Kim, & Lam, 2010), it has been suggested that the acculturation process and acculturative stress may play a role in the development and/or maintenance of mental health conditions. This needs to be studied more.

Arguably the biggest issue that Latinos face is related to immigration status (Benuto, 2017). There are over five million undocumented Latinos in the United States (Krogstad & Passel, 2015) and undocumented Latinos have a diverse range of experiences with regard to how they arrived in United States, how their immigration status impacts their day-to-day lives, and how their immigration status affects their overall functioning in the United States. Indeed, Latinos may have suffered when crossing of the border and likely had to leave key family members behind. Moreover, working as an undocumented immigrant can be dangerous and demoralizing experience as undocumented workers may be subject to abuse and exposure to occupational hazards because of their undocumented status (Arellano-Morales, Liang, Ruiz, & Rios-Oropeza et al. 2016). Documented Latinos may also face issues including worries and concerns about their undocumented parents as well as racism and discrimination. Indeed, regardless of legal status, the chronic experience of racism is a risk factor in the development for depression, isolation, and psychological distress (Arellano-Morales et al., 2016).

Lack of English-language proficiency can also pose a significant problem for Latinos. Because less than half of Latino immigrants residing in the United States have *even* limited English-language proficiency (Patten, 2012), many Latinos face language barriers that make it challenging for Latinos to access healthcare, impacts their ability to be employed, and can impact how others perceive and treat them (Benuto, 2017). Finally, Latinos are disproportionately impacted by poverty and have lower household income than Whites in this country (Feeding America, n.d.). This indicates that Latinos may live in substandard housing, have inadequate nutrition, live in unsafe neighborhoods, and attend under-resourced schools (American Psychological Association, 2016). There is also extensive documentation that Latinos experience barriers to accessing healthcare and the majority of these barriers are related to socioeconomic status (Benuto & Leany, 2011). However, because there is so much heterogeneity in the broad classification of "Latinos" it is also important to say that none of the above may be true: Latinos also comprise middle- and upper-class socioeconomic strata and enjoy all the benefits associated with this.

The Behavioral Health of Latinos

With regard to prevalence rates of mental health disorders among Latinos, in the most comprehensive study of Hispanics/Latinos of different national backgrounds conducted to date (the HCHS/SOL), the prevalence of depression among Latinos was found to 27 % and while the authors did look at anxiety they did not provide an actual prevalence rate but indicated that the rates were similar for anxiety (Wassertheil-Smoller et al., 2014). While this is not higher than what is seen with non-Latinos, this does suggest that, similarly, a large number of Latinos experience depression and anxiety. This study also found that factors such as US-born status was related to prevalence rate with US-born Latinos having higher rates of depression and anxiety than foreign-born Latinos and this highlights some of the intricacies that can be seen with this group. In fact, across the board US-born Latinos experience higher rates of depression, anxiety disorders, and substance use disorders (Alegría et al., 2008). Alegria and colleagues have also noted that lifetime prevalence rates of mental health disorders vary by country of origin with Puerto Ricans experiencing the highest lifetime disorder rate (37.4 %), followed by Mexicans (29.5 %), Cubans (28.2 %) and other Latinos (27 %).

Challenges in Accessing Behavioral Health Services

Latinos experience a number of barriers to accessing behavioral health care, many of which are related to socioeconomic status. Benuto and Leany (2011) have summarized these as consisting of lack of transportation, long waits, inflexible hours, distance between the home and treatment location, lack of health insurance, cost, language, and stigma surrounding the use of mental health disorders. The bulk of the literature on addressing the needs of Latinos is focused on the application of culturally adapted service delivery.

Over the last several decades, two parallel movements have been at play in the field of clinical psychology: the movement toward the use of evidence-based interventions and the cultural sensitivity movement. Indeed, the field of clinical psychology is currently oriented towards evidence-based practice (e.g., Chambless & Ollendick, 2001) and increasingly clients are delivered empirically supported treatments (ESTs: Chambless & Ollendick, 2001). Benuto and O'Donohue (2015) discussed how the focus on ESTs is consistent with the Affordable Care Act, which emphasizes efficient, effective health care interventions in an attempt to improve safety, costs, and outcomes (Wendel, O'Donohue, & Serratt, 2013). With regard to the push towards the provision of culturally sensitive services, the extent to which ESTs generalize to ethnic minority clients has been questioned. Specifically some have alleged that ethnic minorities are underrepresented in the original outcome research (Bernal & Scharró-del-Río, 2001), the majority culture values and assumptions are exclusively represented in these therapies (Benish, Quintana, & Wampold, 2011), and the dependent measures used to assess the outcomes of these therapies were not validated on ethnic minority clients (Cardemil, 2010).

Given these two parallel movements, Benuto and O'Donohue (2015) reviewed the literature to determine what "culturally sensitive" interventions (whereby "culturally sensitive" was defined as any study that included a specific focus on the cultural group of interest) could be considered well-established, beneficial treatments for use with Latinos. They noted that while there are several hundred publications on the general issues related to Latinos and cultural sensitivity, there were only 12 peer-reviewed articles that evaluated empirically supported treatments for the mental health disorders most commonly diagnosed among this population. Benuto and O'Donohue noted that these 12 studies had significant methodological limitations and few employed the "gold standard" designs associated with randomized clinical trials. From this review Benuto and O'Donohue concluded that there is evidence that Latinos may be effectively treated using conventional cognitive behavioral therapy (perhaps translated into Spanish) and that there is little evidence that cultural adaptations result in consistently improved effect sizes. In addition, they noted that the cultural adaptation process was quite variable with different assumptions and assertions across studies regarding what constituted Latino culture. Thus while the majority of the literature has focused on the delivery of culturally sensitivity interventions, there is little empirical support to suggest that such an approach is necessary. However, the barriers to behavioral health services that Latinos experience are substantial and well documented. Thus, it is necessary that a means to address these barriers be established. One possible solution is integrated care.

Integrated Care as a Potential Solution for Latinos

Integrated care is a mechanism of delivering care that attempts to make service delivery more efficient, effective, and client-centered. The basic idea is to collocate and coordinate behavioral health care in a medical setting, particularly primary care.

This allows "one stop" care where both the physical health needs and behavioral health needs can be identified and treated. Part of the rationale for this is that patients' bodies and minds are interconnected and as such cannot be cleanly parsed and treated in two distinct and usually uncoordinated treatment centers. For example, diabetes often has behavioral health components such as comorbid depression, treatment compliance issues, and lifestyle change issues. A coordinated team of medical and behavioral health providers in one treatment center can provide more efficient and effective care than siloed specialty care. In addition, the goals of primary care are not to miss behavioral health problems sand create medical errors in the medical setting as well as to provide prevention services. Interestingly the goals of integrated care match nicely to the needs of Latinos.

Integrated care fits with the needs of Latinos in several ways. First, integrated care is more comprehensive. Specifically, integrated care offers a comprehensive and team-based approach to care so that the patient can have both physical and behavioral healthcare needs met in a single location. It is well documented that Latinos have high-comorbidity between mental health disorders and physical conditions (Sin, 2012). For example, comorbid depression and anxiety and heart disease among Latinos it is well documented in the literature (Wassertheil-Smoller et al., 2014). Given the high comorbidity that Latinos experience, providing comprehensive care in a single location is ideal. Moreover, given the barriers to care that Latinos experience, proving care in a single location can help alleviate some of the challenges Latinos experience in terms of physically accessing care.

Second, integrated care is patient-centered. Patient-centered care places the patient and their families as core members of the care team and actively involves them in treatment planning. Latino culture tends to be focused on the nuclear and extended family (Smith, 2000) so including families as members of the treatment team is consistent with Latino cultural values. Third, integrated care is coordinated across the healthcare system. Given the barriers that Latinos face in accessing care, having care coordinated is critical to removing the barriers that Latinos face in accessing treatment. Lastly, integrated care is accessible. For example in patient-centered medical homes care settings there are enhanced in-person hours so that patients have access to more hours of service. Because issues of access are one of the most pressing issues that Latinos face, flexibility is key.

The Unmet Research Agenda

There is an evidential burden that must be met both with respect to integrated care in general and integrated care with Latino populations. Integrated care delivery models must be evaluated to see to what extent they actually represent a solution to problems encountered by Latinos. The promise of integrated care is just that: a promise and this delivery model must be evaluated in each setting in which it is implemented to actually determine the extent to which this promise is met.

There are reasons to be only cautiously optimistic. Integrated care does not solve the workforce problem in behavioral health but may in fact exacerbate it (O'Donohue & Maragakis, 2016). There are still too few behavioral health professionals with skills in integrated care service delivery and fewer who have these skills and can deliver services in Spanish. This is a key problem in workforce development that there is too little work is done either in a strategic vision or in practical implementation. Also there is the question raised earlier of what cultural adaptations for what problems for what kind of patients need to be developed and evaluated. There is too little research addressing this question for Latinos in the integrated care service model. Of course this question is made more complex by the diverse number of cultural minorities that may present in integrated care. The same lack of evidence is found in screens and other assessment devices for Latinos in integrated care. Similarly, as one of the goals of integrated care is prevention, more prevention research is needed with Latinos in integrated care.

The major problem is that for some integrated care is seen by some as such a "good idea" (as compared to fractionated care)—that too little concern has been placed on the question of demonstrated quality in integrated care. Too many integrated care service delivery settings for any populations hire professionals untrained in integrated care, do not clearly and properly define clinical and operational pathways; do not train medical personnel to work as part of an integrated care team, do not train support staff, do not use appropriate screens, do not utilize psychometrically proper follow up assessment, do not use evidence based treatments, do not use a step care approach, do not properly treat the full range of behavior health problems, do not properly coordinate interventions with the medical teams, do not deliver prevention when called for, miss intervening with important problems like smoking and obesity, do not have the behavioral health provider sufficiently productive, do not show cost reductions, and do not utilize quality improvement procedures to measure and improve key aspects of the integrative efforts. These are many of the problems that also can be found in specialty care in traditional mental health. It is unfortunate and will limit or doom the integrated care movement if the same or similar weaknesses found in traditional mental health also find a place in "new" integrated care settings (see O'Donohue & Maragakis, 2016 for an extended treatment of quality improvement tools in integrated care). Thus, we recommend highly that any integrated care program oriented toward Latinos orient toward these quality issues and not just assume that because the label of "integrated care" is being applied that the program is good.

It is useful to evaluate any program on several quality improvement indices including these 14:

1. Patient satisfaction
2. Physician satisfaction
3. Clinical improvement
4. Use of integrated care interventions vs. Specialty care
5. Medical cost offset
6. Kinds of problems addressed

7. Use of evidence based assessments and interventions
8. Proper use of behavioral health screens
9. Productivity of behavioral health staff
10. Appropriate documentation
11. Prevention
12. Appropriate referrals
13. Comprehensive care
14. Coordination of care

We recommend a quarterly quality improvement report where each of these dimensions is measured and strategies are used to make continual improvements in these.

Summary and Organization of the Book

In sum, integrated care is perfectly positioned to solve many of the issues that Latinos face with regard to behavioral health care. There is some limited research on using integrated care with this population---Bridges and colleagues (2014) found that both non-Latino whites and Latinos had comparable utilization rates and comparable and clinically significant improvements in symptoms when they accessed integrated care. Latinos also expressed high satisfaction with integrated behavioral services. These data provide preliminary evidence suggesting that the integration of behavioral health services into primary care clinics may help reduce mental health disparities for Latinos.

While the field is shifting rapidly towards an integrated care model, discussions on cultural factors and how they interplay with integrated care are largely lacking. This book attempts to fill this gap and provides practical and easy to use solutions to the issues that the behavioral health care specialist is likely to encounter when working with Latinos in a primary care setting. The health disparities among Latinos are vast and this text provides culturally relevant recommendations that could ultimately lead to a reduction in these disparities.

The book is organized so that there are several chapters dedicated to a discussion on working with Latinos who might present with variable circumstances (i.e., immigrants have characteristics and experiences that are fairly distinct from non-immigrants, Cubans and Puerto Ricans both have distinct histories given the relationship with the United States and Cuba and Puerto Rico—thus there are specific chapters on these special populations). Because there are financial elements to healthcare, there is a specialty chapter on community health centers and payment for integrated care. Similarly given recent legislation that has changed the health care system, we also included a chapter on health policy. Finally, there are chapters that focus on the major mental health conditions that are likely to present in an integrated care setting (including presentations such as chronic disease that have important behavioral health implications). Each of these chapters includes recommendations for screening instruments that can be administered to this population in an integrated care setting; how the issue in question (e.g., depression, chronic disease) might present in an integrated care setting; what transpires are the hallway hand-off occurs (i.e., in a primary care setting or patient-centered medical home) and the person is placed in the care of the behavioral healthcare specialist; stepped-care options for the behavioral healthcare specialist; how cultural considerations can be made and applied to evidence-based interventions in an integrated care setting; and how behavioral health care specialists can work in concert with medical professionals to improve the health of Latinos in this country.

References

Alamilla, S. G., Kim, B. S. K., & Lam, N. A. (2010). Acculturation, enculturation, perceived racism, minority status stressors, and psychological symptomatology among Latino/as. *Hispanic Journal of Behavioral Sciences, 32*(1), 55–76. doi:10.1177/0739986309352770.

Alegría, M., Canino, G., Shrout, P. E., Woo, M., Duan, N., Vila, D., … Meng, X. (2008). Prevalence of mental illness in immigrant and non-immigrant U.S. Latino groups. *The American Journal of Psychiatry, 165(3)*, 359–369. doi:10.1176/appi.ajp.2007.07040704.

Arellano-Morales, L., Liang, C. H., Ruiz, L., & Rios-Oropeza, E. (2016). Perceived racism, gender role conflict, and life satisfaction among Latino day laborers. *Journal of Latina/o Psychology, 4*(1), 32–42. doi:10.1037/lat0000049.

Benish, S. G., Quintana, S., & Wampold, B. E. (2011). Culturally adapted psychotherapy and the legitimacy of myth: A direct-comparison meta-analysis. *Journal of Counseling Psychology, 58*(3), 279.

Benuto, L. (2017). Contemporary Issues in Latino Communities. In C. Frisby & W.T. O'Donohue (Eds.). Handbook of Cultural Diversity. New York, NY: Springer.

Benuto, L., & Leany, B. D. (2011). Reforms for ethnic minorities and women. In *Understanding the behavioral healthcare crisis: The promise of integrated care and diagnostic reform* (pp. 367–394). New York, NY: Routledge.

Benuto, L. T., & O'Donohue, W. (2015). Is culturally sensitive cognitive behavioral therapy an empirically supported treatment?: The case for Hispanics. *International Journal of Psychology & Psychological Therapy, 15*(3), 405.

Bernal, G., & Scharró-del-Río, M. R. (2001). Are empirically supported treatments valid for ethnic minorities? Toward an alternative approach for treatment research. *Cultural Diversity and Ethnic Minority Psychology, 7*(4), 328.

Berry, J. W. (2005). Acculturation: Living successfully in two cultures. *International Journal of Intercultural Relations, 29*, 697–712. doi:10.1016/j.ijintrel.2005.07.013.

Bridges, A. J., Andrews, A. R., III, Pastrana, F. A., Villalobos, B. T., Cavell, T. A., & Gomez, D. (2014). Does integrated behavioral health care reduce mental health disparities for Hispanics? Initial findings. *Journal of Latina/o Psychology, 2*, 37–53.

Brittian, A. S., Umaña-Taylor, A. J., & Derlan, C. L. (2013). An examination of biracial college youths' family ethnic socialization, ethnic identity, and adjustment: Do self-identification labels and university context matter? *Cultural Diversity and Ethnic Minority Psychology, 19*(2), 177–189. doi:10.1037/a0029438.

Cardemil, E. V. (2010). Cultural adaptations to empirically supported treatments: A research agenda. *The Scientific Review of Mental Health Practice, 7*(2), 8–21.

Chambless, D. L., & Ollendick, T. H. (2001). Empirically supported psychological interventions: Controversies and evidence. *Annual Review of Psychology, 52*(1), 685–716.

Effects of poverty, hunger, and homelessness on children and youth. (n.d.). Retrieved April 20, 2016, from American Psychological Association website: http://www.apa.org/pi/families/poverty.aspx.

Krogstad, J. M., & Passel, J. S. (2015, November 19). *5 facts about illegal immigration in the U.S.* Retrieved April 20, 2016, from Pew Research Center website: http://www.pewresearch.org/fact-tank/2015/11/19/5-facts-about-illegal-immigration-in-the-u-s/.

Latino hunger facts. (n.d.). Retrieved April 20, 2016, from Feeding America website: http://www.feedingamerica.org/hunger-in-america/impact-of-hunger/latino-hunger/latino-hunger-fact-sheet.html.

O'Donohue, W., & Maragakis, A. (2016). *Integrated primary & behavioral care.* Basel: Springer.

Patten, E. (2012, February 21). *Statistical portrait of the foreign-born population in the United States, 2010.* Retrieved April 20, 2016, from Pew Hispanic Center website: http://www.pewhispanic.org/2012/02/21/statistical-portrait-of-the-foreign-born-population-in-the-united-states-2010/.

Sin, M. (2012). Personal characteristics predictive of depressive symptoms in Hispanics with heart failure. *Issues in Mental Health Nursing, 33*(8), 522–527. doi:10.3109/01612840.2012.687438.

Smith, A. (2000). *Ethnomed: Mexican cultural profile.* Retrieved from http://ethnomed.org/ethnomed/cultures/mexican/mexican_cp.html.

U.S. Census Bureau. (2010). *Hispanic or Latino by type: 2010.* Retrieved from http://factfinder.census.gov/faces/tableservices/jsf/pages/productview.xhtml?pid=DEC_10_SF1_QTP10&prodType=table.

Wassertheil-Smoller, S., Arredondo, E., Cai, J., Castenada, S., Choca, J. P., Gallo, L., … Zee, P. (2014). Depression, anxiety, antidepressant use, and cardiovascular disease among Hispanic men and women of different national backgrounds: Results from the Hispanic community health study/study of Latinos (HCHS/SOL). *Annals of Epidemiology, 24*(*11*), 822–830. Retrieved from http://doi.org.unr.idm.oclc.org/10.1016/j.annepidem.2014.09.003.

Weil, M. (2010). A cultural competency program for psychologists: Clinical and supervisory practices with Latino culture and language. Psychology Distertations, Paper 175.

Wendel, J., O'Donohue, W., & Serratt, T. D. (2013). *Understanding healthcare economics: Managing your career in an evolving healthcare system.* Boca Raton, FL: CRC Press.

Zong, J., & Batalova, J. (2016, April 14). *Frequently requested statistics on immigrants and immigration in the United States.* Retrieved April 20, 2016, from http://www.migrationpolicy.org/article/frequently-requested-statistics-immigrants-and-immigration-united-states.

Chapter 2
Integrated Health Care for Latino Immigrants and Refugees: What Do They Need?

Deirdre Lanesskog and Lissette M. Piedra

Introduction

The idea that health care providers should consider both the health and mental health needs of patients and provide treatment based on an integration of the two is hardly new or novel. Practitioners and scholars have frequently underscored how such an approach would particularly benefit low income and minority clients who frequently turn to health care providers with mental health needs (Sanchez, Chapa, Ybara, & Martinez, 2012). However, the growth of integrated services and the diversity of ways such services can be implemented have created a need for a conversation about best practices. Two tensions frame this discussion. On the one hand, the rising health care costs require an efficient delivery system and integrated services can expedite that mandate. On the other hand, institutional efficacy does not necessarily translate into better service provision for patients, especially those with unique service needs. This chapter explores what immigrants and refugees need in terms of integrated health care. We begin this discussion with a look at the diversity of integrated health care services and the normal tension of crafting service delivery in a way that balances patients' needs for time, attention, and individualized care and providers' needs for expedience and efficiency.

D. Lanesskog, M.P.A., Ph.D. (✉)
School of Social Work, California State University, San Bernardino,
San Bernardino, CA 92407, USA
e-mail: deirdre.lanesskog@csusb.edu

L.M. Piedra, M.S.W., Ph.D.
School of Social Work, University of Illinois at Urbana Champaign,
Urbana, IL 61801, USA
e-mail: lmpiedra@illinois.edu

© Springer International Publishing Switzerland 2016

L.T. Benuto, W. O'Donohue (eds.), *Enhancing Behavioral Health in Latino Populations*, DOI 10.1007/978-3-319-42533-7_2

What Are Integrated Settings?

Immigrants and refugees frequently turn to primary caregivers for their mental health needs (White, Solid, Hodges, & Boehm, 2014). Yet, primary care physicians may be unfamiliar with the relationships between migrants' physical symptoms and underlying mental health problems related to migration. Thus, the integration of mental health and health care services holds particular relevance for these vulnerable groups. However, what is meant by integrated health varies and therefore, merits a brief discussion.

The Hogg Foundation for Mental Health defines integrated health care as the "systematic coordination of physical and mental health care" (2008, p. 7). Such a definition has multiple interpretations, as the *coordination* of services can be quite different from the *integration* of services. For example, services may be coordinated across locations, professions, and providers, or services and providers may be co-located within the same space. However, the integration of health and mental health care includes more than just coordinating or co-locating services, it encompasses the complete integration of treatment so that patients experience seamless, holistic, patient-centered care provided by a multidisciplinary team (Alvarez, Marroquin, Sandoval, & Carlson, 2014; Blount, 2003; World Health Organization, 2008). The World Health Organization (2008) offers a broader definition of integrated health care services that focuses on the "right care" in the "right place," or more specifically, "the organization and management of health services so that people get the care they need, when they need it, in ways that are user-friendly, achieve the desired results and provide value for money" (p. 1).

Although integrated care is often touted for its potential to improve services for patients, a variety of other stakeholders are impacted by its use. Managed health care organizations, public and private insurers and institutions, practitioners across professions, and patient advocates bring distinct and sometimes competing priorities to these efforts (Blount, 2003). In addition to improving patient outcomes, stakeholders' goals likely include some combination of efficiency, cost-containment, provider and patient satisfaction, equity, efficacy, and sustainability. Thus, the ways and extent to which services are integrated can vary accordingly in response. For example, integrated delivery organizations—large networks that provide a highly coordinated continuum of care—may improve patient access to care and streamline processes and costs for providers. However, these systems do not necessarily produce integrated care (Blount, 2003), in which treatment is holistic, is sensitive to patient preferences, and includes one comprehensive treatment plan developed and attended to by a team of professionals who share responsibility for the patient (Singer et al., 2011). These tensions between the needs of patients and the needs of institutions shape the ways integrated care is approached and introduced.

Integrated care is touted as having the potential to improve access to care (World Health Organization, 2008), especially for ethnic, racial, and linguistic minority populations more likely to seek mental health care via a primary care physician

(Sanchez et al., 2012). Alvarez and colleagues (2014) point out that while IHC increases access to mental health services, not much is known about its effectiveness with racial and ethnic groups. Along with other scholars, they underscore the need for cultural-specific strategies to improve minority health outcomes (Bao et al., 2011). This chapter focuses on the potential for integrated care of to meet the unique health and mental health needs of immigrant and refugee clients.

What Do Immigrants and Refugees Need?

The health and mental health needs of immigrants differ from those of the general population. Immigrants and refugees often arrive with better physical and mental health than their non-immigrant peers (Okie, 2007). Over time, difficult migratory experiences and the subsequent stress of adapting to a new country generate rates of health and mental health problems that approach those found in the general public (Kirmayer et al., 2011). Exposure to violence, loss of family and social supports, economic uncertainty, and acculturation stress due to changes in gender roles and intergenerational conflict all contribute to increased prevalence of post-migration health and mental health problems (Kirmayer et al., 2011; Okie, 2007; White et al., 2014). Yet, immigrants and refugees tend to avoid the health care system in general. When they do seek treatment, they are likely to encounter a constellation of barriers to access and appropriate care.

Linguistic and cultural barriers to service access are perhaps the most widely recognized hurdles immigrants and refugees confront when seeking care. Attempts to address these types of barriers have focused on worker practices and institutional policies that facilitate professional behavior and communication across cultures (Alvarez et al., 2014). However, other obstacles exist; poverty and low levels of literacy limit access to institutional structures and processes designed for literate and self-sufficient consumers. Eligibility restrictions for public safety net programs, including Medicaid, relegate immigrants to a loosely connected network of free clinics, public health agencies, and emergency rooms (Frank, Liebman, Ryder, Weir, & Arcury, 2013). Furthermore, immigrants and refugees must navigate these barriers within a hostile political context and across a range of different landscapes; from the large, urban centers with established immigrant communities to the smaller cities, suburbs, and rural areas in which immigrants and refugees are relative newcomers (Gresenz, Derose, Ruder, & Escarce, 2012). Thus, for immigrants and refugees, gaining entrée to appropriate services frequently requires the aid of workers who understand these barriers, have the skills and knowledge needed to overcome them, and who also possess empathy and the will to act on behalf of clients in systems of care not designed to meet their unique needs (Lanesskog, Piedra, & Maldonado, 2015).

Attending to Linguistic and Cultural Barriers

Federal laws mandating language assistance for clients with limited English proficiency (LEP) recognize the importance of a minimum level of communication between provider and client in health and mental health services. Although these laws are unevenly enforced and are often addressed using unreliable and ad hoc methods of interpretation (Partida, 2007; Portes, Fernandez-Kelly, & Light, 2012), they are intended to improve communication, and therefore the quality of care, between immigrant clients and their providers. However, the mere interpretation of words, either by a bilingual practitioner or by an in-person or over the phone interpreter, does not guarantee understanding. Among bilingual professional staff, the lack of standardized assessments of fluency contributes to self-assessments and presumptions of language skills rather than objective evaluation of ability (Engstrom, Piedra, & Min, 2009; Piedra, Andrade, & Larrison, 2011). Similar competency issues, as well as ethical concerns, surround the use of ad-hoc interpreters (e.g. janitorial and clerical staff, friends and family members), who are frequently used in smaller facilities lacking bilingual staff and access to telephone interpreter services. Even the use of telephone interpreters can be problematic, as telephone discussions miss the important cues delivered by body language and facial expression (Portes et al., 2012). These communicative challenges can lead to negative interactions between clients who are sometimes viewed as unwilling or unable to follow instructions, and providers who may be viewed as rude or impatient (Liebert & Ameringer, 2013; Portes, Light, & Fernandez-Kelly, 2009). Particularly in mental health diagnosis and treatment, although also in other health services, the use of trained, in-person, interpreters can improve outcomes and reduce disparities by facilitating patient trust and disclosure (Kirmayer et al., 2011).

Overcoming linguistic and cultural barriers requires workers who can understand clients' words, but also the ways life experiences, attitudes, and traditions impact the meanings behind those words (Gregg & Saha, 2007; Imberti, 2007; Sue et al., 1982). Even within ethnic and racial groups, immigrants may share aspects of culture and language, but their countries of origin, community and familial relationships, and migratory experiences vary greatly. These differences in background and experience shape worldviews, and generate distinct cultural conceptions of health and mental health care. For example, among many Latinos, mental health problems are often viewed as routine life experiences, to be countered by supportive family relationships, rather than by professional treatment (Ruiz, Aguirre, & Mitschke, 2013). Similarly, among many ethnic groups, folk remedies and traditional healers are important sources of care and treatment (Kirmayer et al., 2011; Portes et al., 2009, 2012) as are unlicensed, but trained medical providers who often share the patient's ethnicity, language, or country of origin, but who have not met U.S. licensing requirements (Portes et al., 2012). Reliance on alternative care providers and treatments highlights the importance of trust and familiarity to immigrants seeking care, but also likely stems from unfamiliarity with and lack of access to American systems of care, which were not developed with immigrants in mind (Engstrom & Okamura, 2007; Jones-Correa, 2008).

Addressing Systemic and Institutional Barriers

American health and mental health systems presume that prospective clients possess a basic understanding of how institutions operate and possess the skills and resources to advocate for their own care (Engstrom & Okamura, 2007). Institutions take for granted that clients know where to go to find health and mental health services (Portes et al., 2012) and that they have the transportation and flexible work schedules required to access services during business hours (Liebert & Ameringer, 2013; Portes et al., 2009; Ruiz et al., 2013). Clients are expected to know how to navigate agency websites, appointment scheduling systems, waiting lists, and referral protocols (Engstrom & Okamura, 2007). Once they have gained initial access, immigrant and refugee clients are sometimes compelled to complete intake procedures, including complex forms and medical histories, in English (Liebert & Ameringer, 2013). Yet, immigrants and refugees often need help with all of these processes, let alone with figuring out how to pay for services.

These systems also presume that clients are covered by public or private health insurance, or have the ability to pay for services outright. Federal resettlement programs typically provide refugees with Medicaid coverage and time-limited financial support. Employers usually provide highly skilled, professional immigrants with private health insurance. However, for other immigrants, who are unlikely to have private health insurance, eligibility for Medicaid is limited and is tied to residency status. Legal immigrants are eligible for these programs only after residing in the U.S. for 5 years (Okie, 2007). Undocumented immigrants are barred from such programs almost entirely (Portes et al., 2012). As a result, low-skilled and undocumented immigrants are often underinsured or uninsured, with very limited ability to pay out of pocket (Portes et al., 2012). In fact, half of all Hispanic immigrants and 60 % of undocumented Hispanic immigrants in the U.S. have no health insurance (Brown & Patten, 2014; Livingston, 2009). The inability to pay for care severely constrains service options for immigrant clients. Further, the fear of generating life-altering medical bills often drives poor immigrants to delay seeking care until a crisis (Liebert & Ameringer, 2013), or to use free clinics, many of which require proof of income and residency (Liebert & Ameringer, 2013; Portes et al., 2009, 2012).

For immigrants who lack health insurance and the ability to pay out-of-pocket for care, even getting from the waiting room into the provider's office can be challenging. Many immigrants report receiving high-quality, compassionate care from dedicated providers. However, they must first get past front-desk staff who serve as gatekeepers: protecting the institution from financial concerns and protecting professional staff from the economic and ethical realities of providing indigent care (Portes et al., 2009, 2012). Doctors, nurses, and other health professionals are obligated by professional standards to care for the immigrant patients who reach their exam rooms. Yet, front-desk staff have no corresponding obligation to help immigrant clients fill out forms in English, to schedule appointments around work schedules, or to find ways around providing a social security number, proof of residency, or payment for services. These administrative workers play considerable roles in determining which clients are served and which are turned away, and yet their impact on service access receives limited attention.

Recent health care reforms, including the Affordable Care Act, have improved access and affordability in health and mental health care for millions of low-income Americans. Still, these reforms provide little remedy for immigrants, whose lack of insurance and inability to pay for services often relegates them to a "parallel" system of care comprised of Community and Migrant Health Centers (C/MHCs), Federally Qualified Health Centers (FQHCs), public health departments, pro-bono providers, and emergency rooms (Frank et al., 2013). For example, immigrants can often rely upon free clinic and public health agency programs for cancer screening and detection, as well as for reproductive health care. However, once cancer is detected, immigrant patients find they have few options as these agencies rarely provide specialty care. Emergency rooms are required to treat life-threatening illnesses, but only when the patient's life is in immediate danger. Therefore, this loosely connected health safety net, which operates alongside and sometimes in tandem with mainstream private and nonprofit provider networks, addresses some gaps in health and mental health care for low-income residents. However, it does not approach the level of specialty care and coordination of services one might receive from the type of private or nonprofit networks used by the majority of Americans (Portes et al., 2012).

Overcoming Contextual Barriers

The perception of immigrants residing in centuries-old ethnic enclaves in America's largest cities belies the fact that immigrants are increasingly spread throughout the nation. They reside in cities, suburbs, and small towns of both traditional and new immigrant destinations—places only recently settled by immigrants (Lichter & Johnson, 2006, 2009; Suro, Wilson, & Singer, 2011). As they settle in different communities, immigrants and refugees find themselves immersed in a variety of different contexts. They elicit a range of reactions from established residents who may be unaccustomed to neighbors who look, speak, and act differently. They also encounter variations in political environments across states and localities; some places tolerate or even actively welcome newcomers, while others remain markedly hostile to their arrival. For immigrants and refugees, these variations in place translate into different experiences in employment and quality of life, attitudes and reception, eligibility for social welfare programs, support from ethnic communities, interactions with law enforcement, and access to human services. These contextual variations impact the extent to which immigrant and refugee clients are willing to seek out and are able to find appropriate health and mental health services.

Regardless of the state in which they reside, immigrants have limited access to the federal safety net programs designed to aid the poor (e.g. Medicaid, Foodstamps, cash assistance). Yet, states and localities possess considerable discretion in administering these programs, in determining eligibility (Perreira et al., 2012), and in taking measures to either fill gaps in service delivery or to heighten barriers to service access for immigrants (Portes et al., 2012). One third of states offer medical insurance to residents regardless of immigration status (Derose, Bahney, Lurie, & Escarce, 2009). Other states and localities have developed creative funding initiatives to bolster health services for underserved groups, including immigrants. For example, Miami-Dade County (FL) instituted a half-cent sales tax to fund indigent care, much of which serves immigrants. Conversely, San Diego County (CA) enacted restrictive measures to curtail immigrant access to all public services, including health and mental health care, leading some practitioners to refer their immigrant clients to providers in Mexico (Portes et al., 2012). In order to effectively serve immigrant clients, workers must understand these complex rules and must carefully inquire about the citizenship status of all family members to accurately assess eligibility, especially in families whose members have mixed citizenship status.

In large cities with centuries-old immigrant communities—places like New York City, Chicago, or Los Angeles—recently arriving immigrants can rely upon the support of co-ethnic communities. In these ethnic enclaves, immigrants are often surrounded by established multigenerational families whose members empathize with the challenges of adapting to a new environment and can guide newcomers to local service providers who speak their language, understand their culture, and can help navigate eligibility and cost concerns. However, in new destination cities, and especially in the suburbs of both new and traditional destinations, immigrants are less likely to encounter such entrenched co-ethnic communities and coordinated networks of immigrant service providers (Roth, Golzales, & Lesniewski, 2015). Although suburban communities typically enjoy greater resources than their urban or rural counterparts, the development and funding of suburban safety nets for immigrants have not kept pace with the needs and growth of suburban immigrant populations.

In small-town and rural new destinations, immigrants trade the amenities of more cosmopolitan cities and suburbs for low-skill work and a lower cost of living. These jobs, in agriculture, manufacturing, and food processing, typically do not include health insurance and draw a disproportionate number of undocumented immigrants (Passel & Cohn, 2009) who are largely ineligible for welfare programs. The lower cost of living in rural areas is countered by the presence of fragile human service systems, characterized by fewer institutions with limited resources and little experience serving linguistically and culturally diverse clients (Suro et al., 2011). Further, these communities often lack the bilingual and bicultural professionals needed to provide culturally and linguistically competent care and to negotiate tensions between new and established residents. As a result, immigrants report greater social isolation, fear (Harari, Davis, & Heisler, 2008), and exclusion in new destinations (Jiménez, 2010), as well as more emergency room usage, hospitalization, and medical expenses than their traditional destination peers (Gresenz et al., 2012).

For immigrants and refugees, the bureaucratic and financial challenges of accessing care are often confounded by migratory histories that generate trauma and fear. Refugees are especially likely to have experienced trauma from war, forced migration, and various types of violence inflicted on themselves and their family members. Yet, their traumatic experiences are not likely to be investigated or addressed by the primary care physicians who treat their somatic symptoms (Kirmayer et al., 2011; White et al., 2014). When referred for mental health care, refugees in particular are often reluctant to follow through with either initial visits or follow-up care. Certainly refugees encounter many of the same barriers as immigrants, but these barriers are likely compounded by trauma histories, stigma, and reluctance to disclose mental health problems and to engage in treatment (Kirmayer et al., 2011; White et al., 2014). This specific constellation of barriers refugees experience may require interventions which use integrated care to build trust between refugees and their primary care providers in order to facilitate patient openness and access to mental health treatment (White et al., 2014).

Immigrants are likely to experience the loss of having left behind family members, belongings, and familiar ways of life. Certainly some may have experienced trauma in their home countries or along their migratory journeys; all of these experiences have the potential to inhibit clients' willingness to trust unfamiliar institutions and providers. However, among undocumented immigrants, pervasive fear of detection and subsequent deportation influences immigrants' decisions on if, when, and where they seek care (Portes et al., 2012). In some cases, these fears are unwarranted and emanate from misconceptions about communication or coordination among health care providers and immigration enforcement authorities. However, high profile cases in which health care providers have been targeted for ICE raids, or in which state and local governments engage in staunch efforts to restrict undocumented immigrants' access to care, heighten fears among undocumented immigrants everywhere (Portes et al., 2012).

Providing Integrated Care

Immigrant and refugee clients need the aid of providers who understand the ways linguistic, cultural, systemic, institutional, and contextual factors impede access to care. On a most basic level, they need to be understood by providers who either speak the patient's language or use reliable means of interpretation. Yet, although language skills and cultural knowledge are important, they alone are not enough to facilitate service access and delivery in health and mental health care (Schwartz, Domenech Rodríguez, Santiago-Rivera, Arredondo, & Field, 2010; Schyve, 2007). Immigrant and refugee clients require providers who have the skills and knowledge to overcome communicative and cultural barriers, but who also possess empathy and will to act on their clients' behalf (Lanesskog et al., 2015). For providers, this means taking extra time and care to inquire about patients' cultures: about their beliefs and concerns surrounding mental health treatment, about their migratory experiences, and about their preferences for incorporating family, community, and nontraditional practices into their care.

In accessing systems and institution not designed with them in mind, immigrants and refugees require extra time from staff who can explain appointment and referral systems, help manage paperwork, and follow-up to ensure that clients understand and complete treatment protocols. This necessitates that workers perform extra tasks beyond their usual job responsibilities. For the majority of immigrants who have limited access to health insurance and minimal ability to pay out of pocket, they must rely on providers to inquire, to consider, and to discuss the financial implications of service options. They need providers to have a more thorough and detailed understanding of variations in eligibility criteria, available providers, and costs—across systems, institutions, and geographic locations. Similarly, if providers are to overcome patients' fears—of immigration enforcement, medical bills, or unfamiliar environments—they must be able to differentiate between real and perceived risks. Broadly speaking, immigrant and refugee clients need advocates who are motivated to help clients access the most appropriate, accessible, and affordable care in their communities, but who are also committed to identifying and to changing the systemic structures, institutional processes, and political environments that result in service gaps for immigrants and refugees in the first place. The integration of health and mental health services provides a framework for overcoming many of these barriers. For example, using interdisciplinary, cross-trained teams may improve providers' ability to inquire about, to understand, and to integrate patients' medical and behavioral health needs into treatment. Co-locating services and unifying information systems may help address barriers to referral and follow-up, potentially reducing transportation and time constraints, attending to eligibility concerns, and allowing patients to receive different types of care at one trusted location.

Institution and Provider Perspectives on Integrated Health Care

Regardless of their locations and the types of clients they serve, health and mental health providers throughout the U.S. are increasingly called upon to administer high-quality care while controlling costs. Consequently, institution and provider desires for efficiency are often at odds with immigrants' desires for efficacy. The extra time, attention, and assistance immigrant clients require, whether to build rapport, to explain medical terms, or to arrange for referrals, likely generates indirect costs. These costs are above and beyond those incurred for hiring interpreters and translating written materials into clients' languages. Institutions and providers are simply required to spend more time and money helping immigrant and refugee clients receive appropriate care or accept the possibility that these clients may fall through the cracks. For immigrants, this tension between effectiveness and efficiency can lead to poor health outcomes. For providers, such tension can lead to frustration with immigrant clients' inability to follow through on advice, but also to significant costs associated with poor health outcomes and more expensive treatments in the future.

Integrated health care has the potential to increase access, to improve health outcomes, and to decrease overall health care costs, but the significant costs of implementation fall largely on primary care providers and institutions (Auxier, Farley, & Seifert, 2011). Hiring additional mental health providers, cross-training staff to work as a team, co-locating services, and adopting information systems capable of managing more complex patient records and billing constitute just some of the upfront costs providers are likely to incur. Further, Medicaid and private health insurance billing systems are not designed with integrated care in mind, so providers may be unable to recoup the costs associated with seeing multiple providers during one visit (Auxier et al., 2011; Okie, 2007; Singer et al., 2011), even for refugee and immigrant clients who have health insurance.

Uncompensated care—that which is not reimbursed by either Medicaid or private insurance—presents an even greater challenge to integrated care providers. Hospitals do not routinely collect data on the citizenship status of their patients, so the uncompensated health and mental health costs associated with the care of immigrants, whether in the emergency room or in inpatient settings are largely estimated. These costs, incurred by hospitals that treat indigent patients, some of whom are immigrants, continue to rise (Okie, 2007). Although immigrants tend to use fewer medical services and generate less medical expenditures than their American-born peers, even when they have health insurance (López-Cevallos, 2014), their limited access to preventive and primary care contributes to their overuse of expensive emergency room services (Okie, 2007). The proliferation of immigrants who seek emergency care for conditions that are effectively managed via routine doctor visits in other segments of the population, suggests significant shortcomings in our existing system (Frank et al., 2013).

These costs and their implications for health care providers and the communities in which they reside generate contentious political debates about immigrant access to health and mental health services. For society as a whole and particularly for immigrants, refugees, and the institutions that serve them, integrated care may reduce long-term costs. Yet, overcoming the disincentives to implementing integrated care will likely prove difficult, and measuring the cost-effectiveness of such efforts may be equally challenging (Auxier et al., 2011). As a result, for providers and institutions, integrating health and mental health care may prove quite costly with returns on investments taking many years to materialize, if ever (Burns & Pauly, 2002).

Social Work Perspective on Integrative Health Care

The field of social work was initiated via work helping immigrants in the late nineteenth and early twentieth centuries cope with the myriad of adjustments to life in the United States. Although the field has branched out to serve other vulnerable populations, the profession's central tenets emphasize the importance of attending to the needs of individuals within the contexts in which they are situated: a person-in-environment approach. For immigrants, the integration of health and mental health care attends to their unique needs for linguistically and culturally competent care, while attempting to mitigate institutional, systemic, and contextual barriers to care. The holistic and person-centered approach of integrated care underscores the central role that immigration experience and status play in shaping the life course of immigrants and refugees (Piedra & Engstrom, 2009). Integrated care builds on the resilience of immigrants and refugees, but also leverages the strengths of multidisciplinary providers and institutions who, working in concert, have the potential to positively impact the health of this new century's immigrants.

References

Alvarez, K., Marroquin, Y. A., Sandoval, L., & Carlson, C. I. (2014). Integrated health care best practices and culturally and linguistically competent care: Practitioner perspectives. *Journal of Mental Health Counseling, 36*(2), 99–114.

Auxier, A., Farley, T., & Seifert, K. (2011). Establishing an integrated care practice in a community health center. *Professional Psychology: Research and Practice, 42*(5), 391–397.

Bao, Y. H., Alexopoulos, G. S., Casalino, L. P., Ten Have, T. R., Donohue, J. M., Post, E. P., … Bruce, M. L. (2011). Collaborative depression care management and disparities in depression treatment and outcomes. *Archives of General Psychiatry, 68*(6), 627–636.

Blount, A. (2003). Integrated primary care: Organizing the evidence. *Families, Systems and Health, 21*(2), 121–133.

Brown, A., & Patten, E. (2014). *Statistical portrait of Hispanics in the United States, 2012*. Washington, DC: Pew Research Center. Retrieved from http://www.pewhispanic.org/2014/04/29/statistical-portrait-of-hispanics-in-the-united-states-2012/.

Burns, L. R., & Pauly, M. V. (2002). Integrated delivery networks: A detour on the road to integrated health care? *Health Affairs, 21*(4), 128–143.

Derose, K. P., Bahney, B. W., Lurie, N., & Escarce, J. J. (2009). Immigrants and health care access, quality, and cost. *Medical Care Research and Review, 24*(3), 487–514.

Engstrom, D. W., & Okamura, A. (2007). A nation of immigrants: A call for a specialization in immigrant well-being. *Journal of Ethnic and Cultural Diversity in Social Work, 16*(3-4), 103–111.

Engstrom, D. W., Piedra, L. M., & Min, J. W. (2009). Bilingual social workers: Language and service complexities. *Administration in Social Work, 33*(2), 167–185.

Frank, A. L., Liebman, A. K., Ryder, B., Weir, M., & Arcury, T. A. (2013). Health care access and health care workforce for immigrant workers in the agriculture, forestry, and fisheries sector in the Southeaster U.S. *American Journal of Industrial Medicine, 56*, 960. doi:10.1002/ajim.22183.

Gregg, J., & Saha, S. (2007). Communicative competence: A framework for understanding language barriers in health care. *Journal of General Internal Medicine, 22*(Suppl. 2), 368–370.

Gresenz, C. R., Derose, K. P., Ruder, T., & Escarce, J. J. (2012). Health care experiences of Hispanics in new and traditional U.S. destinations. *Medical Care Research and Review, 69*(6), 663–678.

Harari, N., Davis, M., & Heisler, M. (2008). Strangers in a strange land: Health care experiences for recent Latino immigrants in Midwest communities. *Journal of Health Care for the Poor and Underserved, 19*(4), 1350–1367.

Hogg Foundation for Mental Health. (2008). *Connecting body and mind: A resource guide to integrated health care in Texas and the United States*. Austin, TX: Author.

Imberti, P. (2007). Who resides behind the words? Exploring and understanding the language experience of the non-English-speaking immigrant. *Families in Society: The Journal of Contemporary Social Services, 88*(1), 67–73.

Jiménez, T. R. (2010). *Replenished ethnicity: Mexican-Americans, immigration, and identity*. Berkeley, CA: University of California Press.

Jones-Correa, M. (2008). Race to the top? The politics of immigrant education in suburbia. In D. Massey (Ed.), *New faces in new places: The changing geography of American immigration* (pp. 308–340). New York, NY: Russell Sage.

Kirmayer, L. J., Narasiah, L., Munoz, M., Rashid, M., Ryder, A. G., Guzder, J., … Pottie, K., (2011). Common mental health problems in immigrants and refugees: General approach in primary care. *Canadian Medical Association Journal, 183(12)*, E959–E967.

Lanesskog, D., Piedra, L. M., & Maldonado, S. (2015). Beyond bilingual and bicultural: Serving Latinos in a new growth community. *Journal of Ethnic and Cultural Diversity in Social Work, 24*(4), 300–317.

Lichter, D. T., & Johnson, K. M. (2006). Emerging rural settlement patterns and the geographic redistribution of America's new immigrants. *Rural Sociology, 71*(1), 109–131.

Lichter, D. T., & Johnson, K. M. (2009). Immigrant gateways and Hispanic migration to new destinations. *International Migration Review, 43*(3), 496–518.

Liebert, S., & Ameringer, C. F. (2013). The health care safety net and the affordable care act: Implications for Hispanic immigrants. *Public Administration Review, 73*(6), 810–820.

Livingston, G. (2009). *Hispanics, health insurance, and health care access*. Washington, DC: Pew Research Center. Retrieved from http://www.pewhispanic.org/2009/09/25/hispanics-health-insurance-and-health-care-access/.

López-Cevallos, D. (2014). Are Latino immigrants a burden to safety net services in nontraditional immigrant states? Lessons from Oregon. *American Journal of Public Health, 104*(5), 781–786.

Okie, S. (2007). Immigrants and health care: At the intersection of two broken systems. *The New England Journal of Medicine, 357*(6), 525–529.

Partida, Y. (2007). Addressing language barriers: Building response capacity for a changing nation. *Journal of General Internal Medicine, 22*(Suppl 2), 347–349.

Passel, J. R., & Cohn, D. (2009). *A portrait of undocumented immigrants in the United States*. Washington, DC: Pew Hispanic Center.

Perreira, K. M., Crosnoe, R., Fortuny, K., Pedroza, J., Ulvestad, K., Weiland, C., … Chaudry, A. (2012). *Barriers to immigrants' access to health and human services programs*. Washington, DC: U.S. Department of Health and Human Services, Office of Human Services Policy.

Piedra, L. M., Andrade, F. C. D., & Larrison, C. R. (2011). Building response capacity: The need for universally available language services. In L. P. Buki & L. M. Piedra (Eds.), *Creating infrastructures for Latino mental health* (pp. 55–75). New York, NY: Springer.

Piedra, L. M., & Engstrom, D. W. (2009). Segmented assimilation theory and the life model: An integrated approach to understanding immigrants and their children. *Social Work, 54*(3), 270–277.

Portes, A., Fernandez-Kelly, P., & Light, D. (2012). Life on the edge: Immigrants confront the American health system. *Ethnic and Racial Studies, 35*(1), 3–22.

Portes, A., Light, D., & Fernandez-Kelly, P. (2009). The U.S. health system and immigration: An institutional interpretation. *Sociological Forum, 24*(3), 487–514.

Roth, B. J., Golzales, R. G., & Lesniewski, J. (2015). Building a stronger safety net: Local organizations and the challenges of serving immigrants in the suburbs. *Human Service Organizations: Management, Leadership, & Governance, 39*(4), 348–361.

Ruiz, E., Aguirre, R. T. P., & Mitschke, D. B. (2013). What leads non-U.S.-born. Latinos to Access Mental Health Care? *Social Work in Health Care, 52*(1), 1–19.

Sanchez, K., Chapa, T., Ybara, R., & Martinez, O. N. (2012). *Enhancing the delivery of health care: Eliminating health disparities through a culturally & linguistically centered integrated health care approach: Consensus statements and recommendations*. Washington, DC: U.S. Department of Health and Human Services and Hogg Foundation for Mental Health, Office of Minority Health.

Schwartz, A. L., Domenech Rodríguez, M. M., Santiago-Rivera, A., Arredondo, P., & Field, L. D. (2010). Cultural and linguistic competence: Welcome challenges from successful diversification. *Professional Psychology: Research and Practice, 41*, 210–220.

Schyve, P. M. (2007). Language differences as a barrier to quality and safety in health care: The joint commission perspective. *Journal of General Internal Medicine, 22*(Suppl 2), 360–361.

Singer, S. J., Burgers, J., Freidberg, M., Rosenthal, M. B., Leape, L., & Schneider, E. (2011). Defining and measuring integrated patient care: Promoting the next frontier in health care delivery. *Medical Care Research and Review, 68*(1), 112–127.

Sue, D. W., Bernier, J. E., Durran, A., Feinberg, L., Pedersen, P., Smith, E. J., & Vasquez-Nuttall, E. (1982). Position paper: Cross-cultural counseling competencies. *The Counseling Psychologist, 10*, 45–52.

Suro, R., Wilson, J. H., & Singer, A. (2011). *Immigration and poverty in America's suburbs* (Metropolitan opportunity series, Vol. 20). Washington, DC: The Brookings Institution. Retrieved from http://www.brookings.edu/research/papers/2011/08/04-immigration-suro-wilson-singer.

White, C. C., Solid, C. A., Hodges, J. S., & Boehm, D. H. (2014). Does integrated care affect healthcare utilization in multi-problem refugees? *Journal of Immigrant and Minority Health, 17*, 1444. doi:10.1007/s10903.

World Health Organization. (May, 2008). *Integrated health services – What and why?* Technical Brief No. 1, Geneva: World Health Organization.

Chapter 3
Eliminating Disparities Through Integrated Behavioral and Primary Care: Special Considerations for Working with Puerto Ricans

Nanet M. López-Córdova and José J. Cabiya

According to the latest US census estimate, Hispanics represent the largest minority, with 17.1% of the total estimated population for 2013. Recognizing the diversity within the Hispanic population of the United States in modern times is an important step when integrated behavioral and primary care services are provided. Thus, one important aspect is the recognition of the within-group differences in the Hispanic population and other minority groups. One example is the Puerto Rican population, which has a very particular sociopolitical and biopsychosocial background that should be taken into consideration when quality health services are provided. It is important to recognize these differences because knowledge of the history and worldview of the Puerto Rican population regarding issues of health, disease, health-seeking behaviors, and interaction with health providers among other topics will make it easier for the teams of health professionals to bring better services to the patients being served. This aspect includes the importance of prevention, assessment, and treatment of disease and the development of a professional relationship between the interprofessional/interdisciplinary teams and this population.

General Description of Puerto Ricans

Puerto Ricans are an important group within the growing Hispanic population in the United States because between 2000 and 2010 their number grew by 43 % from 3.4 million to 4.6 million. Although they share some common characteristics with other Latinos, Puerto Ricans are can be distinguished clearly from other Latinos. This diversity could be attributed to differences in cultural and historical backgrounds and how they have assimilated into the mainstream society (Ramos, 2005).

N.M. López-Córdova, Psy.D. (✉) • J.J. Cabiya, Ph.D.
Albizu University, San Juan, PR 00902-3711, USA
e-mail: nlopez@albizu.edu

© Springer International Publishing Switzerland 2016

L.T. Benuto, W. O'Donohue (eds.), *Enhancing Behavioral Health in Latino Populations*, DOI 10.1007/978-3-319-42533-7_3

According to Ramos (2005), Puerto Ricans tend to migrate in circulatory patterns in a back-and-forth movement between the island and the continental United States, as a result of economic factors, including employment conditions in both places. The importance of recognizing, discussing, and teaching the diversity of the Hispanic population results in a better understanding of the four largest Hispanic groups in the United States—Mexican Americans, Puerto Ricans, Cuban Americans, and Dominicans—and their particular characteristics and needs will promote the importance of personalizing health services and reducing the misconceptions and stereotypes that could be factors that hinder the process of seeking health services at all levels.

A 2013 report by the Pew Research Center on the results of the American Community Survey conducted in 2011 by the US Census Bureau with the Puerto Rican community in the United States presents a revealing portrait (Brown & Patten, 2013). An estimated 4.9 million Hispanics (9.5 %) are of Puerto Rican origin and thus are ranked as the second-largest population of Hispanics living in the United States, after the Mexicans, who account for 64.6 %, according to the US Census Bureau's American Community Survey (Brown & Patten, 2013). According to the American Community Survey, their median age is 27 years, well below the average of 37 years for the total population. They are less likely to be married than Hispanics in general, 36 % versus 44 %, among all Hispanics, and they have higher levels of education than the overall Hispanic population, with 16 % older than 25 years having obtained a bachelor's degree. More than 80 % of those aged 5 years or older speak English proficiently. The poverty rate among Puerto Ricans is 27 %, which is higher than both the overall Hispanic rate and the general US rate (25 % and 15 % respectively.) Only 38 % of Puerto Ricans are homeowners, less than the rate for Hispanics overall (47 %) and for the general US population (65 %). Voter turnout among Puerto Ricans was up 3.1 % in 2012 from 2008, with 52.8 % voting, above the 48 % rate for the overall Hispanic population eligible to vote in the United States. Most Puerto Ricans in the United States—3.4 million in all—were born in the 50 states or the District of Columbia. Additionally, about one third (31 %) of the Puerto Rican population in the United States—1.5 million—were born in Puerto Rico. People born in Puerto Rico are also considered native born because they are US citizens by birth (Brown & Patten, 2013).

Moreover, according to the American Community Survey, more than eight in ten Puerto Ricans (82 %) aged 5 years or older speak English proficiently. The other 18 % report speaking English less than very well, compared with 34 % of all Hispanics. Puerto Ricans are concentrated in the Northeast (53 %), mostly in New York (23 %), and in the South (30 %), mostly in Florida (18 %). Puerto Ricans have higher levels of education than the Hispanic population overall but lower levels than the US population overall. Some 16 % of Puerto Ricans aged 25 years or older compared with 13 % of all US Hispanics and 29 % of the US population have obtained at least a bachelor's degree. According to the American Community Survey, Hispanics of Puerto Rican origin aged 16 years or older in the United States had median annual personal earnings of $25,000 in the year before the survey—greater than the median earnings for all US Hispanics

($20,000) but less than the median earnings for the US population ($29,000). The share of Puerto Ricans who live in poverty, 28 %, is higher than the rate both for the general US population (16 %) and for Hispanics overall (26 %). Fifteen percent of Puerto Ricans do not have health insurance, compared with 30 % of all Hispanics and 15 % of the general US population (Brown & Patten, 2013).

A study by Rivera-Batiz and Santiago indicates that Puerto Ricans born on the mainland are improving their economic status, although a significant proportion (30 %) of mainland Puerto Ricans remain in poverty. It is not surprising that the group with the highest rate of psychological distress and disorders is the poorest segment of the population regardless of where they reside as the Puerto Rican mental health profile resembles that of the general US population. Loss of cultural identity is a prominent issue related to Puerto Rican mental health (Flores, 1993). Decades of efforts to Americanize Puerto Rico have taken their toll on the sense of cultural autonomy Puerto Ricans experience relative to other Latino groups, who draw renewal from relatively intact home cultures. The development of a "Nuyorican" culture, although a vibrant force on the mainland, has led to discrimination when migrants return to Puerto Rico to live. The high rates of circular migration have created a subpopulation that is "neither here nor there." Although the implications of these issues are difficult to document in terms of specific mental health outcomes, they provide an important context for understanding the Puerto Rican migrant experience in comparison with that of other Latino immigrants.

Health Service Use and Health Disparities Among Puerto Ricans

Puerto Ricans are relatively high users of health services, particularly the general medical sector (Martinez, Interian, & Guarnaccia, 2013). Access to a widespread public health system in Puerto Rico and eligibility for health benefits and federal health programs on the mainland make financial access issues less of a barrier than for other Latinos. Given the high use of the medical sector both in Puerto Rico and on the mainland, recognition of mental health problems by primary care providers is a significant issue. Recognition of the expressions of *nervios* and *ataque de nervios* as important signs of psychological distress among many Spanish-speaking Puerto Ricans, especially those from working class and poor backgrounds, can contribute to recognition of psychosocial problems in primary care. At the same time, there are not simple translations of these idioms of distress into psychiatric diagnoses; rather they cut across a range of distress and disorders requiring careful assessment of both the symptoms and the contexts of the experience (Martinez et al., 2013). These representations of symptoms have been recognized lately as cultural manifestations in the DSM-5.

Both Espiritismo and Santeria continue to flourish in Latino neighborhoods of New York City. Their presence is more variable in smaller cities in the northeast, where Puerto Ricans have spread. Epidemiological studies with Puerto Ricans (Guarnaccia et al., 2005) report that the use of these alternatives to traditional medicine appears to be more frequent when Puerto ricans seek assistance with their mental health problems. Better educated Puerto Ricans have done well economically and adjusting to the American society mainstream and rely less on folk alternatives while less educated rely more on these alternatives when seeking mental health assistance. Although the role of the Catholic and newer protestant churches, including their clergy and layorganizations, in support of people in psychological distress has been less studied (Guarnaccia et al., 2005), it is equally important as the folk sector.

Puerto Ricans despite being US citizens still experience high levels of discrimination. On arrival many are treated as a foreigner for having a different language and culture. Thus, they have to navigate new and menacing environments, including the health system. Some of their cultural values, such as family values, gender role, and assumption of mental health, have their roots in their Puerto Rican culture and heritage, which often clash with those of mainstream society. Thus, they face the possibility of not achieving full acculturation. At the same time, because of the circulatory nature of the migration of Puerto Ricans mentioned before, some elements of the Puerto Rican culture remain very active as they face the challenges of a very traumatic acculturation experience (Ramos, 2005). From an ecological perspective, acculturation occurs as individuals socialized in one cultural context try to adjust to a different cultural milieu to improve the person–environment fit. This process of adaptation could be conceptualized as very fluid oriented to action and change instead of adjustment to the status quo (Ramos, 2005). For individuals with a separate distinct culture, acculturation can be a source of stress in a society that is strongly influenced by a mainstream culture. Stressors stemming from, for example, language differences and conflicting cultural values disrupt the person–environment fit and, depending on an individual's coping resources, may result in an increased risk of psychological distress. Puerto Ricans who traditionally learn to rely on the family and community and are rewarded for respectful, less assertive behavior may experience conflict and anxiety in a society that discourages passivity and promotes independence and individualism (Martinez et al., 2013). Minority status can inhibit the ability to adjust freely and successfully to the new environment and negotiate mismatches in value systems.

Rates of Behavioral Health Problems Among Latinos and Puerto Ricans

As discussed already, Puerto Ricans have a lower educational and economic status on average. Thus, Puerto Rican children and adults are at a higher risk of mental health problems than other Latino groups, such as Cuban Americans, given their lower educational and economic resources. Puerto Rican Americans reported more sick days due to health disability, more days spent in bed, and more hospitalizations than did Mexican Americans and Cuban Americans, according to Hajat (2000), who conducted interviews in English and Spanish of a nationally representative sample.

Another set of epidemiological studies using diagnostic measures found that Puerto Ricans who reside in Puerto Rico had lower prevalence rates of depression and other mental health disorders than did Mexican Americans who were born in the United States, Mexican immigrants had who lived in the United States for 13 years or more, or Puerto Ricans who lived on the mainland. This consistent pattern of findings across independent investigations, different sites, and Latino subgroups suggests that factors associated with daily living in the United States lead to an increased risk of mental disorders. Some authors have interpreted these findings as suggesting that acculturation may lead to an increased risk of mental disorders. One limitation of this type of research is that the relationship between acculturation and prevalence has never been tested to show that these rates are indeed related. At best, the place of birth and the number of years living in the United States are proxy measures of acculturation. Moreover, acculturation is a complex process; it is not clear what aspect or aspects of acculturation could be related to higher rates of disorders. Is it the changing cultural values and practices, the stressors associated with such changes, or negative encounters with American institutions (e.g., schools or employers) that underlie some of the different prevalence rates.

Lewis-Fernandez et al. examined the clinical risk factors for major depression in US Hispanics in a meta-analysis of previous research on the topic. They noticed that this research has grown significantly during the past two decades. Moreover, Ortega completed an analysis of the National Comorbidity Study and concluded that even after age, income, and education had been controlled for, US-born Hispanics had a significantly higher risk of psychiatric disorder than foreign-born Hispanics. A significant association was observed among separate analyses of Puerto Ricans, Mexican Americans, and other Hispanics. In addition, a comparative study of Puerto Ricans living in poor residential areas in Puerto Rico and New York City revealed similar levels of clinically significant self-reported depressive symptoms in each group. Comparatively, high levels of depressive symptoms were found among Puerto Ricans living in Puerto Rico (29.1 %) and Puerto Ricans living in New York City (28.6 %). These findings suggest that we should not overgeneralize that acculturation increases the risk of depression and suggest a need to examine in greater detail cultural differences between and within Hispanic subgroups and evaluate cultural variation across self-report and structured research interviews of depression.

Although it remains unclear why Puerto Ricans living in the United States have higher rates of mental health problems than other Latinos, researchers have suggested several possible explanations. Research has indicated that the relatively low socioeconomic status of Puerto Ricans could contribute to the risk of worse mental health outcomes (Guarnaccia et al., 2005). According to Sanchez et al., another possible explanation that researchers have postulated for the relatively poor health outcomes for Puerto Ricans is related to the circular migration patterns of Puerto Ricans because of their status as US citizens. In particular, some studies have suggested that many Puerto Ricans come to the United States for treatment of medical problems (Guarnaccia et al., 2005). If that is the case, it might prove useful to examine the comorbidity between mental health problems and physical health problems, which might help researchers understand this pattern. These factors assist us in making better and informed clinical diagnoses and recommendations when working with the Spanish-speaking Puerto Rican population in primary care settings.

Significant Prejudices Experienced by Puerto Ricans and the Behavioral Health Impact

One important aspect of the prejudices that Puerto Ricans living in the United States experience daily could be categorized as multifactorial and thought provoking. This is because this cultural group is not as homogeneous as many would like to think, as will be explained next. Since 1917 Puerto Ricans have been US citizens through the Jones–Shafroth Act, and the opportunities they have to travel, live, and work freely on the US mainland are derived from the rights of being a United States citizen. However, this citizenship is guaranteed only as long as the US Congress determines it so. The US Congress has the power to change laws and in this respect the Jones–Shafroth Act is not dissimilar from other laws. Despite this, Puerto Ricans have to clarify their legal status and even when it has been clarified still receive different social services, in contrast to their Caucasian counterparts.

The main language spoken in Puerto Rico is Spanish and less than half of the population of Puerto Rico is fluent in English. The language barrier when Puerto Ricans are in the United States as a result of migration and/or living on the mainland but not being acculturated or assimilated impacts the mobility of the group in mainstream society (Guarnaccia et al., 2005). According to the Pew Research Center (Brown & Patten, 2013), in the United States more than 82 % of Puerto Ricans aged 5 years or older speak English proficiently. The other 18 % report speaking English not proficiently, which is lower of the 34 % for the rest of the Hispanics (Brown & Patten, 2013). Language fluency is an important factor that could positively or negatively impact most Puerto Ricans in their mobility through North American society, and at the same time this impacts the process of receiving medical and/or mental health services that help reduce the health disparities experienced by the group. Urciuoli (1996) describes how racism and prejudice operate for Puerto Ricans in "English-only America." Urla describes how Urciuoli (1996) in her book describes how the mainstream society's discourse points out that Puerto Ricans speak "bad" or broken English and that if they get rid of their "accent" they will be able to move to mainstream society with all the economic and sociopolitical benefits that represent being part of the "American dream." However, working class, low-income Puerto Ricans who do not speak the language, face exclusion in many aspects, including access to better social services, increasing as a consequence health disparities. The limited number of health providers both in the medical realm and in the mental health realm that speak Spanish and are culturally competent often impacts the active participation of Puerto Ricans in the dynamic of health-seeking behaviors and adhering to treatment.

Another factor is the lack of health insurance because of the nonexistence of provision of insurance by employers of Latinos (Guarnaccia et al., 2005). There is also discrimination against Latinos in mental health services. According to Guarnaccia et al. (2005), this discrimination results from both racial and cultural bias. Although there is more evidence of discrimination for medical conditions (Institute of Medicine, 2002), it is likely these factors operate in the mental health sector as well. Prejudice can also be exhibited by health providers by their having negative attitudes toward minority populations with mental health issues. This could be noticeable by service providers' communication of negative, hopeless, and stigmatizing messages that define people solely by their illness or illness labels (Nemec, Swarbrick, & Legere, 2015). "Microaggression" is a term used by Sue et al. (2007) in the study of cross-cultural communication. According to Deegan (2004), microaggressions tend to be invisible, yet the cumulative effect creates unmistakable tensions between people. For Reidy (1993), patronizing phrases such as "my client," a condescending tone of voice, and dehumanizing language are frequently cited as examples of prejudice. It is for this reason that the most promising approaches for stigma reduction are education and contact (Corrigan, Mueser, Bond, Drake, & Solomon, 2008). The best recommendation to reduce the stigma and prejudice from service provision to minority patients with mental health issues according to Nemec et al. (2015) is the following: education of care staff to guide and shape the work of direct care staff by teaching monitoring, evaluating, and correcting communication skills that express prejudice and discrimination. Teaching and training settings can be structured according to the Nemec et al. to convey a message of hope and recovery rather than focusing on the person served in negative terms, as belligerent, resistant, unmotivated, or disinterested. It is important to model positive and respectful attitudes by use of person-first and culturally sensitive language by the sharing of examples of multidimensional people with strengths, successes, and multiple roles, not just illustrations of illness, failure, and risk. Contact with the population seems to improve attitudes and behavioral intentions toward people with mental illness(es) (Corrigan, Morris, Michaels, Rafacz, & Rüsch, 2012). The influence of the service system impacts the provision of services and perpetuates the stigma toward minorities with mental health issues. For this reason, it is important to change the culture by instilling a sense of hope and optimism by the sharing of achievements and not only the negative aspects of the different interventions (Nemec et al., 2015). Although the system cannot be changed instantly, it is important to have training programs for students, health professionals, and service staff directed at making them aware of the cultural issues experience by the different minority population. Nemec and associates (2015) also proposed that more opportunities to interact with the patients of minority populations need to be provided to service staffs to make them more sensitive to these populations' needs and problems.

Other Stressors Associated with Acculturation

Although acculturation can be stressful for both sexes, Puerto Rican males and females may need to face different types of stressors, specifically, stressors that are the result of having to adapt to the new gender roles and family structure as defined by the new mainstream society. For example, adherence to traditional gender roles in a mainstream society that does not value such roles as machismo can be conflictive and burdensome. Women may also experience role strain as they try to fulfill expected idealized roles of wife and mother while simultaneously working outside the home and adapting to a society with a different set of values and expected roles for women. For traditional men, stressors may relate to role reversal, especially when they are not able to be the main source of income or cannot bring any income at all, which is not unusual given the limited access to employment of many Puerto Ricans in the United States. Ethnic discrimination is associated with poorer mental and physical health, worse health behaviors, and increased mortality, in addition to overall health disparities (Martinez et al., 2013). More specifically, it has been suggested as a possible determinant of the significant race/ethnic differences in the quantity and quality of medical care received by individuals in the United States.

Given the growing diversity in the United States and the prevalence of discrimination, more research regarding the impact on health care utilization is needed. Only when all the factors influencing patient behaviors are better understood will policies and interventions designed to improve them be successful. These are important steps that will help us achieve our national goal of eliminating race/ethnic disparities in health (Schenker et al., 2010) Health disparities need to be diminished in minorities, and the adherence factor is essential to improve their quality of life. Schenker et al. (2010) studied how limitations in English proficiency and concordance between the patient's language and the physician's language negatively impact the treatment of patients with diabetes. They point out the importance of assessing the association of limited English proficiency and physician language concordance with patient reports of clinical interactions is that the provision of services in the native language requires to be improved. Quality and performance assessments should consider physician–patient language concordance.

Nevertheless, Hispanic Americans are the ethnic group least likely to have health insurance coverage, and one third lack a regular source of primary health care Andrés-Hyman, Ortiz, Añez, Paris, and Davidson (2006). Reversing the tide of health disparities for US Hispanics will entail redressing socioeconomic barriers to treatment and improving access, engagement, and therapeutic strategies that operate within specific cultural contexts (Andrés-Hyman et al. 2006). Baig et al. (2014) designed a study that assessed the relationship between community health center providers' Spanish language skills and cultural awareness. They found that providers that saw a significant number of Latinos had good access to interpreter services but that did not have any formal cultural competency training. It is for this reason that Spanish language skills training and better access to cultural competency training with Latinos are needed to provide more effective linguistically and culturally tailored medical care to Latino patients.

According to Ho et al. (2006), more studies are warranted to examine if the acculturated lifestyle, quality of health services, access to health care, and effectiveness in controlling diabetes and its complications are factors associated with the poor health status of mainland Puerto Ricans. This inquiry could be extended to other medical conditions as well as to the provision of mental health services. It is for this reason that we should be aware of the studies available and their findings to help understand the different factors that impact and could impact the provision of primary care services to Puerto Ricans in the United States. For example, Andrés-Hyman et al. (2006) proposed a model where cultural concepts were analyzed from an ecological perspective. They offer practical recommendations that follow from a model based on the specific cultural beliefs of the patients. Although not comprehensive, these recommendations do offer specific approaches for the provision of health services that are consistent with the understanding of Puerto Ricans in their context and consistent with their heritage. This model considers information related not only to the history, value systems, and psychosocial stressors of each patient, but also to the needs of providers and thus demonstrates an appreciation of the patient's and the provider's whole context (Andrés-Hyman et al., 2006).

The literature suggests that treatment of native Spanish-speaking Latinos by bilingual providers is preferable (Comas-Diaz, 1988), even for bilingual clients. As Schyve has reported, the Joint Commission has stated that there are three threats to effective health communication. The health service providers have called this set of threats the "triple threat" to effective health communication; namely, low health literacy, cultural barriers, and limited English proficiency. However, health literacy has often been seen apart from interventions designed to overcome cultural and linguistic barriers. Thus, researchers such as Hahn et al. and DeWalt et al. are working to understand the relationship between health culture, literacy, and language and health outcomes. Despite mastery of a second language, a bilingual client may find that certain feelings or emotions are difficult or impossible to adequately convey in a language other than his or her native tongue. This incompatibility may ensue because emotions are anchored to the first language learned as a child (Guttfreund, 1990), and many words and concepts do not exist or have the same meaning in different languages. In recognition of these issues, many behavioral health agencies have employed bilingual interpreters to translate information. However, several authors have raised misgivings about confidentiality, client discomfort, and the potentially negative impact of third parties on the therapeutic alliance (Altarriba & Santiago-Rivera, 1994; Rivera et al., 2011; Schwartz, Rodríguez, Santiago-Rivera, Arredondo, & Field, 2010). Clients validated these concerns during focus groups, characterizing the use of interpreters in other programs as "no good" (Altarriba & Santiago-Rivera, 1994; Rivera et al., 2011; Schwartz et al., 2010). Moreover, even with interpreters who are carefully selected and trained, information distortion may occur because of differences in dialect and the challenge of matching a client's words with their intended meaning in another language (Altarriba & Santiago-Rivera, 1994; Rivera et al., 2011). Whereas words with concrete referents are easily translated, words that describe abstract concepts (e.g., emotions) are not as readily interpreted (Rivera et al., 2011). Bilingual providers may also be better able to address issues associated with code switching, or reverting to speaking a second language when describing an upsetting event, ostensibly to acquire psychological distance from threatening emotions. Code switching has been proposed as a treatment method to recognize forms of avoidance and to approach difficult topics (Altarriba & Santiago-Rivera, 1994; Andrés-Hyman et al., 2006; Rivera et al., 2011). Therefore, it is crucial that health practitioners familiarize themselves with the cultural values of the Puerto Rican population and other Latino groups.

Puerto Rican Cultural Elements (*Marianismo*, *Familismo*, etc.) and Their Relation to Behavioral Health

The importance of recognizing the importance of cultural elements and/or values in the provision of services in behavioral health and/or in the health-seeking behaviors of individuals provides opportunities to approach the Puerto Rican population from a more culturally competent and culturally sensitive perspective. According to Guarnaccia et al. (2005), examples are the recognition of the idioms/culturally bound syndrome of *nervios* and *ataque de nervios*. Importance should also be given to both Espiritismo and Santeria, and to the role of the Catholic and newer Protestants churches, their clergy, and lay organizations in support of people with psychological distress. Another important aspect within the religion/Espiritismo aspects of religion are that many patients prefer to go first to their religious leaders/community rather than the mental health providers because of the stigma that still permeates the Puerto Rican community seeking help for mental health issues. Given the high use of the medical sector both in Puerto Rico and on the mainland, recognition of mental health problems by primary care providers is a significant issue (Guarnaccia et al. 2005).

Regarding the cultural element of machismo and *marianismo* it is important and relevant to bring it into the process of recruiting Puerto Ricans to behavioral health services by working on eliminating the stigma of men receiving mental health services and not wanting to be seen as "weak" or less of a man and, in addition, by allowing them the space and opportunity to recognize the existence of more adaptive options of masculinity. In regard to the element of *marianismo*, the inclusion of this element provides the opportunity to discuss it and help reduce the pressure of being "perfect" and not vulnerable despite the different stressors of their daily lives. Dignity and respect are important elements to include in the provision of services as a way to retain patients. Providing services in Spanish and recognizing the importance of cultural traditions and nuances could make a difference when mental health services are engaging with patients and increase their sense of trust and will impact adherence. One example of these types of inclusion in treatment would be the recognition of cultural expressions, celebrations of cultural holidays, and cultural beliefs when working with the Puerto Rican population (Andrés-Hyman et al., 2006). Another important aspect is to provide information regarding treatment and the condition/s in the preferred language. The same applies to the labels on the medications. Finally, the inclusion of the element/value of *familismo* is a key factor to engage with, work with, and promote a respectful relationship with patients and their loved ones. Engagement of family members with the patient's authorization in the treatment helps to develop a sense of teamwork that resonates in attendance at appointments, communication with openness to discuss health issues and questions, and adherence to treatment protocols.

By recognizing the importance of the previously mentioned aspects, providers will be able to deliver more culturally sensitive and competent services to the Puerto Rican community taking into consideration the particular characteristics, in addition to not looking at this group as a stereotype but as a group with a lot of diversity from within and as a very important part of the "American collage." The extension of this knowledge to health-related issues for services cannot be the exception.

It is important to not generalize that all Latinos have the same values and in that way perpetuate ethnic stereotypes. Therefore, each value related to Latino values and especially to Puerto Ricans is discussed in the following sections

Dignidad y Respeto (Dignity and Respect)

"Dignity" (honor) and "respect" refer to a cultural value that underscores a reverence for all forms of life, particularly the intrinsic worth of humanity. Accordingly, irrespective of status or wealth, all people merit respect. Respect is also closely associated with a hierarchy of deference in which elders and parents are at the pinnacle (Andrés-Hyman et al., 2006). By convention, youth defers to age, children to parents, women to men, employees to employers, laypeople to experts, and so forth. However, *respeto* promotes "equality, empathy, and connection" in every relationship, even within those perceived as hierarchical (Torres, Solberg, & Carlstrom, 2002, p. 166). The tenets of *respeto* are reinforced through the use of proverbs (*dichos*), which are moral and life lessons recounted in everyday conversation as well as in the instruction of children (Andrés-Hyman et al., 2006).

Beliefs in the intrinsic merit of humanity may be a protective factor and a source of strength. Individuals may avoid discussing problems that compromise dignity. Dissent may be communicated indirectly (e.g., nod as if in tacit agreement). Individuals may seek the provider's advice and recommendations because of her or his professional status. Even if someone does not personally ascribe to the tenets of *respeto*, early learning experiences and enduring cultural expectations may be consonant with these values, and others may anticipate adherence to these mores.

You should attend to the physical environment to communicate respect for the culture (e.g., Hispanic artwork, Spanish reading material, bilingual phone reception), use a formal address before broaching the subject of a person's preferred address, engage in a measured exploration of problems to safeguard dignity, avoid asking personal questions before establishing trust (*confianza*), and explore treatment expectations and offer your view of your role in the helping relationship.

Dignidad y Respeto in Practice

Language barriers were overcome by offering services and forms in Spanish. In addition, the recruitment and retention of bilingual and bicultural staff served to convey esteem and an agency-wide investment in the language and traditions of clients. Bicultural providers also often used *dichos* in their work remind clients of *las condiciones madres* (conditions of the motherland) or of shared cultural experiences and commonly held truths. Admiration of the richness of Hispanic cultural traditions was also communicated through the observance of traditional holidays (e.g., Epiphany) that included the elements of family and community, typical dishes and music, and saying grace before dinner.

Familismo (Family Values and the Value of the Family)

Familismo is an all-centric cultural value related to stressing the centrality of family attachments, reciprocity, and loyalty to family members beyond the boundaries of the nuclear family (Martinez et al., 2013). Allocentrism is a "cultural value by which people understand themselves through others, emphasizing social relationships and highlighting group goals rather than individual ones" (La Roche, 2002, p. 116). Traditionally, the bounds of the family extend far beyond the nuclear family to include extended relatives and close family friends who are assimilated into the family as godparents, conferring an elevated role in the family system somewhat akin to co-parenthood (i.e., *compadrazco*). Families tend to be emotionally close (Comas-Diaz, 1988) and often live together in the same households or neighborhoods and function interdependently. Members of a family may strengthen their bonds by visiting and/or talking with each other daily, celebrating life cycle milestones together (e.g., anniversaries), and proffering financial support and gifts (Falicov, 2005).

Personalismo

Personalismo refers to preferring to relate to others in a personal manner instead of a formal manner. Among the many cultural manifestations of *personalismo* is the permeability of Hispanic households. Relatives and friends commonly drop by one another's homes unannounced for informal conversation. Another implication for social etiquette involves the form of greetings. The most ubiquitous greeting among women is a quick kiss on the cheek and an embrace; among men, a handshake or a pat on the shoulder or back; and among mixed pairs possibly an embrace or kiss. Irrespective of gender, however, physical touch is used more often by Puerto Ricans than Euro-Americans as a sign of warmth and a more personal relationship by the same token, the appropriate physical proximity during a normal conversation for

Puerto Ricans is much closer than for Euro-Americans. Thus, the use of appropriate touch (e.g., handshake) in a greeting or to bid farewell is consistent with the value of personalismo. Thus, it is recommended to introduce clients to new providers when care is being transferred (e.g., from triage).

Moreover, children and parents may continue to have a profound interdependence into adulthood. Immigration and/or family separation may be linked to behavioral health problems, and failure to send money to the family may be a disgrace (Falicov, 2005). Individuals may avoid or feel guilty about disparaging the family in conversation. Professional assistance may be sought as a last resort (after the family or clergy). Parents may leave children with grandparents as they establish financial stability in the United States (Falicov, 2005; La Roche, 2002). If the person is in accord, family members should be integrated into the treatment and the family's troubles (e.g., immigration) should be attended to if these are a priority. Family narratives and photos should be elicited to enhance rapport (La Roche, 2002). The family's treatment expectations, level of adherence to traditional values, and support of recovery goals should be explored. Family problems should be framed constructively to temper guilt about disclosure.

Machismo

Popular lore and the academic literature describe a largely negative and stereotypic conceptualization of Latino machismo, typified by controlling behavior toward women and children, promiscuity, alcohol abuse, stoicism, and aggression (Torres et al., 2002). However, this represents a pathological extension of masculinity observed across ethnicities and cultures, including among Euro-American men, rather than an accurate characterization of a genuine Latino cultural phenomenon (Torres et al., 2002).

Masculinity and gender roles in Puerto Rican culture are alive and well. Despite the stereotype of machismo in Puerto Rican culture both on the island and on the mainland, the cultural value of machismo and gender roles regarding the role of men in society has been evolving. The rapid changes in modern society, women's role in the working world, and gender–role ambiguity among other factors have impacted the "traditional perception" of what machismo is. Traditionally, according to Torres (1998), researchers have focused on the negative connotation of machismo as dominance, aggression, patriarchy, authoritarianism, and oppressive behavior toward women and children, failing to recognize the positive aspects such as emphasis on self-respect and on responsibility for protecting and providing for the family, patience, sensitivity, artistic appreciation, and open verbal communication that exist within the Puerto Rican culture. It is for this reason that Torres (1998) emphasizes the fact that the dominant culture does not permit Latino men to explore adaptive options of masculinity. For example, according to Torres et al., (2002) women's new role as self-sufficient breadwinners impacts their traditional sense of masculinity, but the question for us will be what can they do to change this schema? The schema could be changed by the emphasizing of the positive aspects of being a *machista* (i.e., self-assertiveness) and by the presenting of emotional aspects of themselves. For Gil and Vasquez (1996) the adjustment to the male role also includes a change in the vision of *marianismo*, another cultural value that emphasizes the moral and spiritual superiority of women. At the same time this includes adjustment to changing gender roles in the Puerto Rican family and to the constructs of machismo and *marianismo* and its impact on the different levels of acculturation. Doyle (1983) described that the mainland's societal criteria for manhood are intensified by the psychological stress and role strains stemming from immigration, acculturation, racism, and poverty. According to Torres (1998), one way to address the changes regarding "the new way of doing things" is the adoption of an ecosystemic orientation that takes into account multiple elements such as cultural, linguistic, educational, economic, gender, political, and environmental context engaging the positive aspects of machismo, and other cultural values such as *respeto* and *dignidad*. Another aspect worth mentioning is empowerment of men by facilitative approaches by the societal systems such as providing psychoeducational groups for men and culturally competent providers that emphasize the importance of change for men without diminishing their sense of self but empower them by facilitating their adaptation to healthier roles in their personal and social lives. As a consequence this will impact different areas of their lives, including health-seeking behaviors.

Marianismo

Marianismo, which is rooted in the Roman Catholic adoration of the Virgin Mary, refers to the traditional cultural prescriptive assigned to women. Accordingly, unmarried women are expected to remain chaste before marriage, and the onus for remaining virginal and for transmitting religious and cultural traditions to succeeding generations rests with women. Moreover, women can achieve a higher status of spiritual achievement with motherhood than men and consequently enjoy a commensurate amount of power (Comas-Diaz, 1988). On the other hand, Madonna mothers are expected to embody the virtues of selflessness and to endure suffering with dignity. This value leads to aspirations of humility and kindness and the transmission of norms (for both sexes) to treat others with kindness and display sympathy for others' feelings (i.e., value of *simpatía*; Andrés-Hyman et al., 2006). The pathological extension of *marianismo* is that a woman may become submissive, or a perception of martyrdom may engender conflict with her US-born children.

Religion and Spirituality

Faith, rooted in Roman Catholicism, is generally the cornerstone of Hispanic life (Andrés-Hyman et al., 2006). The rituals of the indigenous peoples of the Americas and of Africans transported to Hispaniola during the slave trade are also evident in the contemporary practices of spiritism and folk healing. In the Hispanic Caribbean, two main forms of spiritism exist: Espiritismo (Mesa Blanca) and Santeria (the worship of saints). As a whole, spiritists attribute problems to either spiritual or material causes, or stated differently, those requiring spiritual or medical intercession, and turn to indigenous healers (*espiritistas* or *santeros*) for aid with problems with spiritual origins, such as being afflicted with and tormented by bad spirits (Andrés-Hyman et al., 2006; Berthold, 1989). Women may avoid appointments that conflict with spending time with their family. Sex may be an improper or private subject, particularly with male providers. Substance abuse may cause or exacerbate feelings of worthlessness. Women may view acceptance of problems and/or suffering as obligatory and proper and hesitate to complain about problems or loved ones. Goals should be framed in line with personal narratives (e.g., helping a mother to assist her family). One should inquire about a potential preference for a woman provider. The level o adherence to traditional gender norms should be explored. Intimate topics should be explored tentatively. One should inquire about a woman's relationship with her family, particularly her children. Socioeconomic concerns should be considered when operating hours are being devised.

Although spiritism is practiced by only a small subset of Puerto Ricans, the belief that the individuals "destiny is at the mercy of God is prevalent across the Spanish-speaking world and is evident in widespread references to God's Will" (Andrés-Hyman et al., 2006; Falicov, 2005). The importance of spirituality and religion in Puerto Rican culture is demonstrated in the structure of the New Life Program of Connecticut: a faith-based agency, composed of a cooperative of churches, formed one arm of the tripartite project. In addition, community spiritual leaders were invited to join advisory boards and other important decision-making bodies. Through these collaborations, a spiritual component was incorporated into each program event.

Culturally Adapted, Tailored Treatment Versus Standard Treatment of Puerto Rican Patients in Primary Care

Culturally competent practices may have a profound impact on treatment access, adherence, and outcomes. These recommendations are intended to serve as a resource for improving the quality of behavioral health care for Puerto Ricans through the use of approaches that are compatible with commonly held cultural values. Additional research is required to examine the effectiveness of these approaches through the use of clinical trials (Sue, 2003). The importance of incorporating a cross-cultural interview in primary medicine has been related to a patient's perception of the illness and any alternative therapies he or she is undergoing and facilitates the development of a mutually acceptable treatment plan (Juckett, 2005, 2013). According to Juckett (2005, 2013), patients should understand instructions from their physicians and be able to repeat them in their own words. Potential cultural conflicts between a physician and a patient include differing attitudes toward time, personal space, eye contact, body language, and even what is important in life.

In addition, many patients use home remedies or traditional healers before seeking conventional medical treatment (Juckett, 2005, 2013). Others return to traditional healers instead of completing an ongoing conventional treatment. Juckett (2005, 2013) reports that the healing traditions of Latinos, including Puerto Ricans, are rich and culturally meaningful but can affect management of chronic medical and psychiatric conditions. For this reason it is important to know the different traditional healing practices and their meanings given by patients and their families. Patients may lose confidence in their physicians if they do not receive prompt, culturally comprehensible treatment. Thus, the practitioner needs to know which non-traditional healing techniques the patient is using and if possible use them complementarily. Efforts directed toward instituting more culturally relevant health care enrich the physician–patient relationship and improve patient rapport, adherence, and outcomes. Clinical success often depends on communicating with these healers and prioritizing tests and treatments (Juckett, 2005, 2013).

Puerto Ricans in comparison with other cultural groups have physical health problems with the worst, or nearly the worst, rates for many diseases when compared with other race and ethnic groups. For example, heart disease rates are 20 % higher for Puerto Ricans than for any other Hispanic group. Also, studies that have used these same data have reported higher levels of overweight and comparable hypertension rates among Puerto Ricans (especially women) than Cubans and Mexican Americans. The rates of mental health problems are no different. It is for this reason that the development of culturally adapted tailored treatments plays an important role in the engagement and process of contacting, engaging, and maintaining adherence in the provision of health services independently if they are for physical or mental conditions or both. Culturally adapted treatments are defined as health care interventions that are tailored to patients' norms, beliefs, and values, as well as to their language and literacy skills. This specific type of care may incorporate language or music preferences, or may delve more deeply into cultural considerations such as social, psychological, and economic factors. Examples of culturally adapted care include matching specialists to patients by race or ethnicity; adapting patient materials to reflect patients' culture, language, or literacy skills; offering education via community-based health advocates; incorporating norms about faith, food, family, or self-image into patient care; and implementing patient involvement strategies.

Kohn-Wood and Hooper provide recommendations for mental health care providers working in primary care settings, while keeping in mind racial/ethnic disparities in mental health, and sustainable solutions to provide culturally tailored solutions. According to these authors, the clinical mental health care providers (psychiatrists, mental health counselors, psychologists, psychiatric nurses, family therapists, and social workers as well as primary care physicians) have a critical need to learn how to improve the treatment they provide to racial and ethnic minorities, given that the current disparities lead to significant rates of untreated mental illness among them.

Finally they emphasized that the most important issues for providers are to (1) recognize factors that underlie disparities in mental health treatment, (2) understand how conceptualizations of cultural competence are evolving, and (3) use and contribute to the literature on cultural tailoring as a way to improve mental health treatment rates for racial/ethnic minority groups in primary care settings.

It is important to mention examples of culturally tailored interventions for Puerto Ricans, such as the brief culturally tailored intervention for Puerto Ricans with type 2 diabetes developed by Osborn et al. Another example with medical conditions is the culturally adapted family asthma management intervention called "CALMA" (an acronym of the Spanish for "take control, empower yourself, and achieve management of asthma") in reducing asthma morbidity in poor Puerto Rican children with asthma developed by Canino et al.

These interventions were conducted with both island and mainland Puerto Rican children. Canino et al. evaluated the effectiveness of the intervention and found it seems promising for the reduction of asthma morbidity. Finally, Duarté-Vélez et al. reported culturally adapted cognitive-behavioral therapy in the case of a Puerto Rican adolescent, who participated in a randomized clinical trial for the treatment of major depression disorder. They maintained fidelity to the treatment protocol, but promoted flexibility addressing cultural values about sexual orientation, spirituality, the family, and identity development as a central part of the treatment. The results evidence that the intervention was successful, being tailored to the particular needs of the patient and taking into consideration the nuances and cultural sensitivity and cultural competence that are required when one is working with the Puerto Rican population, recognizing their similarities and differences under the same scope without losing the importance and respect for the particular characteristics of the individual being treated and that person's ecological surroundings plus a holistic view of the person. These interventions may take more time and effort than the ones with the average population but are worth it considering the increase of the Puerto Rican population in the United States and the importance they play as Hispanics/Latinos in the fabric of that country.

Recommendations on Behavioral Health Screens to Screen for Depression, Anxiety, Pain, and Other Problems Associated with Physical Illnesses in an Integrated Health Care Setting Serving Puerto Ricans

First, to make decisions about implementing systematic depression screening for Spanish-speaking populations, primary care physicians and mental health providers need to know which Spanish language depression-screening instruments are accurate. Reuland et al. reviewed systematically the evidence regarding the diagnostic accuracy of depression-screening instruments in Spanish with primary care populations. They found that the Spanish language version of the Center for Epidemiologic Studies Depression Scale had sensitivities ranging from 76 to 92 % and specificities ranging from 70 to 74 %. The Spanish language version of the Postpartum Depression Screening Scale was 78 % sensitive and 85 % specific for combined major–minor depression (one US study). For depression screening in Spanish-speaking outpatients, fair evidence supports the diagnostic accuracy of the Center for Epidemiologic Studies Depression Scale and the nine-item PRIME-MD in general primary care and the 15-item Geriatric Depression Scale (Spanish) for geriatric patients, meaning that although they a few in number and in more instruments are needed for the Spanish-speaking population in the United States, clinicians could use these instruments in their primary care interventions. On the other hand, Rodero and his team in Spain validated the Chronic Pain Acceptance Questionnaire (CPAQ) for the assessment of acceptance in fibromyalgia. The value of this is that it could be normalized for Spanish-speaking populations in the United States. Analysis of results showed that the Spanish CPAQ had good test–retest reliability (intraclass correlation coefficient 0.83) and internal consistency reliability (Cronbach's α 0.83). The Spanish CPAQ score significantly correlated with pain intensity, anxiety, depression, pain catastrophizing, health status, and physical and psychosocial disability. The Scree plot and a principal components factor analysis confirmed the same two-factor construct as the original English CPAQ. For this reason teams in the United States should work to validate the questionnaire for Spanish-speaking populations. D'Alonzo describes that as Spanish-speaking immigrants participate in and become the focus of research studies, questions arise about the appropriateness of existing research tools, and explains that very little has been written regarding the testing and evaluation of research tools among less educated Latino immigrants. It is for this reason that more culturally appropriate methods should be evaluated for use with the Spanish-speaking population, such as the Self-Efficacy and Exercise Habits Survey, the Latina Values Scale Revised, and the Hispanic Stress Inventory. The tests could be translated and validated to provide a more complete service but also to expand the scope of information to work with the Spanish-speaking population in the United States and particularly in primary care.

The cross-cultural interview proposed by Juckett (2005, 2013) requires time and patience. First, small talk can establish trust (*confianza* in Spanish) between the patient and the physician. According to Juckett (2005), physicians should use a patient's formal name if they are unsure of the appropriate way to address the patient. According to Juckett, patients will sometimes avoid eye contact with physicians out of respect, especially if they are of a different sex or social status. Consequently, the physician should ask the patient what the illness means to him or her and what treatments the patient is currently undergoing. This will allow the physician to explain the different treatment options and find a mutually acceptable treatment plan. The physician should provide instructions, preferably in writing (if the patient or a family member is literate), and ask the patient if the plan is acceptable. Rather than asking, "Do you understand?" the physician should have patients repeat the instructions in their own words.

Time perception and management differ among cultures. For example, many Latinos and especially Puerto Ricans have a relaxed sense of time, and personal relationships are considered more important than schedules. Thus, practitioners should, if a patient is late, tactfully explain the importance of being on time in the US medical setting (Juckett, 2005, 2013; Sue, 2013).

Tseng and Streltzer (2008) mentioned the following as important factors in adherence to prescriptions that need to be taken into consideration to increase adherence to prescriptions recognizing the specific cultural aspects of Puerto Ricans:

1. Patient's concept of the illness, as well as the symbolic meaning of the illness in the patient's culture
2. Medication characteristics, which may be important to the patient
3. The symbolic power and value of the medication in the patient's culture
4. Dietary habits and nutritional interactions with alternative treatments used by the patient
5. The physician–patient relationship, including expectations and symbolic meaning of giving and receiving medication, as well as other transferential aspects of the relationship

According to Levensky and O'Donohue (2006), several variables are extremely important for adherence to treatment:

1. Having a multicultural and multilingual staff
2. Using trained interpreters and receiving training on how to integrate interpreters into clinical practice
3. Providing written instructions in the language spoken by the particular patient/client
4. Training professionals in multicultural awareness
5. Including relevant cultural components in the treatment
6. Consulting, collaborating with, and involving folk healers in the treatment
7. Respecting the client's/patient's culturally based explanations/interpretations
8. Increasing participation by extended family members.

Conclusions and Final Recommendations for Best Practices with Puerto Ricans

An adequate assessment that is culturally sensitive is the basis for promotion of use to health services and adherence to treatment in ethnic minorities, including Puerto Ricans. Ones should always evaluate adherence by taking into account the behavioral, cultural, and environmental factors that affect it. People bring into the consultation their own beliefs and perceptions about the illness, and this may have consequences in the promotion or failure of adherence to treatment that may affect their quality of life (Rodriguez-Gomez, 2006). According to Rodriguez-Gomez, it will be necessary to study the positive short, medium-, and long-term effects that culture-sensitive adherence strategies may have for the survival of minorities so as to diminish physical and mental health disparities (Rodriguez-Gomez, 2006).

One of the most influencing factors on adherence is communication. Patients who do not speak the same language as their clinicians rate their visit with physicians as less participatory as whites (Rodriguez-Gomez, 2006). It is imperative to take into consideration culturally sensitive elements such as the use of folk or home remedies that may have an effect on treatment adherence. Finally, the importance of becoming aware and knowledgeable as providers and teams about how race, culture, and gender affect communication styles is important to provide high-quality services (Sue, 2013). It is important for training programs in primary care and related professions to use an approach that call for openness and flexibility both in conceptualization and in actual skill building (Sue, 2013).

According to Ho et al. (2006), more studies are warranted to examine if the acculturated lifestyle, quality of health services, access to health care, and effectiveness in controlling a chronic illness such as diabetes and its complications are factors associated with the poor health status of mainland Puerto Ricans. This inquiry could be extended to other medical conditions as well to the provision of mental health services. It is for this reason that we should be aware of the studies available and their findings to help understand the different factors that impact and could impact the provision of primary care services to Puerto Ricans in the United States. Primary-care-based interventions that have been effective in non-Latinos could incorporate culturally appropriate elements, and lessons from community-based research and could be applied to Latinos so that their effectiveness can be assessed in this group (O'Malley, Gonzalez, Sheppard, Huerta, & Mandelblatt, 2003). If we recognize these variables and expand the opportunities for teaching, training, supervision, research, and practice with Latinos, in particular with the mainland Puerto Rican population, and exchange information with the treatment and research teams on the island, it should be possible to improve and increase the cultural competence knowledge and skills in the setting of the Puerto Rican population in primary care.

References

Altarriba, J., & Santiago-Rivera, A. L. (1994). Current perspectives on using linguistic and cultural factors in counseling the Hispanic client. *Professional Psychology, Research and Practice, 4*, 388.

Andrés-Hyman, R. C., Ortiz, J., Añez, L. M., Paris, M., & Davidson, L. (2006). Culture and clinical practice: recommendations for working with Puerto Ricans and other Latinas(os) in the United States. *Professional Psychology, Research and Practice, 37*(6), 694–701.

Baig, A. A., Benitez, A., Locklin, C. A., Campbell, A., Schaefer, C. T., Heuer, L. J., … Chin, M. H. (2014). Community health center provider and staff's Spanish language ability and cultural awareness. *Journal of Health Care for the Poor & Underserved, 25*(2), 527–545.

Berthold, M. S. (1989). Spiritism as a form of psychotherapy: implications for social work practice. *Social Casework, 90*, 89–91.

Brown, A., & Patten, E. (2013). *Hispanics of Puerto Rican origin in the United States, 2011*. Pew Research Center Report. Retrieved from http://www.pewhispanic.org/2013/06/19/hispanics-of-puerto-rican-origin-in-the-united-states-2011/.

Comas-Diaz, L. (1988). Mainland Puerto Rican women: a sociocultural approach. *Journal of Community Psychology, 16*(1), 21–31.

Corrigan, P. W., Morris, S. B., Michaels, P. J., Rafacz, J. D., & Rüsch, N. (2012). Challenging the public stigma of mental illness: a meta-analysis of outcome studies. *Psychiatric Services, 63*, 963–973. http://dx.doi.org/10.1176/appi.ps.201100529.

Corrigan, P. W., Mueser, K. T., Bond, G. R., Drake, R. E., & Solomon, P. (2008). *Principles and practice of psychiatric rehabilitation*. New York, NY: Guilford Press.

De La Cancela, V. (1986). A critical analysis of Puerto Rican machismo: implications for clinical practice. *Psychotherapy: Theory, Research, Practice, Training, 23*, 291–296.

Deegan, P. (2004). Mentalism, micro-aggression and the peer practitioner. Retrieved from https://www.patdeegan.com/blog/posts/mentalism-micro-aggression-and-peer-practitioner.

Deyoung, Y., & Zigler, E. F. (1994). Machismo in two cultures: relation to punitive child-rearing practices. *American Journal of Orthopsychiatry, 64*, 386–395.

Doyle, J. A. (1983). *The male experience*. Dubuque, IA: William C. Brown.

Falicov, C. (2005). Emotional transnationalism and family identities. *Family Process, 44*(4), 399–406.

Gil, R. M., & Vasquez, C. A. (1996). *The Maria paradox: how Latina women can merge Old World traditions with New World self-esteem*. New York, NY: Putnam.

Guarnaccia, P. J., Martinez, I., & Acosta, H. (2005). Mental health in the Hispanic immigrant community. An overview. *Journal of Immigrant & Refugee Services, 3*(1/2), 21.

Guttfreund, D. G. (1990). Effects of language usage on the emotional experience of Spanish-English and English-Spanish bilinguals. *Journal of Consulting and Clinical Psychology, 5*, 604.

Ho, G., Qian, H., Kim, M., Melnik, T., Tucker, K., Jimenez-Velazquez, I., … Rohan, T. (2006). Health disparities between island and mainland Puerto Ricans. *Revista Panamericana De Salud Publica, 19(5)*, 331–339.

Institute of Medicine. (2002). *Unequal treatment: confronting racial and ethnic disparities*. Washington, DC: The National Academies Press.

Juckett, G. (2005). Cross-cultural medicine. *American Family Physician, 72*(11), 2267.

Juckett, G. (2013). Caring for Latino patients. *American Family Physician, 87*(1), 48–54.

La Roche, M. J. (2002). Psychotherapeutic considerations in treating Latinos. *Harvard Review of Psychiatry, 10*(2), 115.

Levensky, E. R., & O'Donohue, W. T. (2006). *Promoting treatment adherence: a practical handbook for health care providers*. Thousand Oaks, CA: SAGE Publications.

Martinez, I., Interian, A., & Guarnaccia, P. (2013). Antidepressant adherence among Latinos: the role of the family. *Qualitative Research in Psychology, 10*(1), 63–85. doi:10.1080/14780887.2011.586102.

Nemec, P. B., Swarbrick, M., & Legere, L. (2015). Prejudice and discrimination from mental health service providers. *Psychiatric Rehabilitation Journal, 38*(2), 203–206.

O'Malley, A. S., Gonzalez, R. M., Sheppard, V. B., Huerta, E., & Mandelblatt, J. (2003). Review and special article: primary care cancer control interventions including Latinos. A review. *American Journal of Preventive Medicine, 25*, 264–271.

Ramos, B. M. (2005). Acculturation and depression among Puerto Ricans in the mainland. *Social Work Research, 29*(2), 95.

Reidy, D. E. (1993). *"Stigma is social death": mental health consumers/survivors talk about stigma in their lives*. Holyoke, MA: Education for Community Initiatives.

Rivera, F., López, I., Guarnaccia, P., Ramirez, R., Canino, G., & Bird, H. (2011). Perceived discrimination and antisocial behaviors in Puerto Rican children. *Journal of Immigrant & Minority Health, 13*(3), 453–461.

Rodriguez-Gomez, J. (2006). Adherence in ethnic minorities. In W. T. O'Donohoue & E. Levensky (Eds.), *Promoting treatment adherence: a practical handbook for health care* (pp. 415–420). Thousand Oaks, CA: SAGE Publications.

Schenker, Y., Karter, A. J., Schillinger, D., Margaret Warton, E., Adler, N. E., Moffet, H. H., … Fernandez, A. (2010). The impact of limited English proficiency and physician language concordance on reports of clinical interactions among patients with diabetes: the DISTANCE study. *Patient Education and Counseling 81*(2): 222–228.

Schwartz, A., Rodríguez, M. D., Santiago-Rivera, A. L., Arredondo, P., & Field, L. D. (2010). Cultural and linguistic competence: welcome challenges from successful diversification. *Professional Psychology, Research and Practice, 41*(3), 210–220.
Sue, S. (2003). In defense of cultural competency in psychotherapy and treatment. *The American Psychologist, 58*(11), 964–970.
Sue, D. W. (2013). *Counseling the culturally diverse: Theory and practice*. [serial online]. Retrieved May 20, 2015, from Bibliotheksverbund Bayern, Ipswich, MA.
Sue, D. W., Capodilupo, C. M., Torino, G. C., Bucceri, J. M., Holder, A. M. B., Nadal, K. L., & Esquilin, M. (2007). Racial microaggressions in everyday life: implications for clinical practice. *American Psychologist, 62*, 271–286.
Torres, J. B. (1998). Masculinity and gender roles among Puerto Rican men: a dilemma for Puerto Rican men's personal identity. *American Journal of Orthopsychiatry, 68*, 16–26.
Torres, J. B., Solberg, V. H., & Carlstrom, A. H. (2002). The myth of sameness among Latino men and their machismo. *American Journal of Orthopsychiatry, 72*(2), 163–181.
Tseng, W., & Streltzer, J. (2008). *Cultural competence in health care*. New York, NY: Springer.
Urciuoli, B. (1996). *Exposing prejudice: Puerto Rican experiences of language, race, and class*. Long Grove, IL: Waveland Press.

Chapter 4
Special Considerations for Working with Cubans in Integrated Care: Intergenerational Perspectives on Life-Course Health Promotion

Ester R. Shapiro

Setting the Stage: Cuban Americans, Wellness, and Geopolitics of the Heart

At the time this chapter was being completed, Cuban Americans were prominently in the national news, with President Barack Obama visiting Cuba as part of the first opening of U.S. Cuba diplomatic relations since the 1959 socialist revolution, and two Cuban Americans who had benefitted from preferential immigration treatment were Republican candidates for the Presidential primary, running on anti-immigrant platforms. The polarized, Cold War politics characterizing U.S./Cuba relations have greatly affected family relationships which Falicov (2014) terms "A Geopolitics of the Heart," creating dilemmas of family separations, responsibility, and loyalty both for Cuban Americans living in largest concentrations in South Florida or New Jersey/New York as well as for those of us living outside these enclaves. I am a Cuban American of Eastern European Jewish descent who grew up in South Florida but currently lives and works in Boston, and a clinical psychologist strongly influenced by Cuba's exemplary family medicine-centered health care system and model of integrative care (Shapiro & Louro Bernal, 2014), personal and professional experiences informing the theoretical frameworks, sources of evidence, and clinical practice perspectives informing this chapter.

In exploring treatment recommendations for Cuban Americans in Integrative Care, clinicians discover the specificity by which particular moments in evolving Cuba/U.S. political relationships have marked the shared family life course and dilemmas of politics interwoven with intergenerational differences in acculturation, meaningfully impacting health and mental health care. Those of us with elderly parents of the 1960s immigration immediately post-revolution are struggling to

E.R. Shapiro (✉)
University of Massachusetts, Boston, Boston, MA 02125, USA
e-mail: ester.shapiro@umb.edu

© Springer International Publishing Switzerland 2016

L.T. Benuto, W. O'Donohue (eds.), *Enhancing Behavioral Health in Latino Populations*, DOI 10.1007/978-3-319-42533-7_4

support their care, facing the expectations that family members, particularly daughters, will directly provide or supervise caretakers so that their parents can remain in their homes as long as possible. Others, whose families experienced more time in socialist Cuba, face the scrutiny of earlier immigrants, especially those in the South Florida enclave community, regarding their political opinions, their failure to obey highly valued patriarchal, hierarchical family obligations, or to honor the Catholic Church and its strict prohibitions against abortion, both accepted and publicly funded in Cuba. Cuban immigrants, particularly those of African diaspora descent who are socially identified in the U.S. as Black, experience a different definition of race or racialization in which any visible African features type them for racial stereotyping in absolute terms, in contrast to the Cuban experience of racial categorizing that also includes social class, educational achievement, and professional status (Perez, 2009). Understanding what ails us as Cuban Americans, and how best to evaluate and implement integrative care, requires a highly specific assessment of immigration histories and dislocations, experiences of acculturation, and their impacts on the intergenerational and extended family relationships which are at the heart of Cuban American health and wellness.

Clinicians working with Latino families in general, and Cuban American families in particular, highlight the importance of reflexivity as an element of cultural competence (Kirmeyer, 2012). Reflexivity is defined as critical assessment of personal subjectivity as influenced by intersecting aspects of personal and professional background and social location, to appreciate how these influence interventions both explicitly and implicitly (Bernal & Shapiro, 2005; Comas-Diaz, 2012; Falicov, 2014; Laroche, 2013). This chapter, which draws on an interdisciplinary literature review that includes knowledge of Cuban American contexts of migration and appreciation of the Cuban health care system, addresses both professional and personal perspectives on knowledge as they impact findings and recommendations, encouraging readers to both reflect on and extend personal sources of knowledge in the service of work with Cuban American families. Both professionally and politically, I believe that compassionate, constructive dialogue across differences and societal commitment to equity contribute to health and growth promotion. The following chapter draws from the published research literature as well as personal and professional experiences of negotiating subjectivities and developing partnerships for health promotion on both sides of the divide, striving to learn from both without demonizing either. Clinicians seeking to work with Cuban American families will find that sociopolitical contexts of migration, generating unique circumstances and intergenerational connections and conflicts, have meaningful implications for their lived experience, health/mental health status, and best practices for engaging in treatment within integrative care.

Writers in the fields of integrative health care, arguing for transdisciplinary approaches capable of person-centered care that also contextualizes social determinants of chronic illness care (Cloninger et al., 2014; Juster et al., 2011; Martin & Petersen, 2009) and evidence-based practice (Satterfield et al., 2009), suggest that when health literature reviews cross disciplines they require "reflexive synthesis" sensitive to both societal ideologies and disciplinary perspectives, inevitably shaped by disciplinary assumptions and values as well as economic benefit and societal power inequalities. In arguing for integrative health care in the U.S., practitioners face significant economic and ideological biases favoring fragmented specialty health care and ignoring contexts of inequality (Starfield, 2009). The Affordable Care Act offers new incentives supporting integrative care (Mechanic, 2012), yet due to political compromises was not designed for universal health care access in its global understanding as a human right, but simply expanded access to health insurance, speaking to continuing barriers in delivering quality integrative care to any U.S. population.

Self-awareness of personal subjectivity is particularly important in working with Cuban Americans in family-centered, culturally meaningful integrative health. For Cuban Americans, individual and family lived experiences have been ruptured by Cold War politics that separated families and mandated politically based family loyalties either for or against the Socialist revolution. Clinicians working with Cuban Americans should be aware that the timing and circumstances of Cuban immigration to the U.S. are rooted in very particular political histories as they intersect with intergenerational, family life course processes (Bernal & Shapiro, 2005; Duany, 2011; Eckstein, 2009; Falicov, 2014; Szapocsnik, Schwartz, Muir, & Brown, 2012) with consequences for health and mental health status and access to health resources. Cuban American political identifications affecting individuals and dividing families emerged in the context of embattled, evolving Cold War animosities and changing circumstances as they have impacted immigration and the shared life course. I am a Cuban American of Eastern European Jewish descent, born in Cuba within an immigrant extended family who reluctantly left Cuba in 1960 when I was 8 years old. I was brought up within and enduringly connected through extended family ties and academic networks to the large South Florida Cuban American enclaves, but moved to Massachusetts for college, and clinical psychology training. I now live and work in Boston where the very small Cuban American community is heterogeneous in social class and educational levels as well as politically mixed. I have established strong personal and academic networks supporting engagement with Cuban health and educational institutions and appreciating their accomplishments (Shapiro, 1994; Shapiro & Louro Bernal, 2014), guiding the perspective I bring to all my work. I teach culturally informed clinical and health promotion practice in Boston, emphasizing strengths-based ecosystemic life-course and family-centered social justice perspectives highlighting the societal resources individuals, families, and communities need to maintain "wellness as fairness" (Prilleltensky, 2012). I have preserved ties to both my anti-Castro extended family in South Florida, as well as to family, friends, and colleagues in Cuba and the U.S. who appreciate the values and contributions of the Cuban socialist government to the fields of health and education and to government responsibility in economic equality while recognizing the current system's limitations (Shapiro, 2010a, 2010b; Shapiro & Louro Bernal, 2014). Maintaining this balance requires a critical stance on the strident ideologies and suppression of dissent imposed by both sides of the divide, and sensitivity to the concerns of all members of our expanding Cuban transnational communities. Both the Cuban government and the Cuban exile community have used violence to control dissent. My friends and colleagues in Boston and Miami were targets of Cuban American right-wing terrorism. Many Cuban Americans in the U.S. have enduring memories of the violence during both the socialist revolution and its aftermath, and my Cuban colleagues live in a community where a special police force evaluates their publications to ensure that any critiques of the government fall within an accepted language. A punitive economic embargo (termed a blockade by Cuba) which has helped impoverish Cuba and failed to change Cuban politics remains in place, even though it has failed to meet the political objective of inspiring uprising against Fidel and Raul Castro's socialist government.

For guidance in working with Cuban American families in integrative health settings, the available literature on health and mental health has tended to aggregate data on Latinos, lacking needed specificity on nativity, immigration status, and years in the U.S. This chapter draws on the limited literature focusing on Cuban Americans while including a wider range of studies in migration and cultural studies as well as in integrative health and mental health. Because the literature on health and mental health for Latino populations is only beginning to publish work that disaggregates populations by immigration status and nationality, this chapter reviews the available literature on demographics and contexts of migration, illustrating the impact of these factors through case vignettes. The treatment literature on Cuban Americans is also limited, with a few research teams working in the Miami area collecting health and mental health data and developing and testing treatment protocols based specifically on Cuban Americans. The work of Szapocsnik and colleagues at the University of Miami (Muir, Schwartz, & Szapocznik, 2004; Szapocsnik et al., 2012; Szapocsnik, Muir, Duff, Schwartz, & Brown, 2015) is particularly noteworthy, as this team has studied health and mental health status for Cuban American families focusing on both adolescents and elders. Further, they have developed family-centered interventions to address differential acculturation across generations and develop culturally meaningful strengths-based approaches. Given the limited available intervention literature, the chapter will also draw from Latino-centric approaches to cultural adaptation of health and mental health services (Bernal & Domenech-Rodriguez, 2012), literatures on bridging patient-centered and culturally competent care, particularly for Latinos (Nielsen, Wall, & Tucker, 2016) and a transdisciplinary approach to culturally sensitive integrative care that highlights health equity resources supporting family resilience throughout the life course (Shapiro, 2013a, 2013b). Because most of the current literature on integrative care does not focus specifically on Cuban Americans, the following discussion of clinical considerations draws on a transdisciplinary literature and uses an integrative family life course theoretical approach emphasizing social determinants of integrative health and mental health, and highlighting cultural resources supporting family resilience particularly for families facing challenges of chronic illness (Shapiro, 2013a). This approach can help illuminate both aspects of culture and of circumstances of migration as they shape the presentation of Cuban Americans in health care settings, and inform strategies for effective, culturally sensitive care. Finally, the chapter includes brief case illustrations throughout of clinical services, supervision, and consultations; identifying information in these case illustrations has been altered to protect patient privacy.

Frameworks for Integrative Care with Cuban Americans: Cultural/Ecological Perspectives on Integrative and Evidence-Based Care

A person-centered primary health care perspective has been recommended as an impactful way of reducing disparities by directly addressing social determinants of health as they impact particular patients (Cloninger et al., 2014; Starfield, 2009). Nielsen et al. (2016) tested Tucker's model of patient-centered, culturally sensitive care (Tucker, Marsiske, Rice, Nielson, & Herman, 2011) for Latino patients with both Spanish and English language preference, evaluating the impact of these variables on treatment adherence. Tucker's model of patient-centered culturally sensitive care, developed for racially/culturally diverse populations that included a Latino subsample, focused on how patients perceived their interactions with the clinician in the domains of trust, satisfaction with treatment including cultural and religious sensitivity, and patient sense of personal control/empowerment. The study found that all dimensions of their model's patient-centered, culturally sensitive care enhanced patient satisfaction and treatment adherence for this sample of Latino patients, although effect sizes were considerably larger for the English preferred compared to the Spanish preferred patients. Additionally, the study found that for Spanish language preference Latino patients, patient-perceived Provider Cultural Sensitivity (PCS) also reduced patient sense of control in treatment decision-making. The authors suggested that increasing PCS for these patients may also raise their awareness of barriers due to language differences, lowering sense of personal control. Because the study relied exclusively on patient self-report, and enrolled patients across multiple sites nationally, the research did not directly evaluate whether Spanish-preference Latino patients received linguistically appropriate services whether through a Spanish speaking provider or a trained interpreter. Exploration of Spanish language preference as a dimension of acculturation is especially important to evaluate for Cuban Americans living in ethnic enclaves, and for women within those enclaves, as they may be able to navigate their daily lives with limited use of English. Although the South Florida area, and other areas with larger numbers of Cuban Americans, may also offer more choices for Spanish-speaking health care providers, this study's finding that patient-centered, culturally competent care may actually lower sense of control for Latino patients suggests the complexity and sensitivity of these intersecting language, culture, and relational themes in the health care setting.

Models of integrative care addressing both health and mental health disparities among ethnic minorities further need to take into account the complexity of unique patient characteristics and the characteristics of the health care setting as these vary greatly in their approach to integration and availability of culturally and linguistically competent clinicians. The Cuban values of respeto/respect for authority and personalismo/emphasis on personal networks and relationships offer an excellent bridge to models of primary care that emphasize narrative and storytelling, while linking these to enhanced understanding of person-centered care, leading to enhanced use of evidence-based practice (Silva, Charon, & Wyer, 2011). However, it is also important to critically evaluate constructs from the cultural/ethnographic literature describing cultural characteristics to consider whether patterns attributed to cultural beliefs are interwoven with or confounded by challenges associated with health disparities due to social determinants of health (Lopez, Barrio, Kopelowicz, & Vega, 2012). For example, the construct of "fatalismo" attributed to Latino families, arguing that cultural and religious factors lead to fatalism in the face of illness and will be associated with delayed or avoided care, can be better understood in light of structural barriers such as lack of health insurance, negative experiences with the health care system, or lack of culturally and linguistically trained providers (Abraído-Lanza et al., 2007).

Holden et al. (2014) address the complexity of centering integrative mental health care on cultural factors by arguing for a multi-level approach that addresses both provider cultural competence skills and systemic/organizational competence in integrative care. Their Culturally Centered Model of Behavioral health Care brings together cultural competence skills using a "CRASH" mnemonic of cultural competence skills, with characteristics of a Primary Care Mental Health approach. CRASH includes: **Culture** as shared values and connections in the experience of health and health care and in patient/professional interaction; **Respect** demonstrated with appreciation of cultural expressions; **Assess** to appreciate the wide range of "within-group differences" and inquire about cultural identity, health preferences, beliefs, and understanding of health conditions, language competency, acculturation level, and health literacy; **Affirm** by recognizing that each individual is the world's expert on his/her own experiences, listening for and affirming experiences and identifying cultural strengths in differences; **Sensitivity**, developing awareness of cultural expectations that might cause offense or break down trust and communication; **Self-Awareness**, becoming aware of personal cultural norms, values, and reactivities leading providers to miscommunicate or misjudge others; and **Humility**, recognizing that none of us attains "cultural competence" but commits to a life-time of learning. At the Organizational level, **continuity of care**, a **whole-patient orientation**, **safety and quality**, and **care coordination and integration** support the culturally centered provider/patient relationship. This approach to centering culture within integrative care is especially useful for work with Cuban Americans, as it recognizes the within-family cultural complexity associated with migration status and acculturation levels, the centrality of respect which also includes appreciation of gendered generational roles and acculturation differences, and allows for assessment of migration stories and their impacts.

In integrative care, depending on the setting and the practice model for bridging primary care and behavioral/mental health care, practitioners will need to refer Cuban American patients with specific mental health needs to a mental health practitioner. Because a limited number of empirically validated treatments have been tested for Latinos in general, and Cuban Americans in particular, approaches to cultural adaptation of "empirically supported" or "evidence-based" practice take a broader approach to identifying culturally meaningful adaptations of interventions based on evidence (Bernal & Domenech-Rodriguez, 2012). The Ecological Validity Framework (EVF), proposed by Bernal, Bonilla & Bellido (in Bernal & Domenech-Rodriguez, 2012) is an especially useful guide in evaluating the domains for cultural adaptation of behavioral health/mental health interventions, identifying eight areas of an intervention that may be culturally adapted. Guillermo Bernal, also a Cuban American who left Cuba as a child in the early 1960s migration and who has maintained ties with Cuban psychologists, has developed a body of work on cultural adaptation of evidence-based practices that draws from Cuban perspectives on psychology within socialist health care and cultural values (Bernal, 2016; Bernal & Shapiro, 2005). In the Ecological Validity Framework, **Language** refers to culturally relevant oral and written forms of communication (e.g., translation, specific jargon). The persons dimension captures the client-therapist dyad dynamics (e.g., ethnic match). **Metaphors** include expressing ideas in culturally relevant visual and verbal forms (e.g., role models, sayings). **Content** refers to attending to the client's values, traditions, and interpersonal styles (e.g., familismo, simpatia). The **concepts** about the treatment, the **treatment goals**, and the **treatment methods** also need to be consistent with the cultural values and expectations of the client. Finally, the **context** is taken into consideration in the assessment and intervention (e.g., acculturation, country of origin, family constitution, etc.). Consistent with person-centered care perspectives across disciplines, applying this approach to Cuban Americans emphasizes the importance of starting with a relationship that builds trust and respects cultural values such as gendered hierarchy within family relationships. Discovering culturally meaningful narratives can be best served with a narrative approach, which also allows the emergence of concepts about treatment as well as patient experiences of contexts. Clinicians working within these frameworks also need to become informed about demographic characteristics of the Cuban American population which will be discussed later in the chapter.

In my own clinical and educational practice, I apply a holistic family-centered, ecosystemic life-course perspective sensitive to gender and generation as these intersect with sociopolitical timing and circumstances of migration in both sending and receiving communities (Falicov, 2014; Shapiro, 2013a; Shapiro & Atallah-Gutierrez, 2012). Person- and family-centered inquires begin with how individuals view a presenting problem, their understanding of relevant resources and barriers, their goals for intervention, treatment considerations and constraints in a particular setting, and broader contextual resources and challenges (Shapiro, 2013a, 2013b). Further, I strive to integrate health and growth promotion and problem prevention into treatment, regardless of the setting. When applied to Cuban Americans, this broader approach allows clinicians to assess presenting health and mental health concerns holistically, contextualizing these in light of migration experiences as they contribute to gender and generational differences in experiences of U.S. acculturation, and macro-level social determinants of health and mental health. At the same time, it is important to consider unique circumstances and lived experiences of any individual Cuban American patient, their family and community setting, and cultural resources they bring to their specific health concerns. For this perspective, the chapter turns next to an overview of Cuban Americans in the U.S., their demographic characteristics and conditions of migration, as these create contexts for health and mental health treatment.

Overview of Cuban Americans in the U.S.

Cuban Americans are counted as the third largest group of Latino/a descent in the United States, accounting for 3.7 % of the U.S. Hispanic population, after those of Mexican background (64 %) and Puerto Rican background (9.5). The most recent U.S. census reports an estimated two million self-identified as Hispanics of Cuban origin, meaning they are themselves Cuban immigrants or trace their family ancestry to Cuba. Cuban Americans are the most geographically concentrated of the 14 largest Hispanic origin groups, with 68 % living in Florida, many in ethnic enclaves particularly in the greater Miami area, 78 % living in the South, and smaller groups located in New York, New Jersey, and California (Lopez, 2015; Rothe & Pumariega, 2008). The Cuban-origin population has more than doubled since 1980, with the foreign-born population growing by 78 %, comprising about 58 % of the Cuban American population, compared to 37 % of U.S. Latinos (Lopez, 2015). The Cuban-origin population in South Florida has been dominated economically and politically by the first arrivals in the immediate period following the 1959 Socialist Revolution, self-described "exiles" who considered their stay in the U.S. a temporary one and did not identify as "Cuban American" because they planned on returning (Colona & Grenier, 2010; Gomez, 2016). That first group came of age prior to the revolution, many experiencing significant social and economic privilege but with limited experience of democratic processes (Eckstein, 2009). The first Cuban American exile cohort encouraged a strong sense of Cuban identity among their Cuban-born and U.S. born children, and cultivate a deep sense of outrage and longing regarding the loss of the Cuba they knew as young adults (Eckstein, 2009; Perez, 2013). Compared to other Latino groups, Cuban Americans are more likely to identify as either Cubans or Americans rather than as "Latinos" or Hispanics more broadly (Lopez, 2015).

The Cuban American population continues to be older than both Whites and other Latinos; the median age for Cubans in the U.S. is 40, compared to the Hispanic/Latino median of 27 and the total U.S. median age of 37. More than half of Cuban immigrants arrived after 1990, and Cuban immigrants arriving subsequently are increasingly viewed as economic rather than political immigrants. Cuban Americans continue to receive favored immigration status compared to other Latinos, with fast-track status to residency, U.S. citizenship and public benefits, with no concerns about documentation status which is a significant burden for other Latino immigrant communities (Lopez et al., 2012). Compared to other Latinos, Cuban Americans are more proficient in English, with 60 % reporting proficiency compared to 35 % of the total Latino population (Brown & Patten, 2013; Lopez, 2015). Cuban Americans are less likely to be poor than other Latinos, with 20 % reporting living in poverty compared to 25 % of the overall Latino population (Lopez, 2015). Finally Cuban Americans report higher educational achievement, with 24 % of Cubans 25 and older obtaining at least a Bachelor's degree compared to 13 % of the total Latino population (Brown & Patten, 2013).

Psychologically, Cuban Americans have been described as having highly cohesive, interdependent families with clear roles according to gender and generation and high expectations for family closeness and mutual care (Bernal & Shapiro, 2005; Szapocsnik et al., 2012). Strong emphasis on family cohesion often termed "familismo"/familism, and respect for hierarchical, gender-typed family roles or "respeto"/respect, guide both within-family relationships and relationships in health care settings. It is not unusual to hear U.S. born Cuban young adults with their own established homes and families report that they speak to their mothers at least once daily. When education or employment require relocation away from the family enclave, this is considered a breach of family togetherness. The expectation is typically that once these temporary demands are completed the goal will be to return to the closeness of the extended family setting. There are high expectations for the care of dependents within the family at every age from infancy to elders. Whenever possible a family member will either be expected to provide hands-on care or to supervise care closely, as when an elder can no longer be cared for in the home.

These family-centered psychological processes emphasizing highly gendered family roles, familismo with a strong sense of obligation and hierarchy, and daily expectations of shared lives and interdependence, represent major cultural strengths, but can also create circumstances of intergenerational family conflict leading to mental health concerns (Muir et al., 2004; Szapocsnik et al., 2012, 2015). Szapocsnik and colleagues, conducting research over three decades on Cuban American families with adolescents demonstrating conduct or substance abuse problems, have developed family-centered culturally sensitive interventions including Bicultural Effectiveness Training and Brief Strategic Family Therapy centered on Cuban American family values and cultural strengths while recognizing that within-family generational differences in acculturation and family expectations can result in family conflicts, problematic communication, and maladaptation. More recently, clinical and epidemiological research has focused on challenges for Cuban American elders, an aging population with multiple chronic conditions and high expectations for family-based care particularly from adult daughters with multiple family and work responsibilities in a society that lacks the support for family-based care. Cultural patterns at this stage of the life-course may benefit dependent elders at a high cost to adult daughters. These clinical literatures suggest the importance of sensitively negotiating cultural expectations and health burdens to ensure that all family members are respected and supported in ways that promote positive health outcomes.

For example, Carolina, the middle of three sisters all in their early 70s and living in Miami, approached her primary care physician with complaints of frequent headaches and lack of energy. Her widowed mother had recently died at the age of 96, of complications from pneumonia, with her three daughters and dedicated caretaker of many years all at her side. Carolina had immigrated to Miami from Havana as a young adolescent in the early 1960s. She worked alongside her mother and father in a small clothing store with modest financial success. She kept the business open and worked there 6 days a week far after she would have preferred to sell it, because the store offered her aging parents a place to go to every day, a sense of their own worth as working adults, and a meaningful psychological role and status in the community. Carolina's younger sister had the financial means to provide a home and increasing caretaking for their aging parents, as they grew more impaired by chronic conditions including severe arthritis for her mother and heart disease for her father. However, Carolina, while bringing up two daughters of her own, who married, had children who were now adolescents, and expected her assistance with childcare, was designated as the daughter with the closest bond to both parents and was expected to see them daily, accompany them on doctor's visits and coordinate their daily care. Her father died of a heart attack at 75, but her mother remained active in the business and family affairs into her 90s. While Carolina's headaches and exhaustion were connected to her grief over her mother's death, the loss of her parents was interwoven with the sense of loss for her own possibilities as a woman and a wife. Speaking with her primary physician, she disclosed her regret that now herself in her 70s, with demands on her time as a grandmother, she and her husband had delayed much-desired time to focus on their own lives and marriage. He suggested that she and her husband consult with a family counselor who could help them assess their priorities and possibilities for focusing on their marriage. She accepted a referral for brief marital counseling, along with a referral to behavioral medicine for guided meditation to assist with her headaches. Carolina began to speak to her two daughters about these personal dilemmas, encouraging them to consider their own personal priorities and letting them know she and their father were planning some regular time for themselves as a couple. Carolina also began to reach out to other women of the "sandwich" generation in the extended family, caught between the demands of their children and their aging parents, encouraging them to make time for their marriages and for their personal health, a role which gave her a great deal of satisfaction.

Contexts of Cuban American Immigration and Integrative Health Impacts

Clinical understanding of Cuban American populations and their presentation in a variety of integrative care settings needs to take into account their unique immigration contexts evolving over time, leading to "segmented migration" (Skop, 2001) in which (1) the conditions of departure; (2) the initial resources immigrants bring with them; and (3) the social/economic context that greets immigrants in the host culture have varied within the Cuban immigrant community over time, leading to major waves of migration and corresponding health/mental health contexts. From a clinical perspective, the best framework for understanding immigrant families and Latino families in general, and Cuban American families in particular, is offered by Celia Falicov's Multidimensional Ecological Cultural Assessment (MECA, Falicov, 2014). MECA offers clinicians an assessment tool that incorporates key dimensions of family experience and functioning including circumstances of migration and sociocultural contexts as they impacted both sending and receiving communities, stage of the family life course, and social justice contexts including experiences of discrimination. As a family therapist she highlights family interdependence, though she makes it clear that a family systemic approach can inform work with individuals whose families highly value interdependence.

Cuba's proximity to the U.S., the impacts of the Cuban socialist revolution in 1959, the still evolving Cold War politics enshrined in favored status for Cuban immigrants to the U.S., and earlier attempts to destabilize the Cuban government, have impacted the Cuban American migration story as one in which a group that cherishes extended family connections has been forced to endure unbridgeable family divisions of politics and physical distance (Lemkin & Stug, 2008). Geopolitically, Cuba, the largest island in the Caribbean, has been considered by both colonial-era Spain and later by the United States to have significant economic and military strategic value. Cuban culture and dynamics of Cuban immigration to the U.S. have been deeply shaped by Spanish colonialism and the slave trade, by the 1898 U.S. invasion of Cuba (along with Puerto Rico, Guam, and the Philippines) during the Spanish/American war, and by continued U.S. interference in Cuba's internal politics. At the time Cuba declared independence the U.S. imposed the Platt Amendment giving the U.S. the right to intervene in Cuban internal affairs (repealed in 1933) and established the Guantanamo Bay military base, which remains a highly controversial symbol of U.S. interference in Cuban sovereignty throughout the Caribbean/ Latin American region.

Cubans migrating to the United States have historically received favored status in both entering the country and qualifying for U.S. social benefits, in constant to other immigrants from Mexico, other regions of Central and Latin America, and across the Caribbean. As of this writing, with significant opening of U.S./Cuba relations if not yet the lifting of the economic embargo, U.S./Cuba politics are once again impacting the flow of Cuban immigration to the U.S. The first Cuban immigrants from 1959 to 1965 were predominantly White and from higher socioeconomic classes, locating primarily in Miami, New York, and New Jersey, receiving many federal benefits, and with very limited opportunities for family contact or visits to the island. Initially supportive of the Cuban revolution in its opposition to Batista's dictatorship, this Cuban immigrant cohort sometimes termed the "Golden Exiles" (Eckstein, 2009) left Cuba due to political and economic opposition to both Cuba's socialism and its political suppression of dissent. This aging population, located primarily in South Florida, continues to have disproportionate economic and political power, intensified by the strong culturally based valuing of respect for elders within cohesive extended families.

From a mental health standpoint, this generation has been described as less likely to report mental health concerns when compared to later arrivals (Cisio, Spence, & Gayman, 2010). However, this generation experienced a deep sense of disruption and betrayal, which was intensified by their belief that Castro's socialism was temporary and they would be able to return to their homeland. Their profound sense of outrage and longing over the loss of Cuba remain powerful forces impacting mental health for this aging population (Perez, 2013, 2015), even as this generation has experienced significant economic success and the benefits of strong social and familial ties particularly in the Miami ethnic enclave. However, this generation's insistence on strict control of "exile ideology" has had had powerful impacts on intergenerational family relationships resulting in some vulnerabilities due to family conflicts as documented in the clinical literature (Bernal & Shapiro, 2005; Falicov, 2014; Szapocsnik et al., 2012). As an example, elders of this generation demonize Fidel Castro, and experience a deep sense of betrayal at any sign of negotiation with socialist Cuba, whether it is through personal visits or through political negotiations. Ramon, an 86-year-old elder who immigrated in 1961, whose adult daughter and her husband are both Cuban American academics living in Boston with professional ties to Cuba, threatened to excommunicate them from the family for visiting Cuba and only stopped out of fear that he would lose access to his college aged grandchildren who had also visited Cuba. At a family gathering in Miami, his oldest grandson Julio shared photographs of his family's visit to Ramon's home town in rural central Cuba, where they had met extended family and visited their family home and church. Fighting tears, Ramon said, "I don't like to think about Cuba as it is today, it forces me to remember all I have lost, it is too much sadness." The strategy of complete disengagement, with its geographic, interpersonal, and psychological dimensions, had taken its toll on Ramon's family relationships and added to his own personal health stressors. As an embattled patriarch fighting for dominance he was reluctant to allow his daughter to speak with him about her interests in Cuba, but his investment in his relationship with his grandson allowed for an opening of a more constructive dialogue and greater access to family support.

Additionally, while this group migrated with greater social advantages, it is important to remember that not all were able to establish themselves with high levels of financial success, which can itself become a strain when facing demands of aging with limited economic resources. Perrino, Brown, Mason, and Szapocsnik (2009) conducted the Hispanic Elders Behavioral Health Study, investigating the relationship between neighborhood factors and residents' physical and mental health outcomes in a predominantly Cuban low-income urban Miami community. Their study documented a 35 % prevalence of clinical level depressive symptoms, a rate comparable to, or higher than, prevalence rates reported by most other population-based samples of U.S. older adults, and significantly associated with perceived financial strain. The wide range of economic success experienced within this cohort can itself lead to strains both within extended families and across neighborhood groups in the South Florida Cuban American enclaves. The psychological experience of these aging elders is characterized by a deep sense of loss and grief complicated by the long postponement of the much anticipated return, which Perez conducting qualitative interviews with members of this exile generation discussed using the construct of "ambiguous loss" (Perez, 2013). For this generation, any movement toward reconciliation with the Cuban socialist government embodied in the Castro brothers' dictatorship represents an unacceptable betrayal.

The 1980 Mariel port immigration opened the way for 135,000 Cuban immigrants who had grown disillusioned with the economic privations of the socialist government. The first group immigrating in that era was initially Cubans with relatives from the first wave of migration who were willing to sponsor them, predominantly white and middle class. However, these were followed by a more diverse immigrant group, primarily working class or unemployed with a larger Afro-Cuban descent, and who found it much more difficult to establish themselves in the U.S. Those immigrants termed "Marielitos" were associated in the popular press, especially the *Miami* Herald, with the incarcerated and institutionalized mentally ill, even though those arrivals were not predominantly from criminal or psychiatric populations but were more likely to be poor and to be Afro-descendants. Estimates of the number of Mariel wave immigrants who had been incarcerated were about 10%, but as many as 9% of those had been jailed for black-market infractions such as possession and sale of food and other items. Estimates of "Marielitos" who were either jailed for violent criminal offenses or institutionalized mentally ill were 1–3% (West Duran, 2010). Cuban immigrants from this period had lived much more of their lives within the Cuban socialist experience, and within the Miami Cuban American enclave they were viewed as suspect, stereotyped as having less of a work ethic and accused of disloyalty to the exile identity due to their more nuanced views of the Cuban government. This negative local and national press in turn fueled anti-immigrant sentiment nationally, increased by the economic recession of that time (Eckstein, 2009).

The 1991 dissolution of the Soviet Union and end of economic aid to Cuba resulted in a financial crisis termed the Special Period (Periodo Especial) which created significant hardship on the island and led to an immigration crisis during which many thousands tried to leave the island on rafts. These immigrants, called "balseros" or "rafters" began to be detained and sent to camps in Guantanamo, Cuba, where conditions were crowded with outbreaks of violence, creating highly stressful circumstances and elevated rates of PTSD (Rothe, Lewis, Pumariega, & Martinez, 2002). Nelson, a day laborer who had left Cuba as a "balsero" and was detained in Guantanamo, had been working in Boston doing construction and had established a stable family and working life. However, after a mild cold turned into bronchitis and then pneumonia requiring a week's hospitalization, he became panicked and psychologically destabilized, remembering his traumatic experience in Guantanamo, where he ate dirt and debris to deliberately become ill, hoping to be sent to Miami. With the help of hospital staff, he was able to share these memories with his wife and daughter, and appreciate their enduring impact on his health and mental health. He accepted a referral to brief individual psychotherapy as part of his hospital discharge planning.

In 1996, the Cuban Adjustment Act negotiated between the U.S. and Cuba allowed Cubans who entered the United States to apply for residency after 1 year, and further negotiated 20,000 Cubans a year to legally emigrate through a lottery system. Popularly termed "Wet Foot, Dry Foot," this law allows Cubans seized on the sea to be returned to Cuba, while those entering on land to become eligible for legal residency. Part of the U.S. Cuba agreement was that Cubans who returned would not be subjected to reprisals by the Cuban government, and additionally, Cubans who feared reprisal were permitted a hearing and could be repatriated to a third country (Eckstein, 2009; Skaine, 2004). Emblematic of this cohort of arrivals was the tragic story of Elian Gonzalez, whose mother and stepfather brought him when they left Cuba for Miami on a precarious raft in 1999, the 6-year-old child among the few survivors who washed up on shore. Both Cuban and U.S. governments advocated for Elian's return to his father who had not been informed of the planned flight, while his Cuban American Uncle and extended family in Miami refused to give up a child whose mother had, as they saw it, sacrificed her life for Elian's freedom. Elian was returned to Cuba and his father's family, but only after an armed federal raid on his uncle's home in Miami, compounding the tragic losses on all sides. Research on the mental health of these later arrivals found them to experience significantly higher rates of anxiety and low self-esteem and somewhat more depression, typically associated with their lower levels of SES, education, and family and social support (Cisio et al., 2010). In this study, the authors believed that the poorer mental health outcomes for later arrivals were best explained by English language acquisition, other indicators of acculturation including level of education and employment success, and family support.

Through these multiple migration pathways, the Cuban American community continues to grow, both through the birth of second and third generations closely identified with Cuban identity and the arrival of Cubans through multiple migration pathways have created a growing "transnational" Cuban experience more comparable to the transnational identities of other Caribbean groups (Duany, 2011). These groups have experienced economic challenges in both Cuba and post-recession U.S., and have struggled with the differences in the quality and availability of health and mental health care. The recent opening of U.S. Cuba relations has caused a surge in Cuban immigration through Central America and Mexico, because of fears that this privileged migration status will come to an end. These multiple decades of shifting immigration policies and circumstances have resulted in Cuban families and communities with mixed circumstances of immigration and political views across generations.

Intriguingly, quality of health care and health literacy have been historically of great value in Cuba, both prior to the 1959 socialist revolution and subsequent to it (Shapiro, 2010a; Shapiro & Louro Bernal, 2014). Prior to the revolution, Cuba was considered to have had one of the most advanced health care systems in Latin America and the Caribbean, although with great inequalities in quality and access to care by poverty status, by race, and by region of the country (Shapiro, 2010a). After the revolution, Cuba went through a period where many physicians and nearly all the medical faculty left for Miami. Cuba had an opportunity to build a world-class health care system with universal government funded free access, focused on neighborhood level access to family-centered primary care as the base of operations for entry into a tiered system of collaborative teams offering specialty care including local polyclinics and more specialized care hospitals including those for psychiatric care. Beginning in the 1990s, Cuba reevaluated its integrative health care to address the over-use of psychiatric hospitalizations and fully transformed its mental health system of care (Shapiro & Louro Bernal, 2014). Additionally, Cuba has one of the world's most health literate populations, with health literacy supported by strong science programs in public education and by government controlled media particularly television that delivers health oriented programs. As economic conditions in Cuba have deteriorated, and Cuba has expanded its programs of "medical diplomacy" for both economic and political reasons, deploying Cuban doctors all over the world, the Cuban health care system has experienced challenges in both materials such as equipment and pharmaceuticals and consistent neighborhood level access (Brotherton, 2012). Cuban doctors are paid low wages in national currency (Peso Nacional), when many goods must be purchased with the Cuban foreign currency (CUC, with 1$ equal to 24 Cuban pesos), leading many to hold part-time jobs paid in foreign currency or seek opportunities to work outside Cuba. However, the Cuban health care system continues to excel in all global indicators of quality as measured by morbidity and mortality and patient access to all levels of care from primary to specialty care (Cloninger et al., 2014). The Cuban health system demonstrates globally recognized leadership in areas like maternal and infant health, handling of the AIDS epidemic (Shapiro, 2010a, 2010b), and management of cardiac care and metabolic syndromes. Cuba has left behind health problems of developing countries like infections but with a growing aging population and burdens of chronic diseases, leading Cubans on the island to joke, "We live like the poor and die like the rich." Most of the foreign-born Cubans in the U.S. have lived at least part of their lives with exposure to the Cuban health care system, and the knowledge and expectations of health care quality and access to both primary and specialized services. As I will discuss later in this chapter, the new "transnational" Cuban experience with greater freedom to live in both the island and the mainland and to maintain dual citizenship have created circumstances in which Cubans "shop" for their most favorable location for their health care needs.

Clinical Interventions for Cuban Americans: Family-Centered Life Course Approach to Integrative Health and Mental Health

For providers working in integrated health care settings, these contexts of Cuban American immigration require culturally sensitive assessment of a patient's immigration history and current circumstances, conceptualized in intergenerational terms. In health and mental health research and practice, the terms Hispanic or Latino have most often aggregated data and obscured critical contextual and sociopolitical differences generated by culture of origin, timing and circumstances of migration, and characteristics of sending and receiving communities (Alegria et al., 2007; Lopez et al., 2012). Cuban Americans as a population are more likely to have benefitted from U.S. immigration policies leading to higher economic and educational achievements, associated with better health and mental health outcomes in some domains. These contextual differences are particularly important for practitioners committed to addressing health and mental health disparities by recognizing how societal resources promoting health, and societal burdens interfering with recovery from illness and maintenance of wellness, are not created equal. Yet the Cuban American community, particularly in urban enclave settings like Miami, New York City, Union City, New Jersey, or San Juan, Puerto Rico is characterized by significant diversity, both in economic status as noted earlier in the chapter, and additionally in areas that are unmentioned in the health and mental health or demographic literature. These areas of diversity include the region of Cuba from which they immigrated, particularly as Havana in the West of the island has a larger proportion of White, educated individuals while Santiago de Cuba and the Eastern provinces have a larger proportion of African descendants and less consistent access to education and employment. Racial characteristics, defined differently under racialization in the U.S. as compared to racial definitions in Cuba, can vary widely among Cuban Americans (Perez, 2009), with colorism defined as skin color-based racial bias strong in both countries but "Blackness" defined more elastically in Cuba where a mixture of education, skin color, and hair texture can define racial characteristics where in the U.S. any appearance of mixed-race status more often defines an individual as "Black." Finally, Cubans identify as predominantly Catholic, with 49 % reporting that they belong to this group; 17 % identify as Protestant, evenly divided between Evangelical and Mainline Protestant; 26 % report that they are unaffiliated, and 8 % report religious affiliation as "Other." Cuban Catholicism is deeply influenced by religious syncretism incorporating Afro-Cuban religions into Cuban Catholicism, which some ethnographers suggest has intensified both in Cuba and in the U.S. diaspora as resilience strategies in coping with stressors (West Duran, 2010).

Liliana illustrates some of the complexities of Cuban American experiences regarding diversity across immigration, region, and racial dynamics, as well as both extended family and health seeking behaviors addressing barriers and opportunities in moving between Cuba and Miami. Liliana is a 44-year-old married mother of a 25-year-old daughter who had been in treatment for hyperthyroid disease, and sought a brief consultation for an integrative review of her clinical care. Liliana's 58-year-old husband Carlos had left their rural Eastern province home town of Holguin for Miami during the Mariel migration and had courted and married her during one of his visits home. Although in her home town Liliana considered herself part of a White elite with roots in the landowning history of her region, she found when she came to the United States that her thick kinky hair (termed pelo malo/"bad hair" in Cuban and other Latino communities) and light-coffee-colored skin identified her as having African diaspora ancestry. She commented that her racial heritage had not been much noted in her home town, where it had been common for White landowners to incorporate children from their Black slaves into their household (as a colony of Spain, Cuba ended slavery in 1898), but she felt her race affected her interactions in work and health settings. Liliana, who had worked as a housekeeper in the household of Cuban elders from the first migration for many years, struggled with health and mental health issues focused on family separations, particularly as she had to endure very long separations during critical periods of illness in the family due to Bush administration era punitive restrictions on family visits. Her favorite maternal aunt died of uterine cancer, and her limited opportunities for visiting during that time and her inability to attend her aunt's funeral due to U.S. visa restrictions continued as a source of enduring grief. Her mother was also diagnosed with uterine cancer at an earlier stage, and experienced intensive treatment with a more positive prognosis. For economic reasons, as well as the administrative challenges of receiving travel visas from both the U.S. and Cuban governments, Liliana tended to visit her mother for annual month-long visits. However, her Cuban American employer was reluctant to approve these visits and complained bitterly of these disruptions to their household routines. He believed her first responsibility was to fulfilling her work obligations and such long visits were too disruptive, overlooking the fact that Bush era travel prohibitions at that time only permitted 1 trip every 3 years, so that most Cuban Americans visiting their relatives stayed for the maximum time allowed. The family separations and employment situation caused her a great deal of stress, and she began to notice an elevated heart rate and labile emotions which she associated with these realistic stressors. Her employer did not provide health insurance, but as soon as the Affordable Care Act allowed her to enroll in a plan and visit a primary health clinic she did so. At that time, Liliana was diagnosed with hyperthyroid disease and was treated with a combination of radiation to reduce thyroid activity and medication to bring her thyroid levels to normal range, a process that took many months and was emotionally challenging. However, she refused a mental health referral at that time, preferring to focus on the benefits of a specific diagnosis and treatment plan and improved capacity for mood regulation as her thyroid levels stabilized.

A year after her thyroid treatment, she became particularly alarmed when she began to experience intense pain and severe bleeding during her menstrual cycles, which was diagnosed as due to fibroid tumors. Her insurance plan did not approve her for surgery to remove her uterus, which she believed was the best choice given her symptoms and her family cancer history, and she chose to travel home to Cuba and pay for the surgery there. As part of her treatment in the general surgical hospital in Holguin, she was offered the services of a Health Psychologist associated with that hospital's gynecological services team. A trained Health Psychologist scheduled three individual sessions with her, where she discussed the impact of her surgery while also exploring the deep meaning and sense of loss as she faced the loss of her aunt, the near-loss of her mother, and her fears about her own health and sense of vulnerability compounded by these family separations. Upon her return, her employer volunteered to pay for her surgery as a peace offering (costing $5000 U.S. out of pocket), and to begin to cover her health insurance. In consultation with her primary physician, she resumed physical exercise and enrolled in meditation workshops, both designed to help her manage her experiences of stress. The reconciliation with her employer, and the gradual easing of travel restrictions during the current administration, also relieved her worry that she would be unable to travel to Cuba for an emergency.

The most established area of research on Cuban American mental health services has emerged from the work of Jose Szapocsnik and colleagues (Muir et al., 2004; Szapocsnik et al., 2012, 2015), who first began to document intergenerational acculturation conflicts in Cuban families in the 1980s, and developed a program of research enhancing family communication and negotiation across cultural differences which they termed Bicultural Effectiveness Training. Bicultural Effectiveness Training combined a psychoeducational and family systems/family structural approach, first helping Cuban American adults appreciate the individualistic cultural perspectives and values encouraged by U.S. society in the cultural adaptation of their acculturated children, while also helping these adolescents to better understand the core cultural values of familism and respect that guided their parents. With this foundation of enhanced understanding of different generational experiences of cultural values, they proceeded to focus on reestablishing culturally congruent parental authority, at the same time encouraging greater flexibility in encouraging parents to appreciate their adolescents' experiences in a new societal context. More recently, this work has evolved to inform a broader or transcultural approach to family work with other immigrant families that share these values, which in the Miami community include other families of Latin American, Central American, and Caribbean descent including Haitian families as well as African American/Black families. Brief Strategic Family Therapy (Szapocsnik et al., 2015) was designed to match the value orientations reported by early Cuban immigrants in Miami, but were found in their intervention research to have positive transcultural qualities. BSFT's major therapeutic techniques fall into three major categories: Joining, diagnosing, and restructuring. The therapist joins the family by initially supporting the family structure, by tracking its patterns of interactions, by reflecting the family's style, affect, activity, and mood, and by affirming the family's characteristic interactions and behaviors. Maladaptive behaviors are identified and respectful intergenerational relationships are supported so that the family can address both their clinical challenges and other ongoing problems in culturally meaningful, mutually supportive ways. Even for providers who are not trained as family therapists, attention to family acculturation experiences and sensitive negotiating of mutual understanding regarding these different cultural worlds can greatly enhance family relationships and reduce adolescent behavior problems. Rosita, a 19-year-old Cuban American born in the U.S. to parents who immigrated in the late 1990s during the Special Period, was attending her first year at the University of Miami and living in the dormitory during the academic year. She saw her family physician during her return home for the summer, disclosed that she was sexually active and requested a referral for gynecological services. When she met with her nurse practitioner, she shared that she had truly enjoyed the freedom of having a social life outside of her family's scrutiny, and confessed that her previously excellent grades had suffered as a result. Rosita's parents had been brought up in a more sexually liberated era in socialist Cuba, but the maternal uncle and aunt who sponsored their U.S. residency and had helped support them financially while in Cuba were strict Catholics and closely supervised her cousins who were more socially conservative. A serious family conflict over these different values for sexual health and behavior had intensified when Rosita's cousins told her parents about her social and sexual activities while in school, and her parents had grounded her for the duration of the summer, strictly limiting any social events where she was not supervised by a family member. The nurse practitioner suggested a family consult, and the family agreed to engage in Brief Family therapy with a trained clinician. The six sessions of therapy included support for the parents in setting clear limits not only with their daughter but also with the extended family whose more strict expectations for watching over their daughter's virtue they did not share in the same way. These honest, direct conversations helped reduce intergenerational family conflict, both within the nuclear and extended family. When Rosita returned to school, she found she was more focused on her academic work with greater balance between her social, family, and university life. She decided to pursue brief counseling within her University Counseling Center to help her negotiate greater independence while respecting deep family cultural values of interdependence.

Cuban Americans and Health Disparities: Applying Social/Cultural Health Promotion Frameworks

The Institute of Medicine Report Unequal Treatment (Smedley, Stith, & Nelson, 2009) established the significance of health disparities based on racial discrimination and other forms of social disadvantage as they impacted both health care encounters and equality of opportunities to gain access to resources supporting positive health and mental health outcomes. In a follow-up IOM report (Ulmer 2009), researchers suggested that a "granular approach" would be needed to advance health disparities research by identifying relevant factors impacting disparities. The complexity of these variables is illustrated by Jerant, Arellanes, and Franks (2008), whose research used cross-sectional data from the 1998–2004 National Health Interview Survey (NHIS) and the 1999–2005 Medical Expenditure Panel Survey (MEPS) to compare four Hispanic groups—Mexican (13,522 persons), Cuban (778), Puerto Rican (1360), and Dominican (829) including persons born in the United States and elsewhere—with 45,422 English-speaking Whites born in the United States. On self-rated health and mental health status (using the SF-12) both Mexican immigrants and U.S. born Mexican Americans tended to have better self-reported outcomes than Whites and other Hispanic groups. However, U.S. nativity was associated with worse health and mental health outcomes for Mexican Americans, and better health/mental health outcomes for Cuban Americans. After adjusting for SES and other demographic variables Cuban Americans who immigrated reported the lowest mental health scores, while those of Puerto Rican heritage reported the worst physical health scores. Both self-reported health and mental health status for Cuban, Puerto Rican, and Dominican groups were worse than Whites. This research suggests that the much discussed Latino or immigrant health paradox, in which immigrant groups present with better health and mental health outcomes than predicted by their low economic status, but which are eroded with more time in the U.S. (Garcia-Coll & Marks, 2011; Zambrana, 2011) must be disaggregated by both nation of origin and nativity status. Both these authors suggest that exposure to discrimination by the U.S. born generation erodes the positive benefits of cultural and family protective factors, leading Garcia-Coll and Marks to ask, as in the title of their book: The Immigrant Paradox in Children and Adolescents: Is Becoming American a Developmental Risk?. One way to understand the Cuban American data is that for this community, immigrants experienced more psychological stressors due to family separations and the prohibition of contact, even with their greater privileges with regard to U.S. migration status, education, and socioeconomic status. Additionally, these and other authors noted that life in a Cuban American dominated ethnic enclave reduces discrimination experiences for Cuban Americans.

In a study using data from the National Latino and Asian American Study, Ai et al. (2012, 2013) conducted analyses comparing Latino group health and mental health status, further disaggregating data by gender to suggest some intriguing gender by group differences. She found that Cuban American women reported the highest rates of cardiovascular disease and hypertension, and were the most likely of the Latino groups to seek medical care but not mental health care. While Puerto Rican men reported the poorest health and mental health indicators, Cuban-American men shared similar rates of heart disease and cancer with Puerto Rican-American men as well as similarly low health and mental health utilization rates. Ai (2013) noted that additional variables in addition to gender, class, and ethnic origin need to be considered in making health comparisons across Latino groups. For example, while Cuban Americans have higher SES than Puerto Ricans, both groups tend to reside in cities, generating some areas of comparable health and mental health stressors while also increasing likelihood of access to culturally sensitive health and mental health care.

As an aging population, Cuban Americans are experiencing chronic illnesses requiring both visits to health care providers, compliance with medication protocols to address specific illnesses, and the challenges of health behavior change. Specific challenges embedded in cultural practices are connected to higher rates of smoking than the general population, especially among men (Burroughs Peña, Patel, Rodríguez Leyva, Khan, & Sperling, 2012), higher levels of sedentary behaviors, and preference for a diet high in meat, carbohydrates, and fat and limited variety of vegetables contributing to high rates of metabolic syndrome (Huffman et al, 2009, 2011). Both prior to and after 1959, Cubans in both periods considered rice, beans, viandas (tubers such as potatoes, taros, yams, and sweet potatoes), and meat as the essentials in the national diet (Darias Alfonso, 2012). Further, Darias Alfonso notes the importance of idealized Cuban food practices as part of maintaining cultural identity in the diaspora. While the Cuban government supported food security through a rationing system or monthly "libreta"/coupon book early in the revolution, this practice led to a more restricted/monotonous diet as well as a shrinking of the food ration during the post-Soviet economic crisis, particularly during the "Special Period" in the 1990s when most ordinary Cubans went hungry and some suffered from malnutrition related illnesses including dental and vision loss. Currently, Cubans on the island have access to U.S. dollars, leading to increased access to food for those with work in tourist trade, informal economy, and "Fe"/faith, a joking reference to the fact that these two letters also spell out "Familia en el Extranjero"/Family Abroad who provide foreign currency. Although seldom discussed either in the published literature or among friends and family, I have found that the hunger and scarcity of that period along with the continuing challenges of finding and affording a choice of food in Cuba has led to a mentality for some of eating as much as you can when you can. More documented is the need for creativity and flexibility in the capacity to "resolver"/solve problems and "el invento"/ inventiveness and improvisation, which characterize all aspects of life in Cuba, not only in putting food on the table but also transportation, household repairs, and other material demands of daily life. Further, dependence on family in the diaspora to help pay for essentials in Cuba has created new complexities in extended family relationships. Sergio, an Afro-Cuban student from the far Eastern province of Santiago who was a student in my UMASS Boston Gender Culture and Health Class was participating in a class discussion of healthy eating practices as influenced by culture for a health promotion outreach event, when he suddenly pulled out his phone and showed the class a remarkable family portrait. Sergio's older sister and maternal Aunt had gone to visit their relatives in Santiago the previous year, and had brought foreign currency and other gifts. To celebrate, the family had purchased and roasted a large pig, and the pig on a spit was held across the arms of the gathered relatives like an additional member of the family. While all of us found this photograph charming and amusing, the story behind it, of a long-standing family separation initiated during the Mariel migration of the 1980s and only recently bridged, revealed the mistrust Sergio felt as he wondered if these relatives were only interested in them for their money. Sergio himself had been brought up to think of the Cuban socialist government very negatively, and like his mother, refused to visit, causing conflicts with his sister and Aunt, his only other close relatives in the Boston area. When his mother died suddenly of cardiac disease, he sought treatment at the University Counseling Center, where he explored his loss in light of family separations and migrations, and received help reconciling with his sister and Aunt.

In one of the few studies that reviewed both Cuban and Cuban American health practices, Burroughs Peña et al. (2012) reviewed research literatures compared the life style habits of Cubans on the island and Cuban Americans as they impacted rates of cardiovascular disease. They used available data from multiple sources, noting that the available data on Cuba was more up to date than the Cuban American data, which relied heavily on the Hispanic Health and Nutrition Examination Survey (HHANES), 1982–1984 for national data, considered problematic due to oversampling of higher SES Cuban Americans, supplemented by more recent available research on specific health behaviors. In the area of food consumption, the review found that among Cubans on the island, food preferences for meat and a limited range of vegetables as well as growing access to fast food on the island mirrored Cuban American health practices of high consumption of fast food and a limited diet. The authors concluded that Cuban and Cuban American food practices are highly comparable and problematic for cardiac health. The authors found physical inactivity to be higher in Cuba than for Cuban Americans, with Cuban American men more sedentary compared to White and African American men, but Cuban American women less sedentary than White and African American women. Obesity rates in Cuba were found to be lower than in Cuban American populations, but rising. In the U.S., 9 % Cuban American men and 15 % of Cuban American women were classified as obese, with 30 % of men and 34 % of women as overweight, both rates comparable to other Latinos. Hypertensive Cuban Americans were more likely to be overweight. The authors note that the limited available literature does not associate increased BMI in Cuban Americans with social indicators such as with income, education, acculturation, or socioeconomic status, while emphasizing that the older available data from the HHANES study overrepresented higher SES participants. In examining smoking as a health behavior, tobacco use in Cuba was found to be among the highest in Latin America and the Caribbean, with men's smoking rates higher than women which is a typical finding internationally. The survey identified data estimating that 40 % of all men smoke tobacco daily, with a higher rate of 60 % in middle age men. Elderly Cubans reported smoking at higher rates than the rest of the population, with data from a 2011 study in Havana estimating that 46.5 % of elderly men and 21.5 % of elderly women (over 60) smoked tobacco, a much higher rate than other countries in the region, while an additional 31 % of men and 15 % of women were former smokers. Case control studies in Havana suggest that smoking accounted for one third of the burden of heart attacks. Among Cuban Americans, smoking rates have been declining since the HHANES study with data collected in the 1980s. More recent studies have found smoking rates among Cuban American men ranged from 21.4 to 30.3 %, and in women 11.6–25.9 %. Compared to other Latino groups, Cuban American men who were smokers had the highest mean daily cigarette use of 17.8 cigarettes a day (Perez-Stable, Ramirez, & Villareal, 2001). The authors note that due to Cuban's access to comprehensive primary care as well as neighborhood clinic-based cardiac care, patients have access to medication and follow-up. However, these life style behaviors will continue to compromise patient health outcomes. In the United States, researchers have explored the value of primary care as a setting to reduce health disparities for Latino populations in general, but not for Cuban Americans in particular (Juckett, 2013). Although patients from many cultural backgrounds find it challenging to follow habit change protocols including smoking cessation, increased physical exercise, and dietary change, work with Cuban American patients presents specific challenges of culturally established habits and preferences and of a highly hierarchical family and social structure. Clinical providers can mobilize the authority hierarchy in culturally appropriate ways that can increase motivation and compliance with health promotion recommendations, by working from their own position of expertise, while encouraging male elders to take care of their health so they can maintain their important family roles as providers and guides for the younger generation, while encouraging older women to take care of themselves so they can continue to care for others (Shapiro, 2014).

Family Life Course, Gender, and Generation: Cultivating Resilience

An extensive literature on Latinos in general, and Cuban Americans in particular, identifies family cohesion or "familismo" as a central value guiding intergenerational and extended family relationships (Bernal & Shapiro, 2005; Falicov, 2014). Additionally, family continuity of cultural values including "familismo" and religion/spirituality have been associated with protection from acculturative stressors and both individual and family resilience. A family life course perspective highlighting shared development in linked generations (Shapiro, 2008; 2013a, 2013b) is particularly useful in understanding the health and mental health needs of Cuban American families, who strongly enforce norms of family loyalty and have high, gendered expectations for family connections and caretaking during times of health care needs. A family-centered perspective focused on the family life course also allows the practitioner to identify how immigration experiences have impacted individuals while shaping relationships across the generations.

Bernal and Shapiro (2005) described Cuban American family characteristics associated with gender roles with significant impacts on health and mental health concerns. A traditional family hierarchy with the man as provider is highly valued, and expectations of Respeto/Respect can be a means of reinforcing male authority over women and children. Conflicts may arise when the wife works, shifting the economic basis of the marriage. However, one characteristic of the Cuban American migration has been its capacity to permit women to work outside the home within socially sanctioned gendered settings in family and friend owned businesses, supporting a gendered acculturation process within cultural expectations. Also, as family members acculturate, conflicts emerge from the clash of values between generations. Szapocznik & collaborators (Muir et al., 2004; Szapocsnik et al., 2012, 2015) studied intergenerational conflicts between Cuban American parents and adolescents, particularly over obedience to family-based cultural expectations, finding that "bicultural training" that helped each generation understand the other's needs was associated with improved mental health and reduction of adolescent risk taking.

Cuban American women receive the message, both from their experiences in Cuba and in the U.S., that women are expected to work while at the same time expected to uphold gendered family responsibilities for young children and for family elders. What policy makers in the U.S. are increasingly calling "the triple shift" in women's family responsibilities—work outside the home to help support the family in an economy that often requires two incomes for middle class status; household responsibilities for children's care, family meals and house cleaning; and responsibilities for elderly or disabled kin—have created a great deal of stress that is particularly intense for Cuban American women facing unyielding family expectations for family-based caretaking (Bernal & Shapiro, 2005; Falicov, 2014).

An additional factor of growing importance in the treatment of Latino families is their maintenance of transnational ties (Falicov, 2007). Due to the restrictions on travel and return for both Cubans on the island and in the U.S., Cuban Americans were viewed from more one-directional perspectives on acculturation or "exile" longing for the home country with an emphasis on traumatic loss and without possibilities of maintaining transnational ties through travel or contribution of remittances. Due to internal political restrictions on communications, particularly internet access which remains costly and restricted, Cubans have very limited access to internet communications. Telephone calls which were at one time prohibitively expensive and closely monitored by the government have become more frequent and affordable. Many Cubans now have cell phones which they use like beepers, to signal that someone is trying to reach them, returning the call on a land line to avoid expensive charges. Yet Cubans on the island marshall the creativity of "el invento"/inventiveness and "el resuelve"/the solution to seek ways to stay connected to friends and family on and off the island. By sharing internet connections both at home and in work settings, many Cubans communicate with relatives in the diaspora through Facebook. An affordable pirated service substituting for broadband Internet, the off-the-books El Paquete Semanal ("The Weekly Package") or El Paquete is a one terabyte collection of digital material distributed directly to individual homes where it can be shared by multiple families for a modest payment, circulating since around 2014 on the underground market (though many speculate that it must have some government support or sanction). The most popular content is TV series, soap operas, music and classified ads for local Cuban businesses, as well as films, video clips, Spanish language news websites, computer technology websites, and instructional videos and advertisements for local Cuban businesses. Most buyers request only certain parts of the Package which may sell for as little as $1 US, allowing Cubans to bypass Cuban government controlled television with its limited offerings (Helft, 2015). Further, both travel to Cuba and economic support of relatives on the island have become much more prevalent with changes in Cuban and U.S. policies (Vang & Eckstein, 2012). Cuban family separations due to travel prohibitions on both sides of the divide have been particularly cruel for a culture that is so focused on the centrality of family ties (Lemkin & Stug, 2008). Duany (2011) suggests that Cubans can now be considered as transnational as every other immigrant community of the Caribbean. For example, remittances from U.S. Cuban Americans to relatives in Cuba have become a significant component of the Cuban economy, with estimates ranging from $1 to $3 billion U.S.; estimates vary widely because money is often exchanged through informal as well as formal channels. A great deal of current Cuban small business economic activity, termed "cuentapropista"/self-employed or entrepreneurial is funded by both cash and material contributions by relatives visiting from the U.S. The economic hardships on the island have created truly transnational families with relatives living in the Miami area who host Cuban relatives who come visit for a year, establish residency, and then travel back and forth between Cuba and the U.S. depending on their own needs or the needs of relatives. For example, I met Marina at a Cuban American academic event, where she presented on the challenges of her recent immigration to Miami and her involvement in a local church-based program emphasizing family reconciliation. Marina was a staff member at the Union for Artists and Writers (UNEAC) and a writer of fiction, who accepted early retirement at the age of 64 to move to Miami where both of her adult children, an older daughter and a younger son, had moved to seek employment opportunities. Her husband and elderly mother remained in Cuba. Her daughter had recently gone through a painful divorce, and needed help with the care of her early adolescent children. Marina accepted this responsibility, eager to spend more time with her grandchildren, and disillusioned by the great changes in economic situation and disappointment in the loss of socialist values. However, the adjustment to her life, from a valued professional to a stay at home mother, and the lack of opportunities to speak honestly about her experiences in both Cuba and Miami, made her feel dispirited and frustrated. She was also deeply worried about her husband who was now responsible for coordinating her mother's care which was paid for by a brother living in New York who had migrated during the 1990s Special Period. Unable to return to Cuba for the year she needed to establish her residency, she was invited to attend a special program at her local Catholic church which helped bring together groups from conflicting political backgrounds for dialogues and reconciliation. Marina found attendance to the group supportive as she found other recent immigrants who faced similar dilemmas of Cuban women's lives in divided, transnational families.

Conclusion: Working with Cuban American Families in Integrative Care

This chapter has brought a transdisciplinary perspective drawing across health, mental health, and cultural studies literatures to guide work with Cuban American patients in integrative care. Recognizing the "Geopolitics of the Heart" characterizing Cuban American experience, I have reviewed some of the sociopolitical and demographic contexts shaping Cuban America, including the gradual transformation of a divided community into a more fluid, transnational one. Cuban American families in the U.S. have demonstrated a great deal of economic and educational success and political influence, building on granted immigration advantages to create residential enclaves and family continuity promoting wellness and resilience. The stories of Cuban American families continue to change, and this chapter recommends careful assessment of person- and family-centered health status from a life-course perspective, of within-family differences in acculturation and political affiliations, and clinician reflexivity in assessing personal and professional attitudes and values as they impact patient care. These recommendations, emerging from within the care of Cuban American families, will increase clinician cultural and contextual sensitivity in work with other Latino and other immigrant families.

References

Abraído-Lanza, A., Viladrich, A., Flórez, K., Céspedes, A., Aguirre, A., & De La Cruz, A. (2007). Fatalismo reconsidered: A cautionary note for health-related research and practice with Latino populations. *Ethnic Disparities, 17*(1), 153–158.

Ai, A., Appel, H., Huang B., and Lee, K. (2012). Overall health and healthcare utilization among Latino American women in the United States. J Womens Health, 21(8), 878–85.

Ai, A., Noël, L., Appel, H., Huang B., and Hefley, W. (2013). Overall health and health care utilization among Latino American men in the United States. Am J Mens Health, 7(1), 6–17.

Alegria, M., Mulvaney-Day, N., Torres, M., Polo, A., Cao, Z., & Canino, G. (2007). Prevalence of psychiatric disorders across Latino subgroups in the United States. *American Journal of Public Health, 97*(1), 68–75.

Bernal, G. (2016). Casas, J., Suzuki, L., Alexander, C., and Jackson, M. (Editors), Handbook of Multicultural Counseling (4th Ed.). Multiculturalism: The Final Frontier—Resistance Is Not Futile. Thousand Oaks, CA: Sage, 60–70.

Bernal, G., & Domenech-Rodriguez, M. (2012). *Cultural adaptation of evidence based treatments*. Washington, DC: American Psychological Association.

Bernal, G., & Shapiro, E. (2005). Cuban families. In M. McGoldrick, J. Pierce, & P. Giordano (Eds.), *Ethnicity and family therapy* (3rd ed.). New York, NY: Guilford. 2nd edn. 1996.

Brotherton, S. (2012). Revolutionary Medicine: Health and the Body in Post-Soviet Cuba. Durham, NC: Duke University Press.

Brown, A., & Patten, E. (2013). *Hispanics of Cuban origin in the United States, 2011*. Retrieved from http://www.pewhispanic.org/2013/06/19/hispanics-of-cuban-origin-in-the-united-states-2011/.

Burroughs Peña, M., Patel, D., Rodríguez Leyva, D., Khan, B., & Sperling, L. (2012). Lifestyle risk factors and cardiovascular disease in Cubans and Cuban Americans. *Cardiology Research and Practice, 2012*, 1–6.

Cisio, A., Spence, N., & Gayman, M. (2010). Mental health and psychosocial adjustment of Cuban immigrants in South Florida. *Social Science & Medicine, 71*(6), 1173–1181.

Cloninger, R., Salvador-Carulla, L., Kirmayer, L., Schwartz, M. A., Appleyard, J., Goodwin, N., … Rawaf, S. (2014). A time for action on health inequities: Foundations of the Geneva Declaration on person- and people-centered integrated health care for all. *The International Journal of Person Centered Medicine*, *4*(2), 69–89.

Colona, A., & Grenier, G. (2010). Structuring liminality: Theorizing the creation and maintenance of the Cuban exile identity. *Ethnic Studies Review, 33*(2), 43–51.

Comas-Diaz, L. (2012). *Multicultural care: A clinician's guide to cultural competence*. Washington, DC: American Psychological Association.

Darias Alfonso, I. (2012) We are What We Now Eat: Food and Identity in the Cuban Diaspora. Canadian Journal of Latin American and Caribbean Studies, 37(74), 173–206.

Duany, J. (2011). *Blurred borders: Transnational migration between the Caribbean and the United States*. Chapel Hill, NC: University of North Carolina Press.

Eckstein, S. (2009). *The immigrant divide: How Cuban Americans changed the U.S. and their homeland*. New York, NY: Routledge.

Falicov, C. (2007). Working with transnational immigrants: Expanding meanings of family, community, and culture. *Family Process, 46*, 157–171.

Falicov, C. (2014). *Latino families in therapy* (2nd ed.). New York, NY: Guilford Press.

Garcia-Coll, C., & Marks, A. (2011). *The immigrant paradox in children and adolescents: Is becoming American a developmental risk?* Washington, DC: APA.

Gomez, M. (2016). Cuban American activists connecting to Cuba: Enduring impacts on U.S. Cuba relations. Presentation at the opening of the University of Massachusetts Boston, *Movement in support of Cuba by members of the Cuban diaspora in the US, Puerto Rico & other countries (1960s–1990s)*, Archive collection, Healey Library. Retrieved March 23, 2016, from http://openarchives.umb.edu/cdm/landingpage/collection/p15774coll35.

Helft, M. (2015). No internet? No problem. Inside Cuba's tech revolution. *Forbes/Tech*, July 1. Retrieved March 20, 2016, from http://www.forbes.com/sites/miguelhelft/2015/07/01/no-internet-no-problem-inside-cubas-tech-revolution/#660cb59a76c7.

Holden, K., McGregor, B., Thandi, P., Fresh, E., Sheats, K., Belton, A., … Satcher, D. (2014) Toward culturally centered integrative care for addressing mental health disparities among ethnic minorities. *Psychological Services*, *11(4)*, 357–368.

Huffman, F., Vaccaro, J., Nath, S., & Zarini, G. G. (2009). Diabetes self management: Are Cuban Americans receiving quality health care? *Journal of Health and Human Services Administration, 32*(3), 279–304.

Huffman, F., Vaccaro, J., Zarini, G., & Nath, S. (2011). Coronary heart disease risk in Cuban Americans with and without type 2 diabetes. *The Internet Journal of Health, 12*.

Jerant, A., Arellanes, R., & Franks, P. (2008). Health status among US Hispanics: Ethnic variation, nativity, and language moderation. *Medical Care, 46*(7), 709–717.

Juckett, G. (2013). Caring for Latino Patients. American Family Physician, 87(1), 48–56.

Juster, R., Bizik, G., Picard, M., LaPierre, G., Sindi, S., Trepanier, L., … Lupien, S. (2011). A transdisciplinary perspective of chronic stress in relation to psychopathology throughout life span development. *Devlpmnt & Psychopathol*, *23*, 725–776.

Kirmeyer, L. (2012). Rethinking cultural competence. *Transcultural Psychiatry, 49*(2), 149–164.
Laroche, M. (2013). *Cultural psychotherapy: Theory, methods and practice*. Los Angeles, CA: Sage Publications.
Lemkin, D., & Stug, J. (2008). Psychological distress of Cuban Americans affected by restrictive U.S. travel policies. *Journal of Progressive Human Services, 19*(1), 1–18.
Lopez, G. (2015). *Hispanics of Cuban origin in the United States, 2013*. Washington, DC: The Pew Research Center.
Lopez, S., Barrio, C., Kopelowicz, A., Vega, W. A. (2012). From documenting to eliminating disparities in mental health care for Latinos. *American Psychologist, 67(7)*, 511–523.
Martin, C., & Petersen, R. (2009). The social construction of chronicity: A key to understanding chronic care transformations. *Journal of Evaluation in Clinical Practice, 15*, 578–585.
Mechanic, D. (2012). Seizing opportunities under the affordable care act for transforming the mental and behavioral health system. Health Affairs, 31(2), 376–382.
Muir, J., Schwartz, S., & Szapocznik, J. (2004). A program of research with Hispanic and African American families: Three decades of intervention development and testing influenced by the changing cultural context of Miami. *Journal of Marital & Family Therapy, 30*(3), 285–303.
Nielsen, J., Wall, W., & Tucker, C. (2016). Testing of a model with Latino patients that explains the link among patient-perceived provider cultural sensitivity, language preference and patient treatment adherence. *Journal of Racial and Ethnic Health Disparities, 3*, 63–73.
Perez, L. (2009). Racialization among Cubans and Cuban Americans. In J. Cobas, J. Duany, & J. Feagin (Eds.), *How the United States racializes Latinos: White hegemony and its consequences* (pp. 134–148). New York, NY: Taylor and Francis.
Perez, R. (2013). Paradise lost: Older Cuban American exiles' ambiguous loss of leaving the homeland. *Journal of Gerontological Social Work, 56*(7), 596–622.
Perez, R. (2015). Cuba No; Miami Sí: Cuban Americans coping with ambiguous loss. *Journal of Human Behavior in the Social Environment, 25*(1), 50–66.
Perez-Stable, E., Ramirez, A., & Villareal, R. (2001). Cigarette smoking behavior among US Latino men and women from different countries of origin. *American Journal of Public Health, 91*, 1424–1430.
Perrino, T., Brown, S., Mason, L., & Szapocsnik, J. (2009). Depressive symptoms among urban Hispanic older adults in Miami: Prevalence and sociodemographic correlates. *Clinical Gerontologist, 32*(1), 26–43.
Prilleltensky, I. (2012). Wellness as fairness. *American Journal of Community Psychology, 49*, 1–21.
Rothe, E., Lewis, J., Pumariega, A., & Martinez, O. (2002). Posttraumatic stress disorder among Cuban children and adolescents after release from a refugee camp. *Psychiatric Services, 53*(8), 970–976.
Rothe, E., & Pumariega, A. (2008). The new face of Cubans in the United States: Cultural process and generational change in an exile community. *Journal of Immigrant and Refugee Studies, 6*(2), 247–266.
Satterfield, J. M., Spring, B., Brownson, R. C., Mullen, E. J., Newhouse, R. P., Walker, B. B., & Whitlock, E. P. (2009). Toward a transdisciplinary model of evidence-based practice. *Milbank Quarterly, 87(2)*, 368–390.
Shapiro, E. (1994). Grief as a Family Process: A Developmental Approach to Clinical Practice. NY: Guilford Press.
Shapiro, E. R. (2008). Whose recovery of what? Relationships and environments promoting grief and growth. *Death Studies, 32*(1), 40–58.
Shapiro, E. (2010a). Health and health care: Introduction. In W. Duran (Ed.), *Cuba*. Detroit, MI: Gale.
Shapiro, E. (2010b). HIV/AIDS in Cuba. In W. Duran (Ed.), *Cuba*. Detroit, MI: Gale.
Shapiro, E. (2013a). Chronic illness and family resilience. In D. Becvar (Ed.), *Handbook of family resilience*. New York, NY: Springer.
Shapiro, E. R. (2013b). Culture and socialization in assessment and treatment in thanatology. In D. Balk (Ed.), *Handbook of thanatology* (2nd ed.). Oakbrook Terrace, IL: Association of Death Education and Counseling.

Shapiro, Ester (2014). Translating Latin American/US Latina Frameworks and Methods in Gender and Health Equity: Linking Women's Health Education and Participatory Social Change. International Quarterly of Community Health Education.

Shapiro, E., & Atallah-Gutierrez, C. (2012). Latina re-visionings of participatory health promotion practice: Cultural and ecosystemic perspectives linking personal and social change. *Women and Therapy, 35*(1-2), 120–133.

Shapiro, E., & Louro Bernal, I. (2014). Integrative health and mental health systems of care: The Cuban experience. In S. Okpaku (Ed.), *Global mental health*. London: Cambridge.

Silva, S. A., Charon, R., & Wyer, P. C. (2011). The marriage of evidence and narrative: Scientific nurturance within clinical practice. *Journal of Evaluation in Clinical Practice, 17*, 585–593.

Skaine, R. (2004). *The Cuban family: Custom and change in an era of hardship*. London: McFarland.

Skop, E. (2001). Race and place in the adaptation of Mariel exiles. International Migration Review, 35(2), 449–471.

Smedley, B. D., Stith, A. Y., & Nelson, A. R. (2009). *Unequal treatment*. Washington, DC: National Academies Press.

Starfield, B. (2009). Primary care and equity in health: The importance to effectiveness and equity of responsiveness to people's needs. *Humanity and Society, 33*, 56–73.

Szapocsnik, J., Muir, J., Duff, J., Schwartz, S., & Brown, C. (2015). Brief strategic family therapy: Implementing evidence-based models in community settings. *Psychotherapy Research, 25*(1), 121–133.

Szapocsnik, J., Schwartz, S., Muir, J., & Brown, C. (2012). Brief strategic family therapy: An intervention to reduce adolescent risk behavior. *Couple and Family Psychology, 1*(2), 134–145.

Tucker, C., Marsiske, M., Rice, K., Nielson, J., & Herman, K. (2011). Patient centered culturally sensitive health care: Model testing and refinement. *Health Psychology, 30*(3), 342–350.

Ulmer, C. (2009). Race, Ethnicity, and Language Data: Standardization for Health Care Quality Improvement. Washington, DC: The National Academies Press.

Vang, Z. M., & Eckstein, S. (2012). Toward an improved understanding of immigrant adaptation and transnational engagement: The case of Cuban Émigrés in the United States. *Comparative Migration Studies, 3*(6), 2–20.

West Duran, A. (2010). *Cuba*. Detroit, MI: Gale.

Zambrana, R. (2011). *Latino families in the U.S.: Intersectional perspectives on diversity*. New York, NY: Routledge.

Chapter 5
Latino Trends and Health Policy: From Walking on Eggshells to Commitment

Silvia L. Mazzula and Aileen Torres

Relevant and effective integrated care models require decision-makers who are informed on the general state of the field in addressing the mental health needs of Americans. The National Alliance for the Mentally Ill (NAMI, 2009) highlighted the "dismal" state of mental health services across the nation. The United States received an alarming grade of an overall "D"—only six states received a "B" grade, and these were categorized as top-performing states. According to the report, areas in most need of improvement included funding, consumer/family empowerment, cultural competency, and stigma reduction. In the 2000s, mental disorders were one of the five most costly conditions in the country, with care expenditures rising from $35.2 billion in 1996 to 57.5 billion in 2006 (Agency for Healthcare Research and Quality [AHRQ], 2009). However, the increased costs have not translated to improved budget allocations for public health, which have in general resulted in decreased quantity and quality of care. In fact, NAMI (2015) recently posited that state mental health budget cuts, and the lack of policy enforcement authority, have impaired the efforts to strengthen parity requirements of initiatives such as the Paul Wellstone and Pete Domenici Mental Health Parity and Addiction Equity Act or the Affordable Care Act of 2010.

Nonetheless, these two very important laws represent advancement in public policy that can lead to equality, with the appropriate enforcement of relevant policies. As the national agenda moves towards the ultimate goals of mental health integration and parity, barriers to these goals need to be explicitly detailed, with particular attention to the plethora of diverse consumers in our country. It is well noted that primary care will be the gateway to improving the health of Americans—a large amount of mental health disorders are being treated in primary care settings

S.L. Mazzula
John Jay College of Criminal Justice, New York, NY, USA

A. Torres (✉)
Aileen Torres, Private Practice, Lyndhurst, NJ 07071, USA
e-mail: aileentorres.phd@gmail.com

© Springer International Publishing Switzerland 2016

L.T. Benuto, W. O'Donohue (eds.), *Enhancing Behavioral Health in Latino Populations*, DOI 10.1007/978-3-319-42533-7_5

(Bower & Gilbody, 2005; Unutzer et al., 2006). When considering racial/ethnic differences, racial and ethnic minority populations are more likely to receive mental health care in primary care settings despite the appropriateness of this care (Chapa, 2004). It is also well documented that Hispanic populations, specifically, tend to use primary healthcare services for mental health concerns (Arredondo, Gallardo-Cooper, Delgado-Romero, & Zapata, 2014; Rios-Ellis, 2005) and also tend to use emergency healthcare services instead of having a consistent healthcare provider (Weinick & Jacobs, 2000).

The role of primary care in addressing mental health is also projected to increase significantly in the future. For example, a taskforce created by the American Board of Pediatrics estimated that, by 2020, mental health care would constitute 30 % or more of general pediatric practice (Satterfield & Dover, 2012). Therefore, across the lifespan, primary care is, and will increasingly be, in a unique position to address mental health needs. However, policies must be revisited to integrate structural and sociocultural factors that inform treatments' relevancy to diverse populations. There are several major areas that warrant attention. First, Americans in general continue to experience significant problems in access to good quality care. Yet, there are worst barriers for racial and ethnic minority populations in general, and Latinos specifically. According to the report "Movilizandonos por Nuestro Futuro: Strategic Development of a Mental Health Workforce for Latinos" (USDHHS, 2010), unmet behavioral health needs of the Latino population in the U.S. is a major public health crisis. Second, primary care providers are increasingly challenged to provide treatment that is culturally competent to address the needs of a diverse U.S. population, inclusive of Latinas/os who hold intersections of diverse identities, needs, and challenges. However, we continue to be challenged by a dearth of culturally responsive research (Arredondo et al., 2014; Mazzula & Victoria, 2008; Rios-Ellis, 2005) or a diverse workforce who can contribute diverse perspectives (USDHHS, 2010) to solve pressing health problems of Latinos in the U.S.

Policy-makers, decision-makers, and primary care physicians play an important role in ensuring policies improve the health care of Latino populations. They also have an important role in developing comprehensive plans and policies that are relevant and effective. However, at best, primary care providers may feel like they are walking on eggshells, unsure how to navigate the challenges of addressing the relevant mental health needs of a growing Latino population. As such, there is a strong need for collaboration with practitioners who are experts in mental health and in cultural competent treatment. Whereas integrated emergency care clinical frameworks exist for psychiatric crises, models for standard integrated care are not well-developed. Without assessing how psychological factors may impact client's physical presentation and their treatment adherence, the biopsychosocial model is not being effectively implemented by medical practitioners. Furthermore, while Mind-Body research is being conducted at places like Johns Hopkins University, more translational research on how to implement the knowledge in real-world practices is necessary.

Therefore, the purpose of this chapter is to provide an overview of some of the major challenges that clients with mental health difficulties face. With that in mind, the policy recommendations will focus on how to reduce treatment barriers, improve screening procedures, require cross-cultural translational research, increase mental health coverage by insurance companies and strengthen workforce diversity. First, we provide an overview of the extant literature on barriers to access and service utilization, inclusive of structural and social barriers. Particular attention will be given to documented barriers in access to treatment (e.g., culture, language, medical insurance, etc.) and service utilization (e.g., poor service quality, improper screening and diagnosis). The chapter concludes with recommendations for policy- and decision-makers to implement, re-design, and assess the effectiveness of integrated care with Latino populations. We infuse a psychological perspective to addressing health policy to move from walking on eggshells to commitment to culturally responsive treatment, research, and policies.

Access to Treatment

Although the National Healthcare Disparities Report (USDHHS, 2012) showed that 26.4 % of Americans have difficulties accessing healthcare, there were significant differences when racial and ethnic demographic characteristics were considered—racial and ethnic minorities reported greater barriers than their White American counterparts. While Latinos' access to healthcare has improved, they continue to be one of the ethnic groups with worst access in the United States. In 2011, 35.2 % of Latinos reported barriers to healthcare access (USDHHS, 2012; also see Mazzula & Rangel, 2011 for review). Latino adults in need of mental health care are also less likely than non-Latino Whites to access mental health services, and when they do receive care, it is more likely to be poor in quality (Cabassa, Zayas, & Hansen, 2006; Institute of Medicine [IOM], 2003; USDHHS, 2001). Barriers to access are related to multiple factors, on individual and institutional levels.

Medical Insurance and Coverage: A major barrier to healthcare access among Latinos is lack of medical insurance. Overall rates of insurance coverage for adults are lower for Latinos than for White or African-American populations—nearly one in three Latinos in the U.S. are uninsured (NAMI, 2013). When sub-ethnic groups are examined, disparities become even more heighted. Mexican American populations, for example, have lower rates of public insurance compared to their Puerto Rican counterparts (Bustamante, Fang, Rizzo, & Ortega, 2009; Vitullo & Taylor, 2002). Sub-ethnic groups also experience different barriers to obtaining insurance. For example, while early residency in the United States is a documented barrier among Mexican immigrant groups, language difficulties are more noted among Puerto Rican populations. Accordingly, comprehensive patient-focused needs assessments, that consider structural barriers and the intersections of diverse identities among Latinos, are needed to inform relevant service planning.

From our experience as private practice and community mental health practitioners, it is worth mentioning the impression that low reimbursement rates, coupled with excessive managed care red tape and numerous claims denials, discourage mental health providers from accepting medical insurance reimbursement. This impacts the quality of care provided to the Latino population. It also impacts highly qualified practitioners' ability to practice with this population. The Paul Wellstone and Pete Domenici Mental Health Parity and Addiction Equity Act requires coverage of services for mental health, behavioral health, and substance-use disorders to be comparable to physical health coverage. However, an American Psychological Association (APA) survey found that more than 90 % of Americans were unfamiliar with the mental health parity law (APA, 2014). Additionally, the parity law does not require insurers to provide mental health benefits. Instead, the law states that if mental health benefits are offered, they cannot have more restrictive requirements than those that apply to physical health benefits. A health plan is allowed to specifically exclude certain diagnoses—whether those diagnoses are considered to be physical/medical or behavioral/mental health (APA, 2015).

Medical Insurance and Citizenship Status: While the Affordable Care Act (ACA) promises to help Americans, information on its impact still remains to be developed (Ortega, Rodriquez, & Vargas Bustamante, 2014), particularly when considering citizenship status. Under the ACA, any adult citizen or lawfully present non-citizen who has lived in the U.S. more than 5 years qualifies for insurance. However, many Latino families have mixed residency status (Ortega, Rodriquez, & Vargas Bustamante, 2014). While one member may qualify for services, some Latinos may delay, or refrain from, seeking treatment out of fear of the consequences it will have on their non-citizen family members (Ortega, Rodriquez, & Vargas Bustamante, 2014; Rivera, Rangel, & Mazzula, in press). In addition, the new health law now requires that all individuals have health care insurance—those who do not will be subject to a tax penalty (NAMI, 2013), increasing the financial burden of families already distressed due to mental health concerns.

Moreover, undocumented immigrants, including undocumented children, are not eligible for Medicaid and will not be allowed to buy insurance or request governmental assistance (NAMI, 2013). This creates additional stressors for mixed-status families. It should also be noted that while information provided by applicants or beneficiaries will not be used for immigration enforcement purposes (i.e., it cannot affect their chances of becoming a Lawful Permanent resident or citizen) (USHHS, 2014), emerging studies show undocumented immigrants fear "being found out," and this fear itself increases mental health problems like anxiety and depression (Mazzula, 2014). Accordingly, primary care providers must consider residency and citizenship status of patients, and patients' family members, in addressing access to treatment. Internal processes must also be in place to ensure proper documentation and sensitivity related to issues of residency and citizenship status across different health care providers.

Medical Insurance and Mental Health Conditions: While mental health problems are "shockingly common" according to the President's New Freedom Commission on Mental Health, access to care is significantly associated with disparities in insurance coverage for mental disorders compared to other medical conditions (Mental Health America). In fact, the Surgeon General report in Health Insurance (USDHHS, 1999) noted that insurance plans, from private to Medicare, have a long history of imposing barriers to treatment of mental health problems. Legislation enacted in 2008 indicated that group health plans and employers who self insure were no longer allowed to impose different limitations on mental health and substance abuse coverage (e.g., deductibles, copayments, covered hospital days, and any limits on outpatient treatments) that are not imposed for medical treatment. In other words, limitations should be identical regardless of the condition being medical or psychiatric related. Under this law, insurers could still require that services be medically necessary and medical evidence to support the effectiveness of treatment. Although the Department of Health and Human Services has disseminated rules to implement these requirements (2010), information on the effectiveness of these efforts across systems is scares. We do know, however, that even when insured, individuals with psychiatric conditions have out-of-pocket health care costs that are more than double the costs of other insured conditions—findings that remained after adjusting for socioeconomic factors, health status, and functional limitations (Harman & Keller, 2002). Therefore, policy- and decision-makers must tackle discriminatory practices against people with mental health problems and be willing to assess existing practices, or develop new ones, to ensure anti-discriminatory processes. These also require leadership across systems who are committed to hostile-free environments and who are willing to enforce such policies and practices when necessary for the benefit of maintaining patient-focused integrated care.

Given the long-term consequences of not having insurance, from deteriorating health to financial strains due to out-of pocket expenses (Mental Health America; USDHHS, 1999), we need comprehensive policies and models that adequately assess the diverse needs of Latino families and their children. We believe that given Latinos often experience discrimination based on sociocultural identities (e.g., race, ethnicity, language, etc.), additional experiences of discrimination due to mental illness only exacerbate distress and multiplies barriers to service access. Furthermore, it is well noted that individuals who lack insurance are more likely to seek emergency services than their insured counterparts (USDHHS, 2012). Therefore, lack of insurance is likely to create a significant influx of Latinos in emergency services.

Service Use

Fewer than one in 11 Latinos/as with mental health problems contact mental health specialists, while less than one in five contact general health care providers (NAMI, 2006). Although many Latinos with mental health disorders rarely seek services, recent immigrants have even lower rates of service utilization (Acosta, 2006; NAMI, 2006; USDHHS, 2001)—one in 20 use services from mental health specialists compared to one out of ten who use services from general health care providers (USDHHS, 2001). There are multiple structural barriers that limit service utilization such as lack of health insurance, as noted above. However, the very high drop-out rates are even more concerning—50 % of Latinos who seek treatment never return to a psychologist after the first session, compared to 30 % of their

Caucasian counterparts. Furthermore, despite service need, once clients enter treatment, it is well documented that racial and ethnic minorities receive poorer quality of services (Mazzula & Rangel, 2011; Rivera et al., in Press; USDHSS, 2001, 2012).

Therefore, we need to move from the status quo to really understanding the complex needs of Latinos once they enter treatment. Truly understanding the needs of Latino clients is consistent with a patient-centered approach—that is, the "justification for integrated delivery systems is to meet patients' needs rather than providers" (Rogers & Sheaff, 2000). As psychologists who have seen many clients attend their first "second" session, after years of attending the first session, it is clear that we need to be careful with the oversimplification of the reasons for the high dropout rates. However, we have also learned that for individuals that do not understand the medical system, the more the treatment is integrated, the easier it is for the client to have the space to ask questions. As noted previously, primary care providers will be at the forefront of treating diverse needs, from physical to psychological. Yet, they will be challenged to provide culturally competent treatment to engage and retain Latino populations. When Latino clients, and any other racial or ethnic minority, feel understood, they are more likely to engage in treatment. Below we discuss the extant literature on some of the major problems that we believe need to be address to ensure patient-centered treatment across systems and providers. We infuse a psychological perspective to these barriers, both from scholarship and our own clinical work, and pay particular attention to issues that may not be related to their physical ailment but have been documented to have serious and long term consequences on emotional well-being, and stressors that ultimately impact clients' physical health.

Language: Language perhaps has been the most documented barrier in service utilization and relevant care. Language barriers have predicted, for example, outcomes such as lack of patient satisfaction, poor-quality patient education, and lack of understanding of disorders (Fernandez et al., 2011; Ngo-Metzger, Sorkin, & Phillips, 2009). Specific to integrated care, language barriers, which obstruct effective communication, make it virtually impossible for patients to move smoothly from one provider to another—an important element of integrated care systems (Linenkugel, 2001). Furthermore, language barriers result in an added perception of lack of respect and interest in the patient on the part of the provider (Ida, SooHoo, & Chapa, 2012). From our own clinical work, we have learned that language barriers have also resulted in clients' premature termination from treatment—clients have mentioned comments such as "they [prior clinicians] didn't get it".

Moreover, it has been documented that there are disparities in diagnosis and assessment when language is considered. For example, non-native English speaking patients tend to be misdiagnosed and also perceived to lack awareness of their medical conditions (Sue & Sue, 2008). Often times, providers may misjudge the presence of physical or psychological symptoms, which are simply a result of clients' exhaustion in attempting to communicate with providers in a non-native language (Mazzula & Rangel, 2011). Accordingly, policies must include adequate integration of linguistically relevant assessment and diagnostic tools.

Language barriers also call for inclusion of providers who are well-versed in the clients' language. Recent statistics show over 73 % of Latinos report speaking Spanish at home, only about a third speak only English (Hugo Lopez & Gonzalez, 2013). However, most providers do not speak Spanish (USDHHS, 2001). When providers do speak Spanish, the limited data on this information shows that most only have a high-school level of Spanish language competence (Council of La Raza). However, language competency requires understanding of nuances as terms cannot be simply translated from one language to another without losing their meaning. Moreover, when Spanish speaking providers are not available, facilities often address language barriers by using interpreters, which may not adequately translate the patients' physical and or psychological distress at best—at worst, family members are used to translate. While including members to assist in the translation may appear a collaborative effort, it can disrupt family dynamics, disrupt parent–child structures when children are used as the language-broker and can also increase stress levels for clients do not openly discuss health concerns with their family or cultural community (Sue & Sue, 2008; Rivera et al., in press; Umaña-Taylor, 2003). Including family members as translators also has the potential to increase risk of violence, particularly in cases of domestic violence when a translator is the perpetrator unbeknown to the provider. Scholars, and in some cases policies, have noted that using family members is "not optimal." Including this, and similar statements, however, suggests that it is acceptable when a more appropriate option is not available. However, the USDHHS (2012) has noted, specifically, that language barriers continue to be related to the provision of "suboptimal" care. Therefore, policy- and decision-makers must ensure better systems are in place, from information management to provider-trainings, to ensure Latinos, or any non-native English speaker, receive treatment that is linguistically competent. Polices must also be revised to remove statements such as "not optimal" and enforce linguistically competent services and providers.

Client Worldviews: Understanding how clients' worldviews are related to Latinos' underutilization, premature discontinuation of treatment, or overutilization of emergency services will better inform policies to engage and retain Latino populations. In general, acculturation stressors or loss of family support, as a result of migration, have been cited often as a source of stress for many Latino/a Americans (Arredondo et al., 2014; Rios-Ellis, 2005). For example, studies have noted that Latinos who are second or third generation immigrants have higher risk for mental health problems compared to recent immigrants (Alegria et al., 2007; NAMI, 2006). Latino youth in particular are noted to have increased risk for emotional distress as they adapt in the mainstream American culture. Recent studies highlight this stress may explain, for example, suicide attempts among Americanized Latino adolescent girls—who experience higher rates compared to other ethnic groups in the U.S. (Humensky, Santiago, Gill, Mazzula, & Lewis-Fernández, 2014; Zayas, 2011).

In addition to acculturation, there are other more nuanced values and belief systems that impact treatment seeking and engagement—although these are rarely included in mainstream discussions. It is well documented, for example, that some Latino sub-ethnic groups endorse collectivist values, and therefore tend to first seek support from family and close social support networks (Arredondo et al., 2014; Berdahl & Stone, 2009; Cabassa, 2007; Rios-Ellis, 2005; Sanders Thompson, Bazile, & Akbar, 2004). Yet, most medical and psychological treatment is grounded in Western values of individuality and work under the assumption that each individual client has the sole responsibility to seek services, and to also decide on treatment course without considering his/her family or informal support systems (Arredondo et al., 2014; Mazzula & Rangel, 2011; Sue & Sue, 2008). Other worldviews that have been documented to impact utilization and engagement include values of fatalism (Rios-Ellis, 2005)—that is, the belief that a higher power has control over an individual's future, and consequently ailments (see Gallo et al., 2009; Mazzula & Rangel, 2011; Nadal, 2011). Therefore, policies must include adequate assessment and integration of cultural values, from intakes to treatment plans, to better assist clients in management their illness. However, it should be noted that endorsement of worldviews is not so clear-cut and should not be considered as a simple checklist for primary care providers to use. Studies have documented that worldviews are more complex and include the interplay of other factors such as acculturation or racial cultural identity (Arredondo et al., 2014; Carter, Yeh, & Mazzula, 2008). Therefore, internal processes must be in place with standardized protocols and best practice guidelines to assess client worldviews, for providers across systems, to improve integrated care systems' patient-centered approach and quality of care.

Discrimination and Stigma: Policies to improve quality of care also require attention to experiences of discrimination. Ethnic minority populations continue to experience discrimination on individual, institutional, and system levels (Carter et al., 2013; Carter, Forsyth, Mazzula, & Williams, 2005). Studies show discrimination is directly linked with unhealthy behaviors, such as smoking or noncompliance with medical treatment (Lee, Ayers, & Kronenfeld, 2009), to overall negative outlook on life (Nadal, Mazzula, Rivera, & Fujii-Doe, 2014) and traumatic stress reactions (Carter et al., 2013). Internalized racism, or negative stereotypes about being a racial/ethnic minority, also leads to low self-esteem and mental health problems (Campón & Carter, 2015). Studies also show racial/ethnic minorities may delay seeking services because of the stigma associated with mental health problems, fear of misdiagnosis, or due to perceived burden it may have on their family (Kramer, Kwong, Lee, & Chung, 2002; Nadeem, Lange, Edge, Fongwa, Belin, & Miranda, 2007). Stigma or discrimination experiences are added stressors that primary care providers must be willing to include in their assessment and treatment planning—these are also exacerbated when other factors are considered, such as citizenship or residency status as noted previously. As clinicians who work from a culturally informed framework, we understand discussing issues of discrimination is difficult. Therefore, policies must be in place to train and support providers to engage these conversations. Addressing issues of discrimination or stigma also requires leadership that demonstrates the value of anti-discriminatory practices in policies, mission, and overall culture of the integrated care system. This also includes protocols and procedures that assess patients' experiences with discrimination and stigma within the system, and among providers, to improve patient satisfaction and quality care.

Trauma and Poverty: Policies, protocols, and guidelines are also warranted to prepare providers to address issues of trauma across all levels of care. Various studies have documented the impact of childhood maltreatment on adult health such as higher rates of autoimmune disease, headaches, heart disease, liver disease, and chronic pulmonary disease (Anda et al., 2008; Anda, Tietjen, Schulman, Felitti, & Croft, 2010; Corso, Edwards, Fang, & Mercy, 2008; Dong et al., 2004; Dube et al., 2009). Individuals with histories of trauma are also likely to live in poverty or to lack adequate medical insurance. Accordingly, training on trauma assessment is needed in general, and on intersection of identities and well-being of clients specifically. Adequate training is important given many clients do not present as severely psychiatrically disturbed, making it more a more complex phenomenon to assess. Adequate assessment should also consider noted disparities across racial/ethnic groups. For example, some studies find that while Latino children experience lower rates of sexual abuse or neglect, they experience more domestic or community violence compared to their White counterparts (NCTSN, 2005). In fact, Latinos are three times more likely to experience community violence compared to White populations. Without proper assessment or consideration of traumatic life experiences, clients may continue to develop physical conditions that to not respond well to medical treatment. Accordingly, integrated care must include protocols, guidelines, and policies that ensure adequate assessment, sharing of information across providers and proper referrals.

Recommendations: Beyond the Provider

In general, the Latino population is facing several challenges. We reviewed client-centered barriers that impact access to treatment and quality care, which individual providers can address with proper support, policies, and guidelines. In this section, we attend to more global issues impacting health care, in general, to address systemic barriers related to knowledge, assessment, research, scholarship, and workforce development.

Relevant Knowledge Disseminating

The Latino population is one of the country's largest ethnic minority groups, and the one of the groups with the highest uninsured rates (NAMI, 2013). The ACA is helping reduce this rate. For example, 913,000 Latino young adults (e.g., 19–26 years of age) who would not have had insurance are now covered (USHHS, 2014). Nearly 30 states have also expended their Medicaid programs to extend eligibility, and private plans now have to cover "essential health benefit categories" such mental health and substance use disorder services (USHHS, 2014). A new survey (Barreto & Sanchez, 2013), however, shows there is still considerable work ahead to reach this growing group of consumers, particularly as it relates to knowledge transfer that is relevant and accessible. In a nationally representative study of 800 Latino adult participants, the study (Barreto & Sanchez, 2013) highlighted consumer lack of awareness is a major area of concern. Over half (52 %) of Latinos surveyed felt they were not informed about the ACA (Barreto & Sanchez, 2013). When considering within group differences, the study found that English speakers were more informed compared to their Spanish-speaking counterparts, yet a large number of them were also uninformed. Similarly, they also found that even our college educated are unable to gain a good knowledge base about the ACA. Among Latinos who reported having some knowledge, (69 %) reported that the law was "confusing" and "complicated" (Barreto & Sanchez, 2013).

Despite these limitations, the Latino community appears optimistic about the ACA. The study also found 89 % of Latinos reported interest in learning about the law (Barreto & Sanchez, 2013). Therefore, decision-makers must assess the extent to which knowledge transfer is relevant and accessible, and if it is reaching the intended consumers. For example, Barreto and Sanchez (2013) tested several messaging strategies targeting Latino populations, such s messages that included specific parts of the law (e.g., OB-GYN visits). They found some were more effective than others calling for further assessment and deliberate transfer of knowledge. As noted elsewhere in this document, we also discussed the importance of community involvement in knowledge transfer. Their study supported this noting that participants would be more likely to enroll in the ACA if they were encouraged to do so by their family—Latino doctors were also important in encouraging enrollment. Lastly, Barreto and Sanchez (2013) findings provide evidence on the importance of attending to within group differences (e.g., level of education) among Latinos to effectively reach and understand their needs.

Relevant Screening and Assessment of Mental Health

There are a multitude of health problems, or every-day stressors, that may require mental health treatment and complicate the screening processes for primary care physicians. On one end, the ideal scenario would be polices and protocols that support the inclusion of co-behavioral specialists who can regularly provide consultation on mental health and on working with diverse populations. However, this may not always be possible or cost-effective. At a minimum, it would behoove primary care systems to provide primary care providers, across systems, with introductory training on screening for issues most likely to affect their treatment population. Accurate screening, diagnosis, and treatment, however, are entirely dependent on a linguistically accurate interview or assessment measures. It also requires attention to cultural beliefs and values. For example, some Latino clients may prefer to develop personal relationships that are nurturing and supportive (Arredondo et al., 2014; Marin & Marin, 1991). This focus on the relationship versus on the details/specific symptoms of the presenting problem, may result in socially desirable answers during assessments—that is, to facilitate a perceived nurturing relationship. At other times, these values may mask symptom presentations or may be falsely mistaken by providers as patients' poor boundaries, denial of mental health problems, lack of interest in treatment, or even malingering. Therefore, comprehensive policies and models must be in place to support and train providers to attend to these more nuanced cultural factors.

A degree of basic knowledge is also required to inform the proper use of the screening tools. Generally, as mentioned above, based on psychometric training, psychologists are tasked with the appropriate normed and validated testing procedures necessary for ruling out learning disorders, intellectual disabilities, autism, etc. However, they are not the only practitioners who can effectively provide treatment. While there are many screening measures available, it is important to use screening tools that are already available in Spanish and have been previously utilized for the Latino/a population. Staff should never translate these measures on their own, as there is significant room for grammatical errors by bilingual persons, as well as dialectical biases (Cofresí & Gorman, 2004). Below, we provide a list of sample screening tools available from the American Association of Pediatrics (Satterfield & Dover, 2012) in both English and Spanish, organized by client age and diagnostic area. However, when in doubt, primary care physicians should become more comfortable with referring to mental health specialists. When a positive screen is obtained, there are several different levels of integration, which will require structured and clinically informed responses. Accordingly, it is our impression that behavioral and medical personnel would benefit from co-location or strong referral relationships. Providers should also have knowledge of the local community services available (Table 5.1).

Culturally Responsive Research

With the goals of mental health parity, funding for higher levels of integration is required in general, and more specifically for research and implementation of culturally informed integration. Much of the initial research in this area, however, is focused on the medical elements and oversimplifies mental health disorders. In addition, most of the research that includes mental health focuses on the severely mentally ill or depressed client. Thus, there is a dearth of research on the impact that mental health and primary care integration could have on other diagnoses, such as eating disorders, posttraumatic stress, ADHD, etc. Very often, physicians treat behavioral disorders that may be better treated by a psychiatric provider. Yet, at other times, mental health issues are simply overlooked as these are not physicians' areas of specialty. Co-location of behavioral health or a relevant referral to mental health agency or practitioner would be an easy solution. Community mental health centers are losing funding, fees for mental health treatment are low and, without

Table 5.1 Examples of screening instruments

Screening issues	Measure	Age range	Possible referral
Early childhood developmental delays	Ages and stages questionnaire (ASQ)	Birth–5 years	Early intervention services
Substance use	The CRAFFT screening questions	Adolescent–Adult	Addictions counselor, 12-step programs, therapists
Exposure to alcohol in utero	FAS 4-point diagnostic form	N/A	Hospital-based fetal alcohol syndrome child evaluation centers
Cognitive/memory issues	Mini mental status-MMSE	18–69 years	Neurologist/geriatric psychiatrist
Trauma/PTSD	Trauma PTSD checklist-civilian	18+	Psychologists; licensed clinical social worker/ outpatient mental health agencies
	PCL-C Spanish, also Military version UCLA PTSD Checklist	Children/Adolescent versions	
Pediatric Multi-symptom	Pediatric symptom checklist-35 and youth version available in Spanish	To be completed by parent; Child	Psychologists; licensed clinical social worker/ outpatient mental health agencies
OCD; Hoarding	Yale-Brown obsessive compulsive scale (Y-BOCS)	18+	
		Child version also available 5–17 years	
Adult depression or anxiety	Hamilton depression and hamilton anxiety scales	18+	Psychologists; licensed clinical social worker/ outpatient mental health agencies
Postpartum depression	Edinburgh maternal depression escala Edinburgh para la depresión postnatal	Adolescent–Adult	Psychologists; licensed clinical social worker/ outpatient mental health agencies
Eating disorder	EAT-26	16–35 years	Psychologists; licensed clinical social worker
Autism	M-CHAT autism screener	16–36 months	Autism center, early intervention
Generalized somatic symptoms without medical cause	PHQ-SADS, PHQ-9, GAD-7, and PHQ-15	18+	Psychologists; licensed clinical social worker/ outpatient mental health agencies

Note: Sample screening tools gathered from Satterfield and Dover's (2012) American Association of Pediatrics' Mental Health Toolkit Addressing Mental Health Concerns in Primary Care. A Clinician's Toolkit support from medical professionals, are at risk of collapsing. Research on how to best plan, implement, and assess integrated care is needed.

Some promising culturally appropriate integration research has begun to emerge. For example, Ell and colleagues (2010, 2011) implemented culturally and linguistically competent integrated care models, which addressed depression in Hispanic patients with diabetes and cancer. Yeung and colleagues (2010) also examined a culturally sensitive collaborative treatment model based on Ell's model for the treatment of depression in primary care, but focused on Asian-Americans. The integrated health care intervention designed by Ell and colleagues (2009) addressed systemic barriers by using Spanish-speaking interviewers, adapting study intervention materials for literacy and cultural content, reimbursing patients for completing outcome interviews and paying for transportation expenses. The interventions consisted of bilingual social workers serving as care managers. The intervention also provided training in cultural competency for all staff, with support groups in Spanish and English (Ell et al., 2009). Yeung et al. (2010) implemented similar strategies, however, emphasized the screening and outreach components as stigma was a significant cultural barrier to overcome in the Chinese immigrant community. Finally, in the interventions, by both Ell et al. and Yeung et al., patients were provided their choice in first-line treatment preference, of which psychotherapy alone was an option, instead of antidepressant medication. Patients were also offered the opportunity to include family members in treatment, if preferred, which seemed to capture collectivist values and family loyalty often endorsed by racial/ethnic minority patients.

These models also assessed patients' "illness narrative" to understand how people conceptualized their illness. The illness narrative or illness myth is a very important point to consider in culturally competent services particularly among patients whose health or treatment compliance is impacted by psychological or cultural factors. Benish, Quintana, and Wampold (2011) conducted a robust meta-analysis that found that this very nuanced variable predicted the superiority of culturally modified treatment. Benish and colleagues coined this variable the "illness myth," which appears to support Yeung's mention of the "illness narrative." This "illness myth" refers to the client's beliefs about the etiology, types of symptoms experienced, prediction of the course of illness, consequences of the illness, and what constitutes acceptable treatment—all of which are rooted in the client's cultural worldview, as noted previously in this chapter. Knowing this will help providers to predict barriers and to promote culturally informed dialogues. However, despite these promising data, more research is needed to understand effective integrated care models.

Lastly, we understand, from our own research and clinical work, that engaging in such nuanced patient assessments takes more time than what the managed care model provides primary care physicians. Therefore, integrating behavioral health care specialists who spend longer time with clients could prove quite informative to medical specialists. However, policies that require appropriate reimbursement for these services are also necessary. It may also be beneficial to integrate culturally responsive researchers as consultants in all levels of the system who can provide input, assessments, and recommendations in the design and implementation of evidence-based practices. Yet, lack of a diverse research capital has been noted throughout the country, and across fields of study, which presents a significant challenge for evidence-based integrated care. However, national efforts are on their way to address this shortage. For example, the National Institute of Health's Division of Training, Workforce Development, and Diversity (2015) funds programs that promote the training and development of a diverse research capital—programs that target undergraduate students to postdoctoral and doctoral-level researchers.

Culturally Responsive Scholarship

Similar to the above need for research, lack of scholarship on, or with Latinos, is an additional issue that will impact effective implementation of integrated care models and treatment of Latino/a patients. It is well documented that while the inclusion of racial and ethnic minority populations in psychological research has increased over time, it continues to be limited (Carter & Forsyth, 2007; Delgado-Romero, Glavan, Maschino, & Rowland, 2005; Mazzula, 2013). Latinos also make up a significantly small amount of research samples (Delgado-Romero et al., 2005) thus limiting the generalizability of existing mental health scholarship. In addition to overall poor inclusion of Latinos in psychological research, we know very little about psychological-based cultural factors such as acculturation, racial or ethnic identity—despite evidence to show that these factors are related to important outcomes such as self-esteem, cognitive maturity, psychological adjustment, symptoms of distress, and negative affect (Corenblum & Armstrong, 2012; Jackson, et al., 2012), as well as depression, isolation, and anxiety (Sharkey, Sander, & Jimerson, 2012). For example, in our own review of over 2400 psychological publications in a 16 year timespan, we found most researchers and scholars used global terms such as "Latino" or "Hispanic" without attention to within group differences related to ethnicity, race, or acculturation—in fact, we found only 3 % of publications did so (Mazzula, 2013). Similar findings have been noted across psychology specialty fields. This less optimal state of the scholarship reveals a significant gap in our understanding of mental health needs of Latinos. An alarming finding given most professional ethical boards require providers to ground their treatment and interventions in relevant scholarship.

Therefore, systems must be in place to train providers on how to adequately and critically analyze culturally competent scholarship. With the move toward evidence-based practices, guidelines, protocols, and incentives are also needed to support providers in disseminating culturally relevant scholarship across all systems. Funding support to contract culturally competent scholars and researchers to join inter-disciplinary teams or as consultants may also be helpful in training staff and in ensuring scholarship is relevant to the needs of Latino populations. The mental health needs of Latinos depends on it—the American Psychological Association's "*Guidelines on Multicultural Education, Training, Research, Practice, and Organizational Change for Psychologists*" noted "when research does not adequately incorporate culture as a central and specific contextual variable, behavior is misidentified, pathologized, and, in some cases, psychologists are at risk of perpetuating harm" (APA, 2002, p. 37). Thus, the scholarship that providers read and use to inform their treatment, as well as all material that is disseminated to patients, must be grounded in culturally relevant and competent scholarship.

Workforce Diversity

The last major obstacle to effective integrated care is workforce diversity. In addition to impacting all levels of integrated health, from the values of leadership to the inclusion of diverse perspectives in information management, workforce diversity has been noted to contribute to the persistent racial and ethnic disparities in health. National statistics show providers who treat minority populations are less likely to be board certified than those who treat non-Hispanic White patients (Institute of Medicine, 2003). Minority populations are also underrepresented in most health care professions and limited in high-quality subspecialists and diagnostic imaging. For example, while Latinos account for over 17 % of the US population, they represent less than 3 % of physicians, about 1 % of clinical psychologists, 4.3 % of social workers and 1.7 % of registered nurses in hospital settings (USDHHS, 2010). Their true representation may be even lower, as these published percentages do not incorporate professionals who work specifically in behavioral health. These data also fail to account for levels of cultural competence and providers' bilingual abilities relevant to their treatment populations—skills which are vital to serving non-native English speaking clients.

Considering ethno-cultural factors (e.g., worldviews, experiences of discrimination, stigma, etc.), underutilization of treatment, and high drop-out rates among some Latino/a American groups, it is clear that more relevant health policies are needed to ensure workforce diversity and cultural competence among providers. It should be noted that the Affordable Care Act has attempted to include some recommendations for workforce development. For example, Section 5101 recommends the establishment of a national commission tasked with reviewing health care workforce and projected workforce needs. This inclusion was intended to bridge the alignment of federal health care workforce resources with national needs. In Section 5602, the secretary of health and human services was also directed to establish comprehensive methodology and criteria for designating medically underserved populations and health professional shortage areas. Workforce development policies, or taskforce efforts to assess needs, must consider strategies for retaining diverse populations in health care, from technicians to physicians. These should address issues of proper reimbursement, given documented racial discrimination experienced by minority providers, and for improving cultural and linguistic competency among existing providers.

In addition to workforce development, various efforts are underway to address workforce diversity given the lack of diverse representation of minority populations in the healthcare field, particularly Latinos. Workforce diversity must be addressed, however, across the pipeline. More graduate programs are needed that focus specifically on Latino behavioral health, as well as programs that incorporate cultural competence in graduate curriculum and training programs. Once students enter behavioral health, they must also be supported. Funding and grant support is necessary to develop targeted programs that engage and retain Latino students in behavioral health, particularly in postgraduate education. It is well documented that racial and ethnic minority populations experience discrimination, both on individual and systemic levels. Therefore, organizational efforts must be in place to ensure Latino students are given the opportunity to begin their career on the same level field as their White peers. These include, for example, policies and committed programs that provide access to resources, trainings, scholarships, and mentorship.

In addition, recent developments have shown the importance of mentorship networks to support those who have "made it"—that is, they have entered post-graduate work life—given systemic barriers that impact under-represented clinicians, psychologist, and others such as academics and scholars (Arredondo et al., 2014; Mazzula, 2013; Rivera et al., in press). For example, the recently founded Latina Researchers Network (Mazzula, 2013; www.latinaresearcehers.com) is a multidisciplinary network of faculty members, researchers, clinicians, scholars, and academic leaders across the United States that supports the training, recruitment, and retention of under-represented populations in academia and in advanced research careers. Other mentorship-based networks include the New Connections Program of the Robert Wood Johnson Foundation (www.rwjf-new-connections.org), which provides networking and skill building opportunities for under-represented early to mid-career scholars in health and healthcare research. Similar efforts should be considered in integrated healthcare, and within healthcare systems, to diversify its workforce and support under-represented health care professionals who have shared cultural experiences that impact their career experiences and trajectory. Other efforts are underway, as previously noted, such as the work of the National Institute of Health's Division of Training, Workforce Development, and Diversity (2015) which funds programs that specifically to train and develop a diverse research capital. In fact, the National Institutes of Health (NIH) recently awarded $31 million to academic institutions diversity its grant funded programs (NIH, 2015).

Workforce diversity and development must be addressed if we aim to prepare for our future—both to serve the growing Latino community and to increase the number of health care professionals who are culturally competent or representative of those we serve. In fact, the Report "Movilizandonos por Nuestro Futuro: Strategic Development of a Mental Health Workforce for Latinos" provided five consensus statements we find important to highlight in conclusion:

(1) The Latino population in the U.S. is facing a public health crisis due to poor or unmet behavioral health needs; (2) The lack of a bilingual and bicultural behavioral health workforce plays a significant role in disparities across behavioral health care service delivery; (3) Meaningful access to behavioral healthcare

for Latinos in the U.S. is a social justice issue; (4) Latinos deserve a diverse, multidisciplinary, bilingual, and bicultural behavioral health workforce; and (5) The time for action is NOW! (USDHHS, 2010).

Conclusion

Overall, we can expect the Latino population to continue to use primary care for their mental health needs. We can also expect increased rates of service use given various factors, from culture-bound symptom presentations to lack of insurance to more nuanced worldviews that lead clients to emergency care vs. mental health specialty services. Therefore, a shift in paradigm in the design, planning, and implementation of integrated care must occur to provide culturally grounded services.

More clearly outlined, and enforced, policies that improve language accessibility and screening practices, that support training, funding, and development of culturally competent research and scholarships, and that build a diverse and culturally competent workforce will ensure access and treatment are relevant to Latino populations. Standard practices must be developed to increase awareness of the connection between mental health and chronic disease, as well as overall life stressors experienced by Latino populations (e.g., acculturation, family responsibilities, etc.). Given that stigma and discrimination experiences (whether related to ethnic minority status or mental illness) have a significant impact on help-seeking, stigma awareness trainings with gatekeepers will be a key step in ensuring clients enter the treatment room. Once they enter treatment, the patients' needs to be spoken in a language that they understand and to have adequate time to describe their presenting problems have to be emphasized, valued, and enforced by leadership and decision-makers across systems. In essence, a culturally grounded patient-focused approach must become the culture of the system—valued and celebrated.

Good care must also be taken to support both medical and mental health professionals who continue to be challenged with increasing managed care limitations, despite their efforts and commitment to our clients. Thus, polices must also include trainings and reimbursement—an appropriate and detailed explanation of the enforcement of these policies should also be included in the laws. Medical providers, mental health professionals, and social workers, all bring significant areas of expertise, and must all be at the table—directly involved in the development, planning, and execution of policies, guidelines, and protocols. Therefore, integrated care, as an entity, must also be supported to achieve its goals of serving all clients in general, and Latino patients specifically.

In order to accomplish these challenging, yet manageable goals, we must first advocate for policies that promote social justice, equity, and equality in all systems of care. We hope the recommendations throughout the chapter help to move us from walking on eggshells to commitment to culturally responsive treatment, research, and policies.

References

Acosta, H. (2006). *The current status of Latino mental health in the United States*. Paper session at National Association for Mental Illness' Eliminating Disparities: Multicultural Strategic Summit, Washington, DC.

Agency for Healthcare Research and Quality. (2009). *Program brief: Mental health research findings*. Rockville, MD: Author.

Alegria, M., Mulvaney-Day, N., Torres, M., Polo, A., Cao, Z., & Canino, G. (2007). Prevalence of psychiatric disorders across Latino subgroups in the United States. *American Journal of Public Health, 97*, 68–75.

American Psychological Association (2001). Guidelines on Multicultural Education, Training, Research, Practice and Organizational Change for Psychologists.

American Psychological Association. (2014). *2014 Mental health parity survey*. Washington, DC: Author.

American Psychological Association. (2015). *Consumer guide: What you need to know about mental health coverage*. Washington, DC: Author.

Anda, R. F., Brown, D. W., Dube, S. R., Bremner, J. D., Felitti, V. J., & Giles, W. H. (2008). Adverse childhood experiences and chronic obstructive pulmonary disease in adults. *American Journal of Preventive Medicine, 34*(5), 396–403.

Anda, R., Tietjen, G., Schulman, E., Felitti, V., & Croft, J. (2010). Adverse childhood experiences and frequent headaches in adults. *Headache, 50*(9), 1473–1481.

Arredondo, P., Gallardo-Cooper, M., Delgado-Romero, E. A., & Zapata, A. L. (2014). *Culturally responsive counseling with Latinas/os*. Alexandria, VA: American Counseling Association.

Barreto, M., & Sanchez, G. (2013). New national Latino health care survey results. *Latino Decisions*. Retrieved from http://www.latinodecisions.com/blog/2013/05/01/New-National-Latino-Health-Care-Survey-Results.

Benish SG, Quintana S, & Wampold BE. (2011). Culturally adapted psychotherapy and the legitimacy of myth: a direct-comparison meta-analysis. Journal of Counseling Psycholy V58(3):279–89. doi: 10.1037/a0023626.

Bower P,& Gilbody S. (2005). Managing common mental health disorders in primary care: conceptual models and evidence base. BMJ;330(7495):839–42.

Bustamante, A. V., Fang, H., Rizzo, J. A., & Ortega, A. N. (2009). Heterogeneity in health insurance coverage among US Latino adults. *Journal of General Internal Medicine, 24*(3), 561–566. doi:10.1007/s11606-009-10697.

Cabassa, L. J., Zayas, L. H., & Hansen, H. C. (2006). Latino adults' access to mental health: A review of epidemiological studies. *Administration and Policy in Mental Health, 33*(3), 316–330. doi:10.1007/s10488-006-0040-8.

Campón, R. R., & Carter, R. T. (2015). The appropriated racial oppression scale: Development and validation. *Cultural Diversity & Ethnic Minority Psychology, 21*(4), 497–506.

Carter, R. T., Forsyth, J., Mazzula, S. L., & Williams, B. (2005). Racial discrimination and race-based traumatic stress. In Carter R. T. (Vol. Ed.), *Handbook of racial-cultural psychology and counseling: Practice and training Vol. 2* (pp. 447–476). New York, NY: Wiley & Sons, Inc.

Carter, R.T., Mazzula, S. L., Victoria, R., Vazquez, R., Hall, S., Smith, S., … Williams, B. (2013). Initial development of the race-based traumatic stress symptom scale: Assessing the emotional impact of racism. *Psychological Trauma: Theory, Research, Practice, and Policy, 5*(1), 1–9.

Carter, R. T., Yeh, C. J., & Mazzula, S. L. (2008). Cultural values and racial identity statuses among Latino students: An exploratory investigation. *Hispanic Journal of Behavioral Sciences, 30*(5), 5–23. doi:10.1177/0739986307310505.

Chapa, T. (2004). *Mental health services in primary care settings for racial and ethnic minority populations*. Rockville, MD: U.S. Department of Health and Human Services, Office of Minority Health.

Cofresí, N., & Gorman, A. (2004). Testing and assessment issues with Spanish-English bilingual Latinos. *Journal of Counseling & Development, 82*, 99–106.

Corso, P. S., Edwards, V. J., Fang, X., & Mercy, J. A. (2008). Health-related quality of life among adults who experienced maltreatment during childhood. *American Journal of Public Health, 98*, 1094–1100.

Delgado-Romero, E. A., Glavan, N., Maschino, P., & Rowland, M. (2005). Race and ethnicity: Ten years of counseling research. *The Counseling Psychologist, 33*, 419–448.

Dong, M., Giles, W. H., Felitti, V. J., Dube, S. R., Williams, J. E., Chapman, D. P., & Anda, R. F. (2004). Insights into causal pathways for ischemic heart disease: Adverse childhood experiences study. *Circulation, 110*, 1761–1766.

Dube, S. R., Fairweather, D., Pearson, W. S., Felitti, V. J., Anda, R. F., & Croft, J. B. (2009). Cumulative childhood stress and autoimmune disease. *Psychomatic Medicine, 71*, 243–250.

Ell, K., Katon, W., Cabassa, L. J., Xie, B., Lee, P. J., Kapetanovic, S., & Guterman, J. (2009). Depression and diabetes among low-income Hispanics: Design elements of a socio-culturally adapted collaborative care model randomized controlled trial. *International Journal of Psychiatry in Medicine, 39*(2), 113–132.

Ell, K., Katon, W., Xie, B., Lee, P. J., Kapetanovic, S., Guterman, J., & Chou, C. P. (2010). Collaborative care management of major depression among low-income, predominantly Hispanic subjects with diabetes. A randomized controlled trial. *Diabetes Care, 33(4)*, 706–713.

Ell, K., Xie, B., Kapetanovic, S., Quinn, D. I., Lee, P. J., Wells, A., & Chou, C. P. (2011). One-year follow-up of collaborative depression care for low-income, predominantly Hispanic patients with cancer. *Psychiatric Services, 62*(2), 162–170.

Hugo Lopez, M., & Gonzalez, A. (2013). *What is the future of Spanish in the United States?* Pew Research Center. Retrieved from http://www.pewresearch.org/fact-tank/2013/09/05/what-is-the-future-of-spanish-in-the-united-states.

Humensky, J., Santiago, B., Gill, R., Mazzula, S. L., & Lewis-Fernández, R. (2014). Life is precious: Reducing suicidal behavior in Latinas. *Ethnicity and Inequalities in Health and Social Care, 6*(2), 54. doi:10.1108/EIHSC-10-2013-0027.

Institute of Medicine. (2003). *Unequal treatment: Confronting racial and ethnic disparities in health care*. Washington, DC: The National Academies Press.

Leyro, S. (2015). Legal violence: *Crimmigration and the violent effects of deportation*. Paper session at the 32nd annual Winter Roundtable, Teachers College, NY

Linenkugel, N. (2001). Integrated health networks are not created equal. *Frontiers of Health Services Management, 17*, 41–44.

Marin, G., & Marin, B. V. O. (1991). *Research with Hispanic populations*. Newbury Park, CA: SAGE Publications.

Mazzula, S. L., (2013, August). Chair. *Race and culture in psychology publications: A call to action in research, theory and practice*. Symposium at the American Psychological Association 121st Annual Convention, Honolulu, HI.

Mental Health America (YR). *Position statement 15: Mental health parity in health insurance*.

Nadal, K., Mazzula, S. L., Rivera, D. R., & Fujii-Doe, W. (2014). Racial microaggressions and Latina/o Americans: An analysis of nativity, gender, and ethnicity. *Journal of Latina/o Psychology, 2*(2), 67–78. doi:10.1037/lat0000013.

National Alliance on Mental Illness. (2009). *Grading the states*. Arlington, VA: Author.

National Alliance on Mental Illness. (2013). *New mental health coverage for Latino families*. Arlington, VA: National Latino Behavioral Health Association.

National Alliance on Mental Illness. (2015). *A long road ahead: Achieving true parity in mental health and substance use*. Arlington, VA: Author.

National Child Traumatic Stress Network. (2005). Promoting culturally competent trauma-informed practices. *NCTSN Culture & Trauma Briefs, 1(1)*.

National Institute of Health. (2015). *Current programs in the Division of Training, Workforce Development, and Diversity (TWD)*. Rockville, MD: U.S. Department of Health and Human Services, Division of Training, Workforce Development and Diversity. Retrieved from http://www.nigms.nih.gov/Training/Pages/TWDPrograms.aspx.

New Freedom Commission on Mental Health. (2003). *Achieving the promise: Transforming mental health care in America, Executive summary*. Rockland, MD: Substance Abuse and Mental Health

Services Administration. Retrieved from http://store.samhsa.gov/product/Achieving-the-Promise-Transforming-Mental-Health-Care-in-America-Executive-Summary/SMA03-3831.

Ngo-Metzger, Q., Sorkin, D. H., & Phillips, R. S. (2009). Health care experiences of limited-English proficient Asian Americans. The Patient: Patient-centered Outcomes Research, 2(2), 113–120.

Rios-Ellis, B. (2005). *Critical disparities in Latino mental health: Transforming research into action*. Retrieved from http://www.nclr.org/index.php/publications/critical_disparities_in_latino_mental_health_transforming_research_into_action/.

Rogers, A., & Sheaff, R. (2000). Formal and informal systems of primary healthcare in an integrated system: Evidence from the United Kingdom. *Healthcare Papers, 1*, 47–58.

Sanders Thompson, V. L., Bazile, A., & Akbar, M. (2004). African-Americans' perceptions of psychotherapy and psychotherapists. *Professional Psychology: Research and Practice, 35*, 19–26.

Satterfield, M., & Dover, M. (2012, January). *AAP mental health toolkit addressing mental health concerns in primary care a clinician's toolkit*. Presentation at the NC Center of Excellence for Integrated Care 2010.

Unutzer, J., Schoenbaum, M., Druss, B. G., & Katon, W. J. (2006). Transforming mental health care at the interface with general medicine: Report for the President's Commission. Psychiatric Services, 57, 37–47.

U.S. Department of Health and Human Services (1999). Mental Health: A Report of the Surgeon General. Rockville, MD: U.S. Department of Health and Human Services, Substance Abuse and Mental Health Services Administration, Center for Mental Health Services, National Institutes of Health, National Institute of Mental Health.

U.S. Department of Health and Human Services. (2001). *Mental health: Culture, race, and ethnicity—A supplement to mental health: A report of the surgeon general. Executive summary*. Rockville, MD: U.S. Department of Health and Human Services, Substance Abuse and Mental Health Services Administration, Center for Mental Health Services.

U.S. Department of Health and Human Services. (2010). *Movilizandonos por Nuestro Futuro: Strategic Development of a Mental Health Workforce for Latinos Consensus Statements and Recommendations*. USDHHS Office of Minority Health and the National Resource Center for Hispanic Mental Health.

U.S. Department of Health and Human Services. (2014). *Fact sheets: The affordable care act and Latinos*. HHS.gov/HealthCare, U.S. Department of Health and Human Services. Retrieved from http://www.hhs.gov/healthcare/facts/factsheets/2012/04/aca-and-latinos04102012a.html.

U.S. Department of Health and Human Services Office of Minority Health & Hogg Foundation for Mental Health. (2012). *Eliminating disparities through the integration of behavioral health and primary care services for racial and ethnic minority populations, including individuals with limited english proficiency. A literature review report*.

Umaña-Taylor, A. (2003). Language brokering as a stressor for immigrant children and their families. In M. Coleman & L. Ganong (Eds.), *Points and counterpoints: Controversial relationship and family issues in the 21st century: An anthology* (pp. 157–159). Los Angeles, CA: Roxbury.

Vitullo, M. W., & Taylor, A. K. (2002). Latino adults' health insurance coverage: An examination of Mexican and Puerto Rican subgroup differences. *Journal of Health Care for the Poor and Underserved, 13*(4), 504–525. doi:10.1353/hpu.2010.0653.

Weinick, R. M., & Jacobs, E. A. (2000). Hispanic healthcare utilization: The role of ancestry, language, and duration of residence in the United States. *Abstract of the Academic Health Services Research Health Policy Meeting*.

Yeung, A., Shyu, I., Fisher, L., Wu, S., Yang, H. Y., & Fava, M. (2010). Culturally sensitive collaborative treatment for depressed Chinese Americans in primary care. *American Journal of Public Health, 100*(12), 23972402.

Zayas, L. H. (2011). *Latinas attempting suicide: When cultures, families and daughters collide*. New York, NY: Oxford University Press.

Chapter 6
Community Health Centers and Payment for Integrated Care

Charles Duarte

Community Health Centers (CHCs), which include Federally Qualified Health Centers (FQHCs), have historically provided comprehensive primary care to underserved communities that often include minority populations. Currently, there are over 1200 CHCs with over 9000 health center sites serving over 21 million low-income patients (National Association of Community Health Centers, 2013a). While CHCs serve the entire community, including households with commercial insurance, the main focus of their services are the underserved and publicly insured populations (Medicaid, Children's Health Insurance Program (CHIP) and Medicare) which often makes up 75 % of their patients (The Commonwealth Fund, 2011). Given the mission of CHCs across the U.S., this discussion will focus on the role of CHCs in providing integrated care and the implications for payment reform.

Understanding the state and federal regulatory environment that governs CHCs is essential to understanding the financial opportunities and barriers to integrated care. CHCs operate under a federal regulatory authority detailed in Section 330 of the Public Health Services Act. They are required to provide comprehensive services to patients either by formal referral arrangement, contract, or by providing behavioral health services directly under their federally approved scope of services. These rules also define payment methodologies for Medicaid, CHIP, and Medicare services based on a Prospective Payment System (PPS). Prior to 2000, CHCs were paid using a cost-based reimbursement model. Cost-based reimbursement considered all reasonable costs associated with the mission of the FQHC in developing reimbursement rates for Medicaid and Medicare. In 2000, new federal rules required the use of a PPS rate (BIPA 2000 and CHIPRA). These new federal rules replaced reasonable cost methods with a PPS rate methodology which considered the cost of

C. Duarte (✉)
Community Health Alliance, Reno, NV 89502, USA
e-mail: cduarte@chanevada.org

© Springer International Publishing Switzerland 2016

L.T. Benuto, W. O'Donohue (eds.), *Enhancing Behavioral Health in Latino Populations*, DOI 10.1007/978-3-319-42533-7_6

services paid prior to 2000 and then adjusted for subsequent years for medical cost inflation and changes in the scope of services provided by the FQHC. For FQHCs established after 2000, states use the reasonable cost of services for the prior year adjusted prospectively for medical inflation and changes in the scope of FQHC services. A PPS rate establishes a provider's payment rate for a service before the service is delivered; the rate is not dependent on the provider's actual costs or the amount charged for the service. PPS rates for CHCs are considered "fair payment" from State Medicaid Agencies, and are higher than fees paid to non-CHC providers. PPS reimburses FQHCs at approximately 81 % of their costs to treat Medicaid patients. The PPS also reimburses for comprehensive CHC services, which can include dental, behavioral health, pharmacy, primary care, immunizations, chronic care management, as well as referrals to social services. Medicaid payments to non-FQHC medical practices reimburses them for medical visits only. Under federal rules, PPS rates are guaranteed regardless of whether payments come from the State Medicaid Agency, the Medicare Program, a Medicare Advantage Plan, or a Medicaid Managed Care Organization. Paying for an all-inclusive package of services allows FQHCs to serve as medical homes for Medicaid and uninsured patients (National Association of Community Health Centers, 2013b). A 2013 Texas legislative study reported that the average PPS rate for FQHCs in the state was $174 (Texas Legislative Budget Board, 2014). By comparison, Texas Medicaid currently pays non-FQHC physicians $37 for a routine office visit (Texas Medicaid, 2015).

Federal rules also allow State Medicaid Agencies to establish an Alternative Payment Methodology (APM) with individual FQHCs as long as there is mutual agreement between the FQHC and the State. APMs are subject to approval by the Centers for Medicaid and Medicare Services (CMS) and must reconcile to what the FQHC would have otherwise been paid under a PPS methodology. FQHCs are working with State Medicaid Agencies to develop APMs. A 2014 report by the National Association of Community Health Centers (NACHC) indicated 30 % of responding states offer APM reimbursement models as an alternative to PPS. Nineteen percent of states offered both APM and PPS reimbursement models.

APM reimbursement models are of growing interest to FQHCs as a means of reforming Medicaid reimbursement methods. They are being used to disconnect revenue from the volume patient visits. APMs are also often used to reimburse FQHCs to provide more "in-between" care such as care coordination and case management; services which are essential to their role as a health care home (Buxbaum, 2012).

Many CHCs are also able to take advantage of the favorable prescription drug pricing under Section 340B of the Public Health Service Act. The 340B Drug Discount Program requires drug makers to provide outpatient drugs to eligible health centers, clinics, and hospitals at significantly reduced prices. CHCs are then able to pass on these discounts to their uninsured and underinsured patients as well as State Medicaid Agencies. 340B pricing is a ceiling price, meaning it is the highest price a participating entity can be charged, and it is determined by the CMS. 340B pricing is estimated to be about half of Average Wholesale Price (AWP) and about 20–50 % below true wholesale price (HRSA, 2004). Access to 340B prescription drug pricing gives FQHCs a competitive advantage in providing cost-effective drug therapy to their patients.

Besides use of APMs, State Medicaid Agencies have other regulatory tools at their disposal in order to change health care payment and delivery systems. States can modify their agreement with CMS by amending their State Plan. Medicaid and CHIP state plans are agreements between a state and the federal government. The State Plan describes who will be covered, services provided, methods of payment to providers, and administrative activities conducted by the state. It also gives assurances that a state will abide by federal rules. State Plan Amendments (SPAs) must go through a public review process and require approval by CMS. SPAs are a simple and common method of changing payment and other policies affecting CHC services.

States also use waivers allowed under Section 1915(b) of the Social Security Act (SSA). These "managed care" waivers are used to implement managed care networks, use managed care savings to add services, or restrict the numbers of providers of certain services.

Comprehensive Medicaid reform initiatives are often undertaken using Section 1115 waivers. Section 1115 refers to a section of the Social Security Act (SSA). These waivers, often referred to as Research and Demonstration Waivers, allow the Secretary of the U.S. Department of Health and Human Services (DHHS) to waive certain provisions of the SSA in order to implement Medicaid payment and delivery system reforms. Often these waivers are time limited (3 or 5 years) and must achieve federal budget neutrality within this timeframe. Arizona implemented the nation's most comprehensive 1115 waiver program. On October 1, 1982, the Arizona Health Care Cost Containment System (AHCCCS or Arizona Medicaid) used an 1115 waiver as the regulatory vehicle to implement Arizona's Medicaid program. Since then, it has been exempt from many provisions of the SSA allowing it to utilize managed care networks and other innovative approaches to paying for Medicaid services.

CMS has recently awarded almost $1 billion in planning grants to states to reform their health care systems to test innovations in health care delivery and payment systems. The State Innovations Models (SIM) grants seek to make sweeping changes in payment and delivery systems consistent with the Triple Aim: Improving the patient care experience; improving population health; and reducing the per capita cost of health care.

Still, the simplest regulatory approach to Medicaid reform specifically involving CHCs is through amendments to the Medicaid and CHIP state plans and the use of Medicaid APMs.

Payment Issues Affecting CHCs and Integrated Care

By far, Medicaid is the largest payer of CHC services across the nation. A 2013 report published by the Kaiser Family Foundation State Health Facts found that Medicaid payments represented 40 % of FQHC revenue followed by federal grant funds (21 %). By contrast, Medicare and private insurance made up 6 % and 8 % of revenue, respectively (Kaiser Family Foundation, 2015).

Eligibility for Medicaid services varies from state to state. The saying is "If you've seen one Medicaid program you've seen one Medicaid program." Medicaid is funded with federal and state funds, but administered by states under federal guidelines. As such, states have a great deal of flexibility to design the eligibility criteria as well as the scope of services. While Medicaid has been traditionally focused on covering low-income seniors, individuals with disabilities, and families with children, the Affordable Care Act (ACA) allowed states to expand their Medicaid programs to include low-income adults without children, including many individuals with complex medical and behavioral health conditions.

Increasingly, CHCs are providing mental health and/or substance abuse services as a part of their scope of services. A 2010 assessment conducted by the National Association of Community Health Centers (NACHC) reported that over 70 % of CHCs provided some level of mental health services. In addition, 55 % provided substance abuse services and 65 % met the criteria for integrated care including shared treatment plans and joint decision-making between primary care and mental health providers (National Association of Community Health Centers, 2010).

Besides integrated care, CHCs have been leaders in other areas of health care delivery and patient education including Patient-Centered Medical Homes and Team-Based Care models.

Essential to the concept of the medical home and integrated care is the provision of "in-between care" or wrap-around support services. More CHCs are using Community Health Workers (CHWs) to provide patient education and chronic disease management support between primary care or behavioral health visits. However, the Medicaid regulatory environment has often lagged in its ability to financially support these innovations.

Same Day Billing

Essential to the provision of integrated care are policies that allow CHCs to provide primary care and behavioral health services to patients with complex medical issues on the same day. Unless specifically allowed by a state Medicaid agency through its Medicaid state plan, FQHCs can only bill for one encounter per patient per day. A 2011 report by the National Association of Community Health Centers (NACHC) indicated that 82 % of State Medicaid Agencies allow for more than one CHC visit per day, although many have defined criteria to allow payment for those additional visits (National Association of Community Health Centers, 2011).

An assessment was done in 2011 by NORC at the University of Chicago for the Substance Abuse and Mental Health Services Administration (SAMHSA) and the Health Resources and Services Administration (HRSA). As a part of that survey, CHCs were asked about barriers to the development of patient-centered medical homes and integrated care models. Most of the reporting CHCs saw Medicaid reimbursement as an asset, but more than half reported that restrictions on same-day billing for medical and mental health services were a significant problem. Additionally, respondents indicated that Medicaid reimbursement for substance abuse treatment services was limited and presented a barrier to providing these services (NORC at the University of Chicago, 2011).

Restrictions on same day billing can be readily addressed by State Medicaid Agencies through use of a SPA. Amending the Medicaid and CHIP state plans, and any associated regulations, to allow multiple CHC encounters per day will help to resolve these issues. States may want to impose reasonable restrictions, e.g. allowing one medical, behavioral health, and dental visit per day.

Limits on Qualified Providers

Federal law requires State Medicaid Agencies to cover services provided by certain providers approved under Medicare. These include physicians, physician assistants, nurse practitioners, certified nurse midwives, licensed clinical social workers, and clinical psychologists. Adding additional provider types to this list can enhance the ability of CHCs to expand available behavioral health services. For example, Oklahoma allows licensed professional counselors, licensed marriage and family therapists, licensed alcohol and drug counselors, and licensed behavioral analysts (National Association of Community Health Centers, 2011).

An amendment to the Medicaid and CHIP state plan, and any necessary changes to state regulations, is a simple approach to expanding behavioral health providers available through CHCs.

Medicaid Managed Care Contracting

Many State Medicaid Agencies contract with managed care organizations to provide comprehensive Medicaid benefits to eligible beneficiaries. Based on 2011 report from the Kaiser Family Foundation, over 74 % of the Medicaid beneficiaries were enrolled in managed care plans (Kaiser Family Foundation, 2016). States have increasingly looked to managed care contracts to create savings, increase access to services, and improve quality instead of the traditional fee-for-service Medicaid program. However, the evidence supporting improvements in cost and quality using managed care contracting is mixed. There appears to be little evidence for cost savings from Medicaid managed care on a national level, but some states have been more successful than others. Studies suggest the level of savings depend on how generous Medicaid fee-for-service (FFS) reimbursements are relative to commercial insurance rates. States with higher Medicaid reimbursement rates are able to demonstrate greater savings through Medicaid managed care than states with lower rates. Savings are usually associated with Medicaid managed care contracting at lower rates than FFS Medicaid or from reductions in inpatient bed days through utilization review and prior authorization requirements. Improvements in access and quality are equally mixed depending on each state's level of provider participation in the Medicaid program (Robert Wood Johnson Foundation, 2012).

Medicaid managed care contracts often include comprehensive mental health and substance abuse treatment services. To reduce costs, managed care organizations may limit behavioral health networks that could leave out CHCs. They may also limit assignment of patients to CHCs in favor of less costly contracted providers.

State Medicaid Agencies can address this by including contract requirements for Medicaid managed care plans to include CHCs in their medical and behavioral health networks.

Wrap-Around Support Funding Issues

The Health Resources and Services Administration (HRSA) implemented its Patient-Centered Medical Home (PCMH) Initiative that supports safety-net providers across the country in gaining recognition under the National Committee for Quality Assurance (NCQA) PCMH Program. The PCMH model provides whole person care that is proactive, evidence-based, and coordinated, with attention to high-quality care. To fully achieve whole person care requires an integrated approach to the physical, behavioral, and psychosocial dimensions of the people they serve. The initiative provides grant funding to Federally Qualified Health Centers (FQHCs) to implement this practice model and achieve NCQA PCMH recognition. Recently, NCQA has included more rigorous standards for behavioral health integration in its updated 2014 PCMH Standards.

In 2014, with the growing understanding that integrated behavioral health must be a core principle of the PCMH, six family medicine professional societies put forth joint principles to integrate behavioral health care into the PCMH (SAMHSA-HRSA Center for Integrated Health Solutions, 2014). These principles emphasized inclusion and coordination of behavioral health services in achieving whole person care.

A 2013 paper on integrated care (SAMHSA-HRSA Center for Integrated Health Solutions, 2013) described a continuum of levels of integration going from minimal collaboration and communication to a truly team-based approach focused on holistic care. These highly integrated models are often implemented as a part of PCMHs which provide integrated behavioral health services. These integrated models are also called "health homes."

Besides providing primary medical and behavioral health care, health homes often include "wrap-around" support services provided by professional and paraprofessional team members. These services include: patient and family education; health promotion and chronic disease self-care education; care coordination; transition of care support; referral support services; and use of technology to facilitate these services. The goal is to assist patients and their families in accessing primary care, behavioral health services, and any necessary social services as well as long-term service supports.

There exists as many payment models as there are integrated health care approaches. Payment models also can be described as a continuum from the simple to the complex. Some of the simplest models utilize a Per Member Per Month (PMPM) payment to compensate for PCMH practice transformation costs. These payments are in addition to regular fee-for-service reimbursement or, in the case of CHCs, PPS encounter payments. Payments can vary depending on the complexity of the patient population from $2.50 PMPM for relatively healthy Medicaid beneficiaries to $5.00 PMPM for patients with complex needs (Agency for Healthcare Research and Quality, 2012).

Higher up on the payment complexity continuum are PMPM add-ons adjusted for the PCMH recognition level of the CHC. For example, the National Committee for Quality Assurance (NCQA) uses three levels of recognition for PCMHs. Level 1 is the lowest recognition tier and Level 3 the highest. Some payment models have increasing PMPM payments associated with the increased level of recognition; again to help compensate for the cost of practice transformation and the additional cost of ongoing patient-centered support services. In 2011, Maryland began a 3 year pilot study to test the PCMH model of care, which included 52 primary and multispecialty practices. The model paid PCMH practices between $4.08 and $7.00 depending on their PCMH level of recognition by the National Committee for Quality Assurance (NCQA) and the number of Medicaid patients enrolled in the practice. Results of the pilot study showed improvements in quality, patient satisfaction, and a reduction in costs, but mixed results related to improvements in provider satisfaction and reductions in health disparity (Maryland Health Care Commission, 2015).

A number of State Medicaid Agencies are implementing CHC specific payment models using APMs. A number of these initiatives involve PPS-equivalent capitation payments. In California, a number of CHCs are involved in a pilot within the Medi-Cal managed care program. Managed care plans will pay health centers a PMPM based on the equivalent of one-twelfth of the PPS revenue per enrollee. Payments are stratified based on the aid category of each Medi-Cal enrollee, with higher payments for seniors and persons with disabilities. Reconciliation to PPS payments, usually a requirement when using APMs, is only done at the request of the CHC, which reduces the administrative cost for Medi-Cal and the CHCs. The pilot methodology includes the ability of the CHC to request a change in service scope, as well as annual adjustments based on the Medicare Economic Index (MEI) (National Association of Community Health Centers, 2013).

Other states including Colorado, Maine, Washington, Minnesota, Oregon, Maryland, and Vermont are moving forward with APMs in order to help compensate for practice transformation costs as well as align incentives to improve the quality of care and reduce per capita costs. Oregon recently launched an APM demonstration where participating FQHCs no longer earn revenue based on the volume of patient encounters, but instead get paid a monthly PMPM payment based on the size and composition of their patient population. The goal is to shift the paradigm from paying for medical visits to paying for the provision of high-quality, team-based care that improves health and reduces cost (Hostetler, Sisulak, Cottrell, Arkind, & Likumahuwa, 2014).

Special Billing Issues

Group and Family Therapy Sessions

State Medicaid Agency rules often preclude billing for group sessions using the FQHC PPS payment methodology. While group and family therapy is often the most cost-effective treatment method, many state Medicaid programs either do not allow it or do not address it. If a group includes a number of Medicaid beneficiaries, the total cost of the session under PPS would exceed what a state may normally pay for group therapy. A 2010 survey indicated that 51 % of state Medicaid programs paid FQHCs for group mental health sessions and 53 % paid for group substance abuse sessions (National Association of Community Health Centers, 2014). The State of Nevada recently passed regulations allowing CHCs to bill for group sessions outside of the PPS system. Qualified behavioral health providers bill for group sessions as a non-CHC provider and the CHC is paid using standard Medicaid rates.

Screening, Brief Intervention, Referral to Treatment (SBIRT)

Despite its proven effectiveness, SBIRT is not routinely covered by State Medicaid programs. The 2010 survey by McKinney also reported that only 25 % of responding states paid FQHCs for SBIRT services. It is unclear why states have been unwilling or unable to cover these services.

Conclusion

State Medicaid Agencies have not yet universally embraced integrated care models in FQHCs. A 2014 NACHC report indicated that only 30 % of states have implemented APMs (National Association of Community Health Centers, 2014). Of those states using APMS, it is unclear how many are using this approach to support integrated care. However, there is evidence from early pilots to suggest the models improve quality and reduce costs. The availability of APMs also allow states to move forward with FQHC payment reform without having to implement cumbersome and costly waiver initiatives. States could learn from these early innovator states and design programs to take advantage of their experiences to expand integrated care in FQHCs.

References

Bailit, M. (2011). *Payment rate brief. Patient-centered primary care collaborative*. Washington, DC: Patient-Centered Primary Care Collaborative.

Buxbaum, J. (2012, August 29). *Helping FQHCs get off the treadmill*. Retrieved from https://www.statereforum.org/weekly-insight/helping-fqhcs-get-off-treadmill.

Harris, I., Marsteller, J., Kiptanui, Z., Pederson, S., Perlmutter, D., Franey, C., … Emery, D. (2015). *Evaluation of the Maryland multi-payor patient centered medical home program*. Columbia, MD: Maryland Health Care Commission.
Heath, B., Wise-Romero, P., & Reynolds, K. A. (2013). *A standard framework for levels of integrated healthcare*. Washington, DC: SAMHSA-HRSA Center for Integrated Health Solutions.
Hostetler, C., Sisulak, L., Cottrell, E., Arkind, J., & Likumahuwa (2014, April 14). *Origins in Oregon: The alternative payment methodology project*. Retrieved from http://healthaffairs.org/blog/2014/04/14/origins-in-oregon-the-alternative-payment-methodology-project/.
Kaiser Family Foundation. (2015). *Distribution of revenue by source for federally-funded federally qualified health centers*. Retrieved from http://kff.org/other/state-indicator/fqhc-revenue-by-source/.
Kaiser Family Foundation. (2016). *Total medicaid managed care enrollment*. Retrieved from http://kff.org/medicaid/state-indicator/total-medicaid-mc-enrollment/.
Kidney, R. (2013). *Health care payment reform: State initiatives to meet the triple aim*. Washington, DC: National Association of Community Health Centers.
Lardiere, M., Jones, E., & Perez, M. (2011). *NACHC 2010 assessment of behavioral health services in federally qualified health centers*. Washington, DC: National Association of Community Health Centers.
McKinney, D., Ertle, L., & Wong, W. (2014). *2014 update on the implementation of the FQHC prospective payment systems (PPS) in the states*. Washington, DC: National Association of Community Health Centers.
McKinney, D., Kidney, R., Xu, A., Lardiere, M. R., & Schwartz, R. (2010). *Health center reimbursement for behavioral health services in medicaid*. Washington, DC: National Association of Community Health Centers.
McKinney, D., Kidney, R., & Burns, K. (2011). *Update on the status of the Medicaid prospective payment system in the states*. Washington, DC: National Association of Community Health Centers.
National Association of Community Health Centers. (2013a). *Key health center data by state: Federally funded health centers only*. Washington, DC: NACHC.
National Association of Community Health Centers. (2013b). *FQHC prospective payment system: Essential to the health center model*. Washington, DC: NACHC.
NORC at the University of Chicago. (2011). *National Association of Community Health Centers assessment of FQHC's integrated behavioral health services*.
Rich, E., Lipson, D., Libersky, J., & Parchman, M. (2012). *Coordinating care for adults with complex care needs in the patient-centered medical home: Challenges and solutions*. Rockville, MD: Agency for Healthcare Research and Quality.
Richardson, K. (2004). *The bridge to 340B comprehensive pharmacy services solutions in underserved populations*. Washington, DC: HRSA.
Rosenbaum, S., Zakheim, M. H., Leifer, J., Golde, M. D., Schulte, J. M., & Margulies, R. (2011). *Assessing and addressing legal barriers to the clinical integration of community health centers and other community providers*. New York, NY: The Commonwealth Fund.
Sparer, M. (2012). *Medicaid managed care: Costs, access and quality of care*. Princeton, NJ: Robert Wood Johnson Foundation.
Steinberg, J. (2014). *Advancing behavioral health integration within NCQA recognized patient-centered medical homes*. Washington, DC: SAMHSA-HRSA Center for Integrated Health Solutions.
Texas Legislative Budget Board. (2014). *Federally qualified health centers prospective payment systems for medicaid services (ID: 1326)*. Austin, TX: Author.
Texas Medicaid. (2015, April 14). *Static fee schedules*. Retrieved from http://public.tmhp.com/FeeSchedules/StaticFeeSchedule/FeeSchedules.aspx.

Chapter 7
Using a Translator in Integrated Care Settings

Jose Ribas-Roca and Pracha Eamranond

Failure to address limited English proficiency (LEP) is one of the main reasons leading to health disparities among Latinos. Translators in the clinical setting facilitate communication between providers and patients with LEP. In this chapter we talk about the effect of choosing to utilize a translator or not and its relationship to the quality of communication, patient/physician satisfaction, and health-related outcomes.

We describe the different types of interpreters available and compare the advantages and disadvantages of each type, patient and physician preferences, and the quality of interpretation they provide. Our hope is to provide a framework from which the provider will be able to decide the form of interpretation most appropriate for each particular circumstance.

We also explore specific themes on using a translator for mental health encounters. We will provide some information relevant to everyday interpreter use and tips to make more effective use of interpreters in integrated care settings.

We then comment on different policies and systems approaches that have been tried in order to improve communication with Hispanic patients and improve interpreter utilization. Finally, we share some insights found in the literature from the translators themselves about improving communication with Latino LEP patients.

J. Ribas-Roca • P. Eamranond (✉)
Lawrence General Hospital, Lawrence, MA 01841, USA
e-mail: jose.ribasroca@lawrencegeneral.org

© Springer International Publishing Switzerland 2016

L.T. Benuto, W. O'Donohue (eds.), *Enhancing Behavioral Health in Latino Populations*, DOI 10.1007/978-3-319-42533-7_7

Problems Latinos Face Related to Limited English Proficiency

Disparities in health care services between Latinos and non-Hispanic whites in the United States are well documented. Several of those disparities could be improved by having better access to interpreter services.

Latinos with fair and poor English proficiency reported approximately 22 % fewer physician visits than non-Latinos whose native language was English. The magnitude of the association between limited English proficiency and number of physician visits was similar to that for having poor health, no health insurance, or no regular source of care (Derose & Baker, 2000). Not being able to speak English proficiently also results in more difficulty obtaining appointments: 25 % of the Spanish-speaking patients reported regularly having problems getting an appointment in a primary care setting compared to 17 % among English-speakers (Welty et al., 2012). Disparities are even higher in the Emergency department, where 22 % of Spanish-speaking patients reported an interpreter was not used but should have been used (Baker et al., 1996).

Another problem leading to miscommunication is that patients and providers often misjudge their level of English proficiency. This could mislead them into believing an interpreter is not needed during an encounter. One study by Zun et al. administered standardized tests to clinic patients who stated they spoke English. 66 % of the self-proclaimed English speakers scored at or above a seventh grade reading level. Additionally, they found physicians and nurses overestimated their assessments of the patients' English competency (Zun, Sadoun, & Downey, 2006). Physicians may also overestimate their own ability to speak in Spanish, and assume they are communicating at an acceptable level (Lion et al., 2012), and the patient may choose to politely nod rather than express their difficulty following what the physician is trying to say (Haffner, 1992).

Two different studies involving pediatric and psychiatric residents found that there are conflicting perceptions around the usefulness of an interpreter. Patients often found the interpreter as helpful and expressed preference towards using them again in future visits, whereas the clinicians did not appreciate a significant impact in the interview (Cunningham et al., 2008; Kline et al., 1980).

Poor health literacy is also a major barrier to healthcare among Latinos. Leyva et al. evaluated how Latino parents with LEP understand written instructions accompanying a routinely prescribed medication for their young children. In their study of 100 participants, 22 % correctly demonstrated understanding of the dosing and frequency of the medication. Of subjects comfortable speaking English, 50 % correctly demonstrated the amount of medicine to give. Higher education and comfort speaking English were associated with better medication dosing (Leyva, Sharif, & Ozuah, 2005).

Communication during the clinical encounter is remarkably impaired for Latinos with LEP. Compared to English-speaking patients, Spanish-speaking patients made less attempts to describe their symptoms, feelings, expectations, and thoughts. Spanish-speaking patients also were less likely to receive responses from their physicians that facilitate further discussion and were more likely to have their comments ignored (Rivadeneyra et al., 2000). It is not surprising then, that Latinos were less likely to report having their medical problems resolved at the end of a medical visit (Welty et al., 2012). Additionally, LEP Latinos reported significantly more dissatisfaction about feeling listened by the medical staff, receiving reassurance and support from their doctors, having their questions answered and receiving explanations about prescribed medications, medical procedures and test results (Morales et al., 1999). Clinicians reported difficulties eliciting exact symptoms, explaining treatments, and eliciting treatment preferences. Clinicians perceived that lack of knowledge of a patient's culture hindered their ability to provide quality medical care yet only 18 % felt they were unable to establish trust or rapport (Karliner, Perez-Stable, & Gildengorin, 2004).

Greater Spanish language fluency by physicians was strongly associated with optimal elicitation and responsiveness to patients' problems and concerns. Higher cultural competence also improved explanation of the patient's condition and patient empowerment (Fernandez et al., 2004). Patients randomized to language-concordant encounters reported higher comprehension and satisfaction than patients using usual and customary modes of interpretation (Gany et al., 2007a). When patients are assigned language-concordant physicians, they were more likely to be counseled on diet and physical activity compared to patients with language-discordant physicians (Eamranond et al., 2009). In summary, the majority of the literature indicates that the ability to speak Spanish with a LEP Latino patient, whether directly by the provider or through an interpreter, improves the quality of care.

Types of Interpreters

The art of interpreting involves many particular challenges above verbatim "word for word" translation. Interpretation requires an absolute command of two languages, in-depth knowledge of cultural context, and the ability to manipulate registers ranging from formal to casual, including slang. It also requires appropriate disposition to facilitate evoking from the LEP patient without feeling rushed or creating a burden. Interpreters are obligated to apply their best skills and judgment to preserve the meaning of what is said, including the style and register of the speech. That may include statements that appear nonsensical, obscene, rambling, or incoherent (Gonzalez, Vasquez, & Mikkelson, 1991; Hewitt & Lee, 1996).

The interpreter's presence makes the typical dyadic interaction of the clinical setting into a triad, adding considerable complexity to the social situation and generating operational and technical challenges. Aranguri et al. found that speech was significantly reduced and revised by the interpreter, and visits that included an interpreter had virtually no rapport-building "small talk" (Aranguri, Davidson, & Ramirez, 2006).

Every consultation with LEP patients requires clinical judgement as to the type of interpretation needed. The clinician needs to assess the complexity of the interpreted encounters, as well as potential advantages and disadvantages that come with each type of interpreter. The clinician should always keep in mind the goal of having an interpreter is to optimize effective communication between provider and patient (Gray, Hilder, & Donaldson, 2011).

Untrained (Ad-Hoc) Interpreters

Interpreter guidelines warn against the use of untrained interpreters, yet the lack of uptake of interpreter services likely means that they are still often used. Gray et al. found that 49 % of all interpreted consultations used untrained interpreters (mostly family), with more used in the same day clinic setting (Gray et al., 2011). If the patient chooses to communicate in English or use a family member as an interpreter, it would be a good idea to confirm their understanding of the language by using open-ended questions, and asking them to repeat in their own words information you have provided (Gray, Hilder, & Stubbe, 2012).

One of the most significant disadvantages of using untrained interpreters is the decrease in technical quality of interpretation. Laws et al. evaluated the number or errors or omissions during clinic encounters (Laws et al., 2004). 66 % of segments in which translation should have occurred had substantial errors. In 30 % of segments, the interpreter engaged in speech unrelated to interpretation. Quality of interpretation was inversely associated with the word count per segment and, independently, whether the interpreter engaged in speech acts which did not consist of interpretation.

Many clinics use their bilingual support staff for translation, as they may share Hispanic ethnicity. They present the same technical limitations as untrained interpreters, but may still provide a cultural bridge between the patient and the clinician. They may be better situated to serve as interpersonal mediators, system mediators, educators, and advocates. They have also received training in patient confidentiality and may provide some degree of continuity for patients who are frequently seen at the clinic (Gray et al., 2012). However many studies confirm that the quality of trained interpretation, whether in-person or video conferencing, is higher than ad hoc interpretation (Napoles et al., 2010).

The evaluation of LEP psychiatric patients through an untrained interpreter can be inaccurate and misleading. The most common errors that untrained interpreters make include omission, addition, condensation, and substitution. Misinterpretation in mental health assessments can have significant consequences such as minimization of a patient's suicide attempt or exaggeration of a patient's passive suicidality (Vasquez & Javier, 1991).

Factors to keep in mind when assessing the appropriateness of an untrained interpreter include: complexity of the clinical presentation, the wishes of the patient, especially around trust and confidentiality, patient's need for advocacy or ongoing support and continuity of care, familiarity of the clinician with the patient and ad hoc interpreter, patient's health literacy, and clinician's familiarity with the ethnic group. A family member/friend can be considered acceptable when the untrained interpreter has enough English proficiency to effectively interpret, is over 18 years of age, is known to the clinician to be reliable and in good relationship with the patient, and when the consultation is a fairly straightforward, nonsensitive one (Gray et al., 2012).

Family Members

Several elements that interfere with effective communication in the primary care setting include lack of trust, intense pressure with regard to time constraints, mismatch of agendas (biomedical versus lifeworld) and firm expectations of a specific outcome (e.g. referral, prescription) (Greenhalgh, Robb, & Scambler, 2006). Having a family member provide interpretation provides advantages such as general trust from the patient, sharing of the lifeworld agenda, and shift the power balance in the patient's favor (Greenhalgh et al., 2006). They may also facilitate continuity of care and bypass the resistance patients may have to an unknown interpreter (Gray et al., 2012).

At the same time, when using family members as translators, the clinician may need to work harder in eliciting patient's concerns and differentiating them from the concerns of the family member. In integrating care settings, having a family member translate may interfere with the accurate assessment of a patient's mental status and delay diagnosis and recognition of mild cognitive impairment and dementia, as relatives may attempt to cover their deficits, or answer questions for them. In particular, Latino women are often reluctant to reveal personal or private problems if their children interpret (Haffner, 1992).

Certain topics related to mental health also carry stigma for family members who are translating. Domestic violence will likely be missed if the family member serving as interpreter is the abuser, or may be normalized and ignored if it is congruent with the cultural norm. Men will likely have more difficulty expressing emotions such as fear and sadness in front of their wife or children, as children are commonly taught "men don't cry." Patients with high stigma around depression will be less likely to disclose that diagnosis to their family (Vega, Rodriguez, & Ang, 2010). The use of children is never appropriate, as they lack the emotional and maturity level to cope with difficult situations and sensitive content will likely not be offered or translated accurately (Gray et al., 2012).

Both patients and medical residents demonstrate the highest level of satisfaction for professional interpreters compared to ad-hoc and family interpreters. Patients were significantly more satisfied than providers with using family members and friends (85 % vs. 60 %) (Kuo & Fagan, 1999). Patients were also more concerned than providers about the ability of the interpreter to assist them after the physician visit (94 % vs. 45 %).

In-Person Trained Interpreters

In-person trained interpreters are regarded as the ideal method of translation, as they provide the highest degree of accuracy, confidentiality, and ethical behavior. However, even in locations where such interpreters are readily available, providers choose not to use them for every encounter (Schenker et al., 2007). Trained interpreters may not be used due to clinicians perceiving ad-hoc interpreters work well most of the time (Gray et al., 2011). Clinicians may also hold misperceptions of interpreters resulting in increased interview time (Fagan et al., 2003) or patients preferring family members to professional ones (Kuo & Fagan, 1999). Trained interpreters also result in additional cost, not currently reimbursed by insurance payors. However certified trained medical interpreters remain the gold standard to provide highest quality care.

Trained interpreters should always be used to obtain informed consent. Any consent gained without the use of a trained interpreter cannot be adequately informed and would not stand up in court if challenged (Gray et al., 2012). A trained interpreter would also be preferred when discussing sensitive issues, complex clinical presentations, or caring for vulnerable population, such as refugees and patients presenting with mental health problems.

Fagan et al. studied the impact of interpretation method on clinic visit length. They found that compared to those not requiring an interpreter, the duration of encounters for patients using certain forms of interpreter had longer mean provider times by 6.4 min and clinic times by over 10 min. This effect was present with both telephone interpreter and patient-supplied interpreters. In contrast, patients using a trained medical interpreter did not have significantly different mean provider times (26.8 min vs. 28.0 min) or mean clinic times (91.0 min vs. 82.4 min) than patients not requiring an interpreter. Even though the difference didn't reach statistical significance, the trained interpreter group had almost 10 min longer clinic time, which could be accounted for by the time it took for the interpreter to be called and arrive into the room (Fagan et al., 2003).

Telephone Interpreters

Using telephone interpreting services makes professional interpreters readily available. The preferred device is a dual-headset telephone, as it allows both parties to talk and hear the interpreter with the highest fidelity. Traditional phones may be used instead, but may provide limited help if the patient is hard of hearing, and it may be more difficult to assure confidentiality when the phone is set on speaker mode.

Cunningham et al. surveyed a cohort of almost 100 women after encounters with pediatric residents, where half were randomized to ad-hoc or no interpretation and the other half to a phone interpreter. The intervention cohort overwhelmingly rated telephonic interpretation as "very helpful" (94 %), indicating the visit would have been "harder" without the service (98 %). Significantly more intervention cohort mothers were "very satisfied" with the clinic overall (85 % vs. 57 %). Almost all intervention cohort mothers (96 %) reported a preference to use telephonic interpretation at their subsequent visit; however, only one-third of residents believed their patients would prefer to use the telephonic interpreter in the future. These findings are especially important, because most Latino patients will not be aware they have the right to an interpreter or that such service may be readily available in the form of phone interpretation. It should be the provider's duty to inform the patient about those services and encourage their use when LEP is suspected (Cunningham et al., 2008).

Locatis et al. found that the duration of interviews using phone interpreters was 7.4 min shorter than both video and in-person interpreting. Providers in the study liked telephone interpreter the least, considered it the most distracting method due to poor audio quality, lack of visual communication and restriction on the use of their hands (Locatis et al., 2010). These results differ from the earlier study by Fagan, who reported using telephone and ad hoc interpreters both increased the length of the interview by a mean of 6.4 min compared to those who did not need an interpreter (Fagan et al., 2003).

Video Conferencing Interpreters

Napoles et al. surveyed clinicians to compare quality of interpretation, visit satisfaction, degree of patient engagement, and cultural competence during visits using three different methods of interpretation. The quality of interpretation for in-person and video conferencing modes were rated similarly in all categories; both methods were superior to ad-hoc interpreting. Video conferencing only scored lower than in-person interpretation for cultural competence. The authors concluded that video conferencing increases access without compromising quality and that cultural nuances are better addressed by in-person interpreters (Napoles et al., 2010).

Locatis et al. did not find a significant difference in the duration of video interviews compared to in-person interpreting. Providers and interpreters in this study showed a distinct preference for video over phone interviews. Both rated in-person interpreting significantly higher in quality than video conferencing (Locatis et al., 2010).

Readily available handheld devices may be appropriate for remote interpreting. Wofford et al. studied the impact of audio and video technology included in handheld devices. Most patients rated overall quality of videoconferencing as good/excellent. Most patients favored using videoconferencing during future visits. The 18 clinicians that participated in the study reported similar results.

Remote Simultaneous Medical Interpreting

Remote-simultaneous medical interpretation (RSMI) is performed by interpreters trained in simultaneous interpretation. The interpreters are linked from a remote site by headsets worn by the clinician and patient. Compared to in-person consecutive interpretation, RSMI demonstrated an increase in the number of physician and patient utterances in the visit, improved quality of interpretation, and higher preferences by physician, interpreter, and patients (Hornberger et al., 1996).

A more recent study by Gany et al. found that patients randomized to RSMI were more likely than those with usual and customary methods of interpretation to think doctors treated them with respect. RSMI resulted in fewer medical errors and was faster than all other methods of interpreting. Patients randomized to RSMI were also more likely to think the interpreting method protected their privacy (Gany et al., 2007a, 2007b).

Remote simultaneous interpreting is often employed at the United Nations and at major international conferences. However in the medical setting, superior clinical outcomes of RSMI are still to be determined (Gany et al., 2011). RSMI is not readily available in clinical practice at this time, likely due to higher technical complexity, higher implementation costs including headset equipment, and lack of reimbursement for interpreting services.

Utilization of Interpreters in Clinical Practice

Trained interpreters are underutilized despite the advantages and quality improvement with professional interpretation. A survey of pediatric residents serving a population in which 10–20 % are Spanish-speaking with LEP revealed they rarely use professional interpreters. 75 % of nonproficient residents reported use of hospital interpreters "never" or only "sometimes." Instead, they tend to rely on their own inadequate language skills, seek interpretation from their proficient colleagues, or avoid communication with Spanish-speaking families with LEP. Proficient residents estimated that they spent a mean of 2.3 h/week interpreting for other residents (Burbano O'Leary, Federico, & Hampers, 2003). Schenker et al. found that despite the availability of on-site professional interpreter services, charts of hospitalized LEP patients were less likely to contain full documentation of informed consent for common invasive procedures (53 % vs. 28 %) when compared to English-speaking patients (Schenker et al., 2007).

Interpreter utilization varies depending on the physician's level of Spanish proficiency: those with low proficiency report frequent use of ad-hoc interpreters for all information-based scenarios. For difficult conversations and procedural consent, most used professional interpreters. Medium proficiency physicians reported higher rates of using their own Spanish skills for information-based scenarios, lower rates of professional interpreter use, and little use of ad-hoc interpreters. They still relied on trained interpreters for difficult conversations. Those with high-level Spanish proficiency almost uniformly reported using their own Spanish skills (Diamond, Tuot, & Karliner, 2012).

Guidelines have emerged in order to direct the decision of whether to obtain an interpreter and which type may be most appropriate, as using trained interpreters may not always be possible due to cost and logistics involved. The judgement of when to use trained versus untrained interpreters is a complex decision that needs careful consideration and evaluation of all the issues involved: clinical, ethical, practical, social, and financial (Gray et al., 2012).

Recommendations to improve communication with LEP start at the policy level for every practice. Practices should have an idea of the percentage of LEP patients they serve and therefore have policies that will allow them to effectively respond to those needs. Recommendations include assigning a budget for employment of interpreters, allocating longer encounter times for LEP patients, having a medical record capable of flagging which patients need to be seen with an interpreter, having patient information available in common languages of the practice, and providing staff with training on how to determine the need for an interpreter and how to work with one (Gray et al., 2012; Roat & CAFP, 2005).

When asking about language preference, clinicians should avoid leading questions, or nonverbal language hinting that using an interpreter would be burdensome to them or the practice. Rather than asking patients whether they need or want an interpreter, it is recommended to ask: "In what language would you prefer to receive your health care?" (Roat & CAFP, 2005).

Additional factors that will make a case for obtaining a trained interpreter include the complexity of the clinical presentation, the sensitivity of the content to be discussed (applies to all mental health encounters), the vulnerability of the patient (refugee or background that includes high likelihood of trauma), and urgency of the situation (which may limit available options) (Gray et al., 2012; Roat & CAFP, 2005).

Interpreter Use and Mental Health

Diagnostic Challenges During Evaluation in Patient's Non primary Language

The common errors that untrained interpreters make during primary care encounters may present severe unintended consequences in the integrated care setting. Misinterpretation has a marked impact on the quality of care, such minimization of a suicide attempt or conversely exaggeration of suicidality (Vasquez & Javier, 1991). Untrained interpreters in the patient-provider relationship can also lead suboptimal rapport building and prevents a strong therapeutic alliance required for management of behavioral health.

Interviewing patients in a language different than their native one may have greater impact on the quality of psychiatric care than in other specialties. Psychiatric evaluation hinges on observations from a detailed history and many key diagnostic symptoms that may only be obtained through the clinical interview, since laboratory and imaging data have limited added value. Additionally, patients are less likely to disclose psychological symptoms compared to physical symptoms (Bischoff et al., 2003).

A literature review by Bauer et al. elaborates on ways in which language barriers may interfere with the mental status examination. Disorders of speech and language such as aphasias, pressured speech, and neologisms may be missed. Abnormal thought processes including flight of ideas, disorganization and tangentiality, and abnormal thought contents such as delusions, grandiosity, obsessions, and magical thinking may not be identified (Bauer & Alegria, 2010).

Psychiatric assessments performed without interpreters tend to have more closed-ended questions and elicit brief responses, limiting the assessment of spontaneous thought content (Drennan & Swartz, 2002; Marcos et al., 1973a). Furthermore, when a patient with LEP tries to communicate in English, speech delays may be confused for thought blocking, word finding difficulty and delayed thought process (Marcos et al., 1973b). The quality of neuropsychological testing may also be affected for LEP patients. Interpreter use may significantly improve scores for verbally mediated tests such as Vocabulary and Similarities (Casas et al., 2012).

During psychiatric evaluations, ad hoc interpreters make more errors when translating psychotic content. When patients provided lengthy or convoluted replies, omissions are especially likely, as interpreters may have difficulty registering and remembering a patient's statement if they cannot discern its meaning (Price, 1975). Ad hoc interpreters are less likely than professional ones to report they cannot follow the patient's abnormal thought process (Drennan & Swartz, 2002). Trained interpreters may also bring to the provider's attention subtle signs of depression such as poor eye contact, decreased spontaneity, delayed responses and restricted affect.

Use of professional interpreters is associated with increased disclosure of traumatic events and psychological symptoms, as well as increase psychiatry referrals compared to ad-hoc interpreters (Eytan et al., 2002). Spanish-speaking patients seen with an interpreter for an initial therapy interview reported that they found they felt understood and helped, and subsequently wanted a return visit. In contrast, the therapists felt they provided less help to patients seen with interpreters and very few thought those patients wanted to return (Kline et al., 1980).

The Impact of Cultural Differences on Mental Health Encounters

Language barriers may also have important effects in mental health care and treatment outcomes beyond those of impaired communication and diagnostic accuracy. Language discordance may hinder the identification of important factors such as stigma, shame, patient's explanatory model of illness, patient's acceptance of the diagnosis and treatment, and fostering of a therapeutic alliance (Bauer & Alegria, 2010).

Patients reporting higher levels of perceived stigma are less likely to disclose their depression diagnosis to their family and friends and also less likely to be taking antidepressant medication. Patients with high stigma are less likely to attend scheduled appointments and follow through with referrals to mental health providers (Vega et al., 2010). Interpreters in integrated care settings may have the unique opportunity to serve as cultural ambassadors for mental health concerns. They may help providers understand more about the common preconceptions Latinos have around psychiatric diagnoses and psychotropic medications.

Villalobos found that use of interpreters in integrated behavioral health care patients did not have a significant impact on patient's rating of the therapeutic alliance. However, patients expressed a strong preference for bilingual providers, citing greater privacy, sense of trust, and accuracy of communication as the main advantages (Villalobos et al., 2015). Among older Latino clients receiving mental health services, the degree in which the health care organization matches the cultural needs of the patient had a predictive effect in treatment outcomes (i.e., reduction of symptomatology) independent of treatment (Costantino, Malgady, & Primavera, 2009).

Treatment preferences related to Latino culture should also be taken into consideration if treatment is to be successful. Compared to non-Hispanic white responders, Spanish-speaking Hispanic but not English-speaking Hispanic respondents had a lower preference for antidepressant medications. Older age and history of depression were found to predict for antidepressant-inclusive treatments. All responders who endorsed a biomedical explanation of depression demonstrated preference for antidepressant-inclusive options (Fernandez et al., 2011).

Alternative treatments should be discussed with every patient. Sleath et al. found that 36 % of patients reported talking with a minister or other religious person about feelings of depression or sadness. 17 % of patients had used herbal remedies or nonprescription medications, and 5 % had seen a curandero for feelings of depression or sadness. Overall, Hispanic ethnicity and language were not significantly related to patient use of alternative treatments for depression (Sleath & Williams, 2004).

Clinical Pearls for Interpreter Use

The decision about whether an interpreter is needed is often made by the patient or by his or her relatives. However, some patients can speak some English but are not fluent enough to for appropriate communication during an encounter, or may not be aware that an interpreter is available. It falls to the provider to suggest an interpreter be used and subsequently how to utilize the interpreter, particularly if discussing important test results or treatment options such as surgery or other treatments (Juckett & Unger, 2014).

Before meeting with the patient, review with the interpreter the purpose of the interview. Mention any potentially delicate or distressing issues that will be covered and ask the interpreter if there are any specific cultural factors that may have direct bearing on the interview. If using an untrained interpreter, the provider should emphasize the absolute need for confidentiality and the requirement to translate as precisely as possible what is said.

Seating should be arranged as a triangle, allowing patient and doctor to look at each other directly and for the interpreter to be perceived as neutral. Talk directly to the patient, addressing him/her in second person. Appear attentive when patient responds and respond to patient's nonverbal cues. Keep control of the consultation. Feel free to stop the patient if he/she is not allowing enough time for effective translation.

During physical examinations, it's preferable to have the interpreter present, but the patient should be asked for his or her preference. If the interpreter will not be present, extra care needs to be taken to explain beforehand to the patient what will happen during the examination.

For psychiatric interviews, the interpreter should be told that the encounter will be longer than average and more emotionally challenging. If psychosis is suspected, the interpreter should be told that the patient may say things that don't make immediate sense. Abnormal mental status findings may be more accurately evaluated by using simultaneous interpretation. This method will make it easier for the interpreter to keep up with rapid speech, tangentiality, disorganization, flight of ideas, and looseness of associations. It is strongly preferred to keep using the same interpreter for future encounters whenever possible, more so if trauma narratives have been discussed.

Consider discussing a strategy in case the patient needs to get in touch with you after the encounter. Patient may experience side effects of medications, worsening of symptoms, or the need to reschedule an appointment. Reassure the patient that an interpreter can be obtained for post-visit encounters, such as by phone or at an urgent care setting if available.

Closing the Cultural and Language Gap

Improving Provider's Spanish Level Proficiency

Offering options for physicians serving LEP Hispanic populations to improve their Spanish may have significant impact in patient care. Physician self-rated language ability and cultural competence are independently associated with Hispanic patients' reports of care. Greater language fluency was strongly associated with optimal elicitation and responsiveness to patients' problems and concerns. Higher cultural competence was associated not only with higher elicitation and responsiveness, but also to improved explanation of the patient's condition and patient empowerment (Fernandez et al., 2004).

The first step towards improvement is having a reliable measurement of non-English language proficiency. Using self-report measures can result in providers overestimating their proficiency. Standardized testing can also provide immediate benefits: after being tested on their Spanish skills, nonproficient residents reported a decrease in the comfort level using Spanish in straightforward clinical scenarios from 56 to 39% (Lion et al., 2012). Such awareness may be used to increase motivation for more frequent use of interpreters and may encourage the provider to pursue further improvement of his/her Spanish proficiency.

Proposals for improving medical care towards LEP patients with are becoming available at all levels. Escott et al. describe the development, organization, and evaluation of a workshop for medical students designed to develop their skills using trained bilingual simulated patients (Escott, Lucas, & Pearson, 2009). Surveys of fourth year medical students in a US university hospital found that 68 % had at least rudimentary Spanish skills. 85 % of them reported that they would probably or definitely participate in further individual language training, 70 % expressed at least possible willingness to have their Spanish formally evaluated, and 80 % predicted that it is at least possible that they will use their Spanish as attending physicians (Yawman et al., 2006).

Language immersion training is an option for some residency programs and faculty. After 2 weeks of language immersion, pediatric faculty demonstrated an increase from their baseline proficiency score of 28 % to a post-intervention score of 55 %, which was sustained at 6 and 12 months (Barkin et al., 2003). In one family medicine program, interns are offered a pre-residency 10-day immersion program at a nearby language institute, which includes thrice-monthly classroom instruction and personal instruction during continuity clinics by a teacher/translator for a year. All residents demonstrated significant improvement in Spanish language proficiency thru independent examiner testing (Valdini et al., 2009).

A 10-week medical Spanish course for pediatric ED physicians was associated with decreased interpreter use and increased satisfaction among Spanish-speaking-only families. The course was conducted for 2 h weekly. The class emphasized medical history taking and Hispanic cultural beliefs. Surveys found post-intervention families were significantly more likely to strongly agree that the physician was concerned about their child, made them feel comfortable, was respectful, and listened to what they said (Mazor et al., 2002).

Improving Use of Interpreters

In addition to improving cultural competency and provider's Spanish language skills, working effectively with interpreters may also require specific training. A survey of clinicians in outpatient settings found that previous training in interpreter use was associated with increased use of professional interpreters and increased satisfaction with medical care provided (Karliner et al., 2004).

In an acute psychiatry ward, a standard training package and a policy promoting interpreter use improved communication opportunities. The intervention included: (a) a survey of the multilingual skills of 80 clinical staff; (b) recording of patients' ethnic background and proficiency; (c) tracking of communications with patients in a language other than English and (d) staff training and active encouragement in interpreter use. Following the intervention, interpreter bookings and booking duration increased significantly (Stolk et al., 1998).

Interpreter Training, Standards, and Certification

Despite documented risks, the U.S. health care system lacks a required standardized certification for medical interpreters. In her recent commentary, VanderWielen makes a case for standardized certification for medical interpreters (VanderWielen et al., 2014). She illustrates lessons learned from the Federal Court system, where studies revealed interpreter's politeness could affect juror perception of witness testimony, and individuals had been found wrongfully convicted on the basis of inaccurate interpretation. As a result, the U.S. Congress passed the Federal Court Interpreters Act, which mandates that U.S. courts institute a system of qualified interpreters for judicial proceedings. Certified court interpreters must pass a written and oral examination.

For medical interpreters, the only national requirement is to demonstrate satisfactory abilities to interpret in a medical setting. Such a vague definition allows current use of family members and other ad hoc interpreters. In healthcare, two organizations have created certification processes for medical interpreters: the National Council on Interpreting in HealthCare (NCIHC) and the International Medical Interpreters Association (IMIA). These certifications include oral and written examinations to assess health care terminology, linguistic proficiency, interactions with health care professionals and cultural awareness and responsiveness (VanderWielen et al., 2014).

The NCIHC and IMIA provide the code of Ethics by which certified medical interpreters abide. Stipulations include protecting confidentiality, accurately rendering the message, taking into consideration its cultural context, striving to maintain impartiality, and refraining from projecting his/her own personal biases and beliefs. They also encourage advocacy when the patient's health, well-being, or dignity is at risk.

Insights from Interpreters

Medical interpreters offer additional insights into the complexities of translating for Latinos with LEP. Highly educated and affluent Latinos have attitudes and beliefs about healthcare reasonably comparable to those of similarly educated and wealthy Americans. Translating to Latinos who are poor, come from rural areas, have little or no schooling, and have little or marginal fluency in English pose additional challenges. Providers must recognize that the situation is bicultural and not merely bilingual (Haffner, 1992).

Latino family members often try to hide the seriousness of medical situations from ill relatives, especially if the patient may be dying. Family members feel providing encouragement is more beneficial and prefer that the doctor also convey hope, even if it is unrealistic. The head of the family is expected to make the decisions regarding any family member. These desires and cultural practices are directly opposed to the Western notion of informed consent. Latinos feel they should agree with physicians out of politeness and respect, even when they really disagree or do not understand the issues involved (Haffner, 1992).

Hudelson identifies two additional domains where physicians and patients were likely to differ (Hudelson, 2005):

Ideas About the Patient's Health Problem

Patients may have their own ideas about what caused certain medical problems, especially for psychological diagnoses. They may experience getting a mental health diagnosis as a sign of defection and disbelief on the part of the physician. They may attribute their problems to spirits or evil eye, but feel ashamed to reveal these beliefs and their recourse of traditional healing practices to doctors, for they me be perceived as ignorant. They may feel their illness was God's will, and only God could decide to heal them. They may hide beliefs and treatment noncompliance from doctors for fear of ridicule.

Expectations of the Clinical Encounter

Appointment scheduling systems may not exist in many home countries of LEP Latinos. They are seen using a walk-in system and would normally seek the doctor only when feeling sick, rather than at previously scheduled time. This difference translates in patients often arriving for appointments too early, too late, or not at all, which often causes frustration to physicians. Patients may expect an authoritative, high-tech medical encounter, usually ending with blood or imaging studies, and not something that could be obtained over the counter. They are not familiar with the bio-psycho-social model and may be weary of answering questions about their personal life, migration, or traumatic experiences.

Interpreters are usually reluctant to offer insight or suggestions to the provider without first being asked. It is the physician's role to initiate such discussions and clarify if strict translation is expected, and the amount of cultural brokering that would be welcome (Norris et al., 2005). Clinicians may be unaware of the emotional toll that interpretation of bad news can take on the interpreter. Some interpreters feel that to use them as only a conduit, and not think of them as a member of the health care team, does them a disservice. Debriefing after a difficult or trauma-related conversation may be helpful for the interpreter (Norris et al., 2005).

Although patient and provider differences in social and cultural background and education create the potential for misunderstanding, it is the lack of awareness of these differences that is at root of the problems (Hudelson, 2005). When important communication problems occur, they are more commonly due to problems understanding the social construct of illness from the perspective of the patient, than a result of poor translation in the linguistic sense (O'Neil, Koolage, & Kaufert, 1988).

Summary

Medical interpreters facilitate communication between providers and Hispanic patients with Limited English Proficiency (LEP) who face multiple health disparities in the U.S. The art of interpreting involves many particular challenges beyond word for word translation. The clinician needs to assess the complexity of every consultation with LEP patients and make a clinical judgement as to the type of interpretation needed. A trained interpreter should always be used to obtain informed consent and would also be preferred when discussing sensitive issues, complex clinical presentations or caring for population with mental health problems. Despite their advantages in accuracy and confidentiality, professional interpreters are underutilized in clinical practice. Patient's limited English proficiency and different cultural background pose unique diagnostic challenges during a mental health assessment and treatment. Interpreters may also function as cultural brokers to help bridge these differences. Several programs are becoming available to improve use of medical interpreters, and increase Spanish fluency of clinicians serving significant Latino population. For medical interpreters, the only national requirement is to demonstrate satisfactory abilities to interpret in a medical setting, which allows for untrained interpreters and family members to be used. The National Council on Interpreting in HealthCare (NCIHC) and the International Medical Interpreters Association (IMIA) provide certification for medical interpreters, which includes oral and written examinations. Interpreters also offer insights for clinicians to improve their communication with LEP Latinos.

References

Aranguri, C., Davidson, B., & Ramirez, R. (2006). Patterns of communication through interpreters: A detailed sociolinguistic analysis. *Journal of General Internal Medicine, 21*(6), 623–629.

Baker, D. W., Baker, D. W., Parker, R. M., Williams, M. V., Coates, W. C., & Pitkin, K. (1996). Use and effectiveness of interpreters in an emergency department. *JAMA, 275*(10), 783–788.

Barkin, S., Balkrishnan, R., Manuel, J., & Hall, M. A. (2003). Effect of language immersion on communication with Latino patients. *North Carolina Medical Journal, 64*(6), 258–262.

Bauer, A. M., & Alegria, M. (2010). Impact of patient language proficiency and interpreter service use on the quality of psychiatric care: A systematic review. *Psychiatric Services, 61*(8), 765–773.

Bischoff, A., Bovier, P. A., Rrustemi, I., Gariazzo, F., Eytan, A., & Loutan, L. (2003). Language barriers between nurses and asylum seekers: Their impact on symptom reporting and referral. *Social Science & Medicine, 57*(3), 503–512.

Burbano O'Leary, S. C., Federico, S., & Hampers, L. C. (2003). The truth about language barriers: One residency program's experience. *Pediatrics, 111*(5 Pt 1), e569–e573.

Casas, R., Guzmán-Vélez, E., Cardona-Rodriguez, J., Rodriguez, N., Quiñones, G., Izaguirre, B., et al. (2012). Interpreter-mediated neuropsychological testing of monolingual Spanish speakers. *The Clinical Neuropsychologist, 26*(1), 88–101.

Costantino, G., Malgady, R. G., & Primavera, L. H. (2009). Congruence between culturally competent treatment and cultural needs of older Latinos. *Journal of Consulting and Clinical Psychology, 77*(5), 941–949.

Cunningham, H., Cushman, L. F., Akuete-Penn, C., & Meyer, D. D. (2008). Satisfaction with telephonic interpreters in pediatric care. *Journal of the National Medical Association, 100*(4), 429–434.

Derose, K. P., & Baker, D. W. (2000). Limited English proficiency and Latinos' use of physician services. *Medical Care Research and Review, 57*(1), 76–91.

Diamond, L. C., Tuot, D. S., & Karliner, L. S. (2012). The use of Spanish language skills by physicians and nurses: Policy implications for teaching and testing. *Journal of General Internal Medicine, 27*(1), 117–123.

Drennan, G., & Swartz, L. (2002). The paradoxical use of interpreting in psychiatry. *Social Science & Medicine, 54*(12), 1853–1866.

Eamranond, P. P., Davis, R. B., Phillips, R. S., & Wee, C. C. (2009). Patient-physician language concordance and lifestyle counseling among Spanish-speaking patients. *Journal of Immigrant and Minority Health, 11*(6), 494–498.

Escott, S., Lucas, B., & Pearson, D. (2009). Lost in translation: Using bilingual simulated patients to improve consulting across language barriers. *Education for Primary Care, 20*(2), 93–98.

Eytan, A., Bischoff, A., Rrustemi, I., Durieux, S., Loutan, L., Gilbert, M., et al. (2002). Screening of mental disorders in asylum-seekers from Kosovo. *The Australian and New Zealand Journal of Psychiatry, 36*(4), 499–503.

Fagan, M. J., Diaz, J. A., Reinert, S. E., Sciamanna, C. N., & Fagan, D. M. (2003). Impact of interpretation method on clinic visit length. *Journal of General Internal Medicine, 18*(8), 634–638.

Fernandez, A., Schillinger, D., Grumbach, K., Rosenthal, A., Stewart, A. L., Wang, F., et al. (2004). Physician language ability and cultural competence. An exploratory study of communication with Spanish-speaking patients. *Journal of General Internal Medicine, 19*(2), 167–174.

Fernandez, Y., Garcia, E., Franks, P., Jerant, A., Bell, R. A., & Kravitz, R. L. (2011). Depression treatment preferences of Hispanic individuals: Exploring the influence of ethnicity, language, and explanatory models. *Journal of the American Board of Family Medicine, 24*(1), 39–50.

Gany, F., Leng, J., Shapiro, E., Abramson, D., Motola, I., Shield, D. C., et al. (2007a). Patient satisfaction with different interpreting methods: A randomized controlled trial. *Journal of General Internal Medicine, 22*(Suppl 2), 312–318.

Gany, F., Kapelusznik, L., Prakash, K., Gonzalez, J., Orta, L. Y., Tseng, C. H., et al. (2007b). The impact of medical interpretation method on time and errors. *Journal of General Internal Medicine, 22*(Suppl 2), 319–323.

Gany, F., Leng, J. C., Winston, G., Tseng, C. H., Qin, A., & Changrani, J. (2011). Diabetes care and language discordance among Chinese and Latino primary care patients. *Ethnicity & Disease, 21*(4), 473–479.

Gonzalez, R., Vasquez, V., & Mikkelson, H. (1991). *Prerequisites for court interpreting*. Durham, NC: Carolina Academic Press.

Gray, B., Hilder, J., & Donaldson, H. (2011). Why do we not use trained interpreters for all patients with limited English proficiency? Is there a place for using family members? *Australian Journal of Primary Health, 17*(3), 240–249.

Gray, B., Hilder, J., & Stubbe, M. (2012). How to use interpreters in general practice: The development of a New Zealand toolkit. *Journal of Primary Health Care, 4*(1), 52–61. A1-8.

Greenhalgh, T., Robb, N., & Scambler, G. (2006). Communicative and strategic action in interpreted consultations in primary health care: A Habermasian perspective. *Social Science & Medicine, 63*(5), 1170–1187.

Haffner, L. (1992). Translation is not enough. Interpreting in a medical setting. *The Western Journal of Medicine, 157*(3), 255–259.

Hewitt, W. E., & Lee, R. J. (1996). Behind the language barrier, or "You say you were eating an orange?". *State Court Journal, 20*(1), 23–31.

Hornberger, J. C., Gibson, C. D., Jr., Wood, W., Dequeldre, C., Corso, I., Palla, B., et al. (1996). Eliminating language barriers for non-English speaking patients. *Medical Care, 34*(8), 845–856.

Hudelson, P. (2005). Improving patient-provider communication: Insights from interpreters. *Family Practice, 22*(3), 311–316.

Juckett, G., & Unger, K. (2014). Appropriate use of medical interpreters. *American Family Physician, 90*(7), 476–480.

Karliner, L. S., Perez-Stable, E. J., & Gildengorin, G. (2004). The language divide. The importance of training in the use of interpreters for outpatient practice. *Journal of General Internal Medicine, 19*(2), 175–183.

Kline, F., Acosta, F. X., Austin, W., & Johnson, R. G., Jr. (1980). The misunderstood Spanish-speaking patient. *The American Journal of Psychiatry, 137*(12), 1530–1533.

Kuo, D., & Fagan, M. J. (1999). Satisfaction with methods of Spanish interpretation in an ambulatory care clinic. *Journal of General Internal Medicine, 14*(9), 547–550.

Laws, M. B., Heckscher, R., Mayo, S. J., Li, W., & Wilson, I. B. (2004). A new method for evaluating the quality of medical interpretation. *Medical Care, 42*(1), 71–80.

Leyva, M., Sharif, I., & Ozuah, P. O. (2005). Health literacy among Spanish-speaking Latino parents with limited English proficiency. *Ambulatory Pediatrics, 5*(1), 56–59.

Lion, K. C., Thompson, D. A., Cowden, J. D., Michel, E., Rafton, S. A., Hamdy, R. F., et al. (2012). Impact of language proficiency testing on provider use of Spanish for clinical care. *Pediatrics, 130*(1), e80–e87.

Locatis, C., Williamson, D., Gould-Kabler, C., Zone-Smith, L., Detzler, I., Roberson, J., et al. (2010). Comparing in-person, video, and telephonic medical interpretation. *Journal of General Internal Medicine, 25*(4), 345–350.

Marcos, L. R., Uruyo, L., Kesselman, M., & Alpert, M. (1973a). The language barrier in evaluating Spanish-American patients. *Archives of General Psychiatry, 29*(5), 655–659.

Marcos, L. R., Alpert, M., Urcuyo, L., & Kesselman, M. (1973b). The effect of interview language on the evaluation of psychopathology in Spanish-American schizophrenic patients. *The American Journal of Psychiatry, 130*(5), 549–553.

Mazor, S. S., Hampers, L. C., Chande, V. T., & Krug, S. E. (2002). Teaching Spanish to pediatric emergency physicians: Effects on patient satisfaction. *Archives of Pediatrics & Adolescent Medicine, 156*(7), 693–695.

Morales, L. S., Cunningham, W. E., Brown, J. A., Liu, H., & Hays, R. D. (1999). Are Latinos less satisfied with communication by health care providers? *Journal of General Internal Medicine, 14*(7), 409–417.

Napoles, A. M., Santoyo-Olsson, J., Karliner, L. S., O'Brien, H., Gregorich, S. E., & Pérez-Stable, E. J. (2010). Clinician ratings of interpreter mediated visits in underserved primary care settings with ad hoc, in-person professional, and video conferencing modes. *Journal of Health Care for the Poor and Underserved, 21*(1), 301–317.

Norris, W. M., Wenrich, M. D., Nielsen, E. L., Treece, P. D., Jackson, J. C., & Curtis, J. R. (2005). Communication about end-of-life care between language-discordant patients and clinicians: Insights from medical interpreters. *Journal of Palliative Medicine, 8*(5), 1016–1024.

O'Neil, J. D., Koolage, W. W., & Kaufert, J. M. (1988). Health communication problems in Canadian Inuit communities. *Arctic Medical Research, 47*(Suppl 1), 374–378.

Price, J. (1975). Foreign language interpreting in psychiatric practice. *The Australian and New Zealand Journal of Psychiatry, 9*(4), 263–267.

Rivadeneyra, R., Elderkin-Thompson, V., Silver, R. C., & Waitzkin, H. (2000). Patient centeredness in medical encounters requiring an interpreter. *The American Journal of Medicine, 108*(6), 470–474.

Roat, C., & CAFP. (2005). *Addressing language access issues in your practice: A toolkit for physicians and their staff members*

Schenker, Y., Wang, F., Selig, S. J., Ng, R., & Fernandez, A. (2007). The impact of language barriers on documentation of informed consent at a hospital with on-site interpreter services. *Journal of General Internal Medicine, 22*(Suppl 2), 294–299.

Sleath, B. L., & Williams, J. W., Jr. (2004). Hispanic ethnicity, language, and depression: Physician-patient communication and patient use of alternative treatments. *International Journal of Psychiatry in Medicine, 34*(3), 235–246.

Stolk, Y., Ziguras, S., Saunders, T., Garlick, R., Stuart, G., & Coffey, G. (1998). Lowering the language barrier in an acute psychiatric setting. *The Australian and New Zealand Journal of Psychiatry, 32*(3), 434–440.

Valdini, A., Early, S., Augart, C., Cleghorn, G. D., & Miles, H. C. (2009). Spanish language immersion and reinforcement during residency: A model for rapid acquisition of competency. *Teaching and Learning in Medicine, 21*(3), 261–266.

VanderWielen, L. M., Enurah, A. S., Rho, H. Y., Nagarkatti-Gude, D. R., Michelsen-King, P., Crossman, S. H., et al. (2014). Medical interpreters: Improvements to address access, equity, and quality of care for limited-eEnglish-proficient patients. *Academic Medicine, 89*(10), 1324–1327.

Vasquez, C., & Javier, R. A. (1991). The problem with interpreters: Communicating with Spanish-speaking patients. *Hospital & Community Psychiatry, 42*(2), 163–165.

Vega, W. A., Rodriguez, M. A., & Ang, A. (2010). Addressing stigma of depression in Latino primary care patients. *General Hospital Psychiatry, 32*(2), 182–191.

Villalobos, B., Bridges, A. J., Anastasia, E. A., Ojeda, C. A., Rodriguez, J. H., Gomez D. (2015). *Effects of language concordance and interpreter use on therapeutic alliance in Spanish-speaking integrated behavioral health care patients*, University of Arkansas.

Welty, E., Yeager, V. A., Ouimet, C., & Menachemi, N. (2012). Patient satisfaction among Spanish-speaking patients in a public health setting. *Journal for Healthcare Quality, 34*(5), 31–38.

Yawman, D., McIntosh, S., Fernandez, D., Auinger, P., Allan, M., & Weitzman, M. (2006). The use of Spanish by medical students and residents at one university hospital. *Academic Medicine, 81*(5), 468–473.

Zun, L. S., Sadoun, T., & Downey, L. (2006). English-language competency of self-declared English-speaking Hispanic patients using written tests of health literacy. *Journal of the National Medical Association, 98*(6), 912–917.

Chapter 8
Enhancing and Improving Treatment Engagement with Hispanic Patients

Ana J. Bridges and Elizabeth A. Anastasia

In the United States, Hispanics both use health and mental health care services at lower rates and receive lower quality care than do non-Hispanic Whites (Alegría et al., 2008; U.S. Department of Health and Human Services, 2001; Young, Klap, Sherbourne, & Wells, 2001). For example, among people with a depressive disorder, 63.7 % of Hispanics did not access mental health care (defined as having at least one visit to a mental health or general medical provider in the past year), compared to 40.2 % of non-Hispanic Whites (Alegría et al., 2008). Also, of those who did access care, 22.3 % of Hispanics received adequate treatment (defined as comprising at least four visits to a specialty or general health care provider in the past year and use of antidepressant medications for 30 days), compared to 33.0 % of non-Hispanic Whites (Alegría et al., 2008). In addition, when care is sought clinical outcomes are often worse in Hispanic patients, in large part because they are more likely to drop out of treatment prematurely compared to non-Hispanic Whites (Olfson et al., 2009). However, studies have generally suggested that successful engagement in treatment leads to comparable outcomes for Hispanics and other ethnic or racial groups (Miranda et al., 2005; Sue, 1988; Tonigan, 2003; Voss Horrell, 2008). This suggests that an important way to reduce the current health disparities experienced by Hispanics is to increase their engagement in health-related treatment services.

Integrating behavioral health services into primary clinics shows promise for increasing treatment engagement and reducing health disparities experienced by Hispanics (Bridges et al., 2014; Sanchez, Chapa, Ybarra, & Martinez, 2012). Hispanics and non-Hispanics alike seek behavioral health services more frequently from primary care providers than any other professionals, including specialty mental health providers (Bridges, Andrews, & Deen, 2012; Vega, Kolody,

A.J. Bridges, Ph.D. (✉) • E.A. Anastasia, M.A.
Department of Psychological Science, University of Arkansas,
Fayetteville, AR 72701, USA
e-mail: ana.bridges@gmail.com

© Springer International Publishing Switzerland 2016

L.T. Benuto, W. O'Donohue (eds.), *Enhancing Behavioral Health in Latino Populations*, DOI 10.1007/978-3-319-42533-7_8

Aguilar-Gaxiola, & Catalano, 1999; Wang et al., 2005). Bridges and colleagues (2014) found Hispanic patients accessed integrated behavioral health services at comparable rates to their representation in the general clinic population, engaged in follow-up behavioral health sessions at comparable rates, and experienced clinically significant improvements in their overall well-being comparable to their non-Hispanic White counterparts.

At their core, integrated care models involve the embedded of behavioral health specialists into the primary health care team (Blount, 1998; Robinson & Reiter, 2007; Strosahl, 1998). These specialists collaborate with medical providers to deliver whole person care. The structure of behavioral health sessions in integrated care differs from more traditional care. Sessions tend to be shorter in duration (e.g., 20–30 min) and quantity (typically 2–4 sessions to address the acute behavioral health need). Integrated behavioral health services are typically used episodically for acute problems and the emphasis is on enhancing patient functioning rather than symptom amelioration (Robinson & Reiter, 2007). Typically, behavioral health specialists accept same-day referrals and frequently conduct sessions in the same medical examination room utilized by the other health care providers. Medical providers will typically introduce the behavioral health specialist using a "warm-handoff" that includes a brief description of the patient's presenting concern(s) and the role of the behavioral health specialist on the medical team. Behavioral health specialists typical use brief screening tools rather than conduct comprehensive assessments, and adapt components of evidence-based interventions to be suitable for the pace and structure of primary care (Bridges et al., 2014; Bryan et al., 2012; Corso et al., 2012; Hunter, Goodie, Oordt, & Dobmeyer, 2009; Ray-Sannerud et al., 2012).

Any integrated care clinic that wishes to serve their Hispanic patients in a culturally competent manner potentially faces numerous challenges. In this chapter, we begin by delineating the set of challenges facing integrated care providers. We follow this with recommendations for how primary care clinics can better respond to the specific cultural needs of their Hispanic patients so as to enhance treatment engagement. In so doing, we first consider policies and procedures that may be employed at the administration level, thereby articulating system-level factors that could enhance or impede treatment engagement. We then turn to the specific activities of members of the primary care team, from medical providers and assistants who may be involved in screening patients for behavioral health concerns to the specific assessments and interventions behavioral health specialists may deliver in primary care. We also describe the importance of community partnerships and outside referrals. Throughout, we weave in cultural considerations and address how language and cultural values may shift the specific practices of providers. We turn finally to a brief discussion of the focus of integrated care services—that of improving the overall health of a population—and what this focus means for reducing health disparities in Hispanic patients.

In making all suggestions, the authors use their experience with designing, supervising in, and consulting for an integrated behavioral health care program at Community Clinic, a Federally Qualified Health Center (FQHC) located in Northwest Arkansas. Community Clinic has four free-standing primary care clinics, seven school-based health clinics, and two free-standing dental clinics. In 2013, the clinic served nearly 30,000 patients. Approximately half of the clinic's patients are ethnic and linguistic minorities and over 90 % are at 200 % or below the federal poverty level (ACHI, 2015; see also http://www.communityclinicnwa.org/about). Accordingly, half of the clinic's staff is bilingual and bicultural. The free-standing primary care clinics are staffed with myriad health service professionals, including medical doctors, doctors of osteopathy, advanced practice nurses, nurse practitioners, registered nurses, licensed practical nurses, physician's assistants, nutritionists, patient advocates, case managers, and medical assistants. Medical assistants typically serve as trained interpreters for both medical and behavioral health visits. Community Clinic welcomed licensed clinical social workers and licensed clinical psychologists as part of their health care team when they expanded to integrated medical and behavioral health services in 2009.

Challenges to Engagement in Health Services Treatment

Research showing that Hispanics are less likely to seek services for mental health problems and more likely to terminate therapy prematurely than members of other ethnic groups highlights existing challenges to the engagement of Hispanic patients in traditional mental health care (e.g., Alegría et al., 2008; Olfson et al., 2009). For example, in a study conducted by Alegría and colleagues (2008), 63.7 % of Latinos who met diagnostic criteria for a depressive disorder in the past year did not seek any mental health treatment, as compared to non-Latino white participants with a depressive disorder in the past year, of whom only 40.2 % failed to seek treatment. Using data from the National Comorbidity Study Replication, Olfson et al. (2009) found that Latinos were three times more likely to prematurely terminate therapy than non-Latinos. Both internal and external factors limit engagement. Internal factors include attitudes and beliefs patients may have about behavioral health services and help-seeking. They may also include problem recognition and health literacy. Many of these internal barriers are influenced by culture. External factors include limited availability of Spanish speaking providers or lack of culturally congruent care centers, cost and insurance barriers, and the structure of health services in the United States. These challenges are reviewed more fully below. For the purposes of this chapter, we refer to research regarding the Hispanic population overall, as there is limited relevant research comparing these factors among Hispanic subgroups.

Internal challenges. Limited mental health literacy may serve as an obstacle for treatment seeking by Hispanics and can contribute to premature termination of services. For example, Cabassa, Lester, and Zayas (2007) found that only 55 % of participants in a Latino-only sample (80 % Mexican, 14 % Central American, 5 % Caribbean) used the words "depression" or "depressed" to describe a standardized vignette of an individual who meets diagnostic criteria for major depressive disorder. Similarly, López et al. (2009) found that only 2 % of participants in a Latino-only sample were able to identify psychotic symptoms in a case vignette involving delusions and auditory hallucinations. Some empirical evidence suggests that Hispanic individuals who are experiencing psychological distress are more likely to conceptualize their symptoms as somatic and present to primary care for their problems than Whites (e.g., López, 2002; Varela et al., 2004). In a meta-analysis, Benish, Quintana, and Wampold (2011) found that the incorporation of illness myth into culturally adapted treatments resulted in better outcomes compared to unadapted bona fide therapy. Bona fide therapy was defined as involving a therapeutic relationship tailored to fit the individual client with at least two of the following: use of an established therapeutic approach, inclusion of psychological processes, use of a manual or training guide, and identification of the active components of therapy. Studies were included as culturally adapted if the purpose of the adaptation was to provide a more effective treatment to racial/ethnic minority clients; examples of adaptations include language and/or ethnic matching, inclusion of cultural values, consultation with members or experts of a cultural group, cultural sensitivity training for therapists, and adaptation of illness myth. Because a framework that fits cultural beliefs about illness is often absent in traditional mental health care, some Hispanic patients may seek help for psychological difficulties through folk healers whose methods fit more closely with their beliefs about illness (e.g., Bridges et al., 2012).

Certain Hispanic cultural values may discourage the engagement of Hispanics in traditional mental health services (e.g., Kouyoumdjian, Zamboanga, & Hansen, 2003). *Machismo*, a value of traditional masculinity, may translate into the belief that help-seeking is weak, supported by findings that *machismo* and help seeking attitudes are inversely correlated (Andrés-Hyman, Ortiz, Añez, Paris, & Davidson, 2006; Davis & Liang, 2015). As in some other cultures, *marianismo* depicts women as self-sacrificing in order to prioritize the needs of others; as such, Hispanic women may be too busy caring for others to attend to personal mental health needs, which could be perceived as selfish (Andrés-Hyman et al., 2006). *Familismo*, which places the family at the center of the individual's life and experience, encourages Hispanics to attempt to solve mental health problems within the family and not seek services from outsiders or share personal information about oneself or family members during therapy sessions (Antshel, 2002). Consistent with this possibility, Chang, Natsuaki, and Chen (2013) found that Hispanics with strong family bonds were less likely to seek mental health services and Villatoro, Morales, and Mays (2014) found that Hispanics with high endorsement of *familismo* were more likely to seek informal or religious assistance than traditional mental health services for mental health problems. Hispanic cultural values ascribe importance to friendly, personal relationships even in professional domains (*personalismo*); a businesslike style of interaction with mental or medical health professionals may be more unwelcoming or bothersome to Hispanic patients than to patients who expect formal interactions in these settings (Antshel, 2002). *Simpatía* refers to the importance of maintaining a pleasant demeanor and repressing anger or sadness in interactions with others (Antshel, 2002). If patients are reluctant to share unpleasant emotions in therapy, this could present challenges for establishing therapeutic alliance, conceptualizing the patient's difficulties, and determining an appropriate treatment strategy. The prospect of sharing these emotions may even deter some Hispanic patients from seeking mental health services at all. Many Hispanics ascribe to strong religious and spiritual values (*fatalismo*, *espiritualismo*) and may be more likely to seek assistance for psychological problems from religious leaders than mental health professionals (Andrés-Hyman et al., 2006). The interference of certain cultural beliefs in the engagement of Hispanic patients in traditional mental health services is likely lower as acculturation increases.

Stigma likely constitutes a significant deterrent from treatment seeking and engagement for Hispanics experiencing mental health problems as for others. Gary (2005) theorizes that mental illness is doubly stigmatizing for ethnic minorities, who may not want to add to the discrimination they already experience by seeking services for their problems. Interian, Martinez, Guarnaccia, Vega, and Escobar (2007) found stigma was a common concern for participants of a Latino-only sample who were prescribed antidepressant medication. Research with a Hispanic sample showed views of mental illness as stigmatizing discouraged participants from seeking services (Hirai, Vernon, Popan, & Clum, 2015).

Some (e.g., Kouyoumdjian et al., 2003) have speculated that low rates of mental health service use by Latinos are in part due to negative attitudes about the effectiveness of mental health care for their problems. In addition to negative attitudes about the effectiveness of psychological treatment in general, concerns about the cultural competence of such services can deter Latinos with mental health problems from seeking treatment. These beliefs are likely strengthened when the few Latinos who do seek mental health services receive inadequate and insufficiently culturally competent care. Recent studies suggest that overall, Hispanics do not have more negative attitudes about the helpfulness of mental health services than members of other ethnic groups (Gonzalez, Alegría, & Prihoda, 2005); Cabassa et al. (2007) found that 84 % of participants in a Hispanic sample believed that therapy improves depressive symptoms, with 75 % of the sample endorsing therapy as equally effective as medication for treating depression. However, one study did find that in a Hispanic-only sample of adults aged 60 and above, older age was associated with more negative attitudes about the effectiveness of therapy for addressing mental health problems, consistent with trends for members of other ethnic groups (Jang, Chiriboga, Herrera, Martinez Tyson, & Schonfeld, 2011; Kinoshita, Sorocco, & Gallagher-Thompson, 2008).

In a sample of Mexican American families, McCabe (2002) found that parents who believed they should be able to overcome their child's health problem on their own, who perceived more barriers to treatment, and who expected their child to recover quickly were more likely to terminate prematurely.

External challenges. Latinos also face external barriers that interfere with engagement in mental health services. The Hispanic population in the United States continues to grow (with 37.6 million Spanish speakers identified in 2011), yet Spanish-speaking mental health professionals remain limited (Ryan, 2013). In many studies, Hispanic participants have identified language as a significant barrier to the receipt of appropriate mental health care in traditional settings (e.g., Bridges et al., 2012; Kim et al., 2011; Rastogi, Massey-Hastings, & Wieling, 2012; Sentell, Shumway, & Snowden, 2007; Shattell, Hamilton, Starr, Jenkins, & Henderliter, 2008). Rastogi and colleagues (2012) found that Hispanic participants in their qualitative study cited low availability of interpreters as a barrier to receiving appropriate mental health services. Another study found that the availability of professional interpreter services increased medical service use by patients with limited English proficiency; however, the associated cost may pose another barrier, as interpreter services can be expensive (Jacobs et al., 2001).

Multiple studies have identified cost of traditional mental health services and lack of health insurance as significant obstacles to service utilization for Hispanics with mental health problems (e.g., Bridges et al., 2012; Kim et al., 2011). These difficulties are likely related to lower levels of full-time employment, lower salaries, and poorer benefit packages for Hispanics as compared to members of other ethnic groups (Bridges & Lindly, 2008; Kouyoumdjian et al., 2003). Wells, Lagomasino, Palinkas, Green, and Gonzalez (2013) found that many Latinos who were employed worked long hours, which they reported interfered with their ability to initiate and maintain therapy. Hispanics have also reported significant difficulties obtaining transportation to therapy appointments, which may be exacerbated in areas with few mental health providers nearby (Kouyoumdjian et al., 2003; Wells et al., 2013). In several research studies, Hispanics have reported that fear of deportation hampers their ability to receive mental health care (Bridges et al., 2012; Rastogi et al., 2012; Shattell et al., 2008; Wells et al., 2013).

Impersonal staff and culturally incongruent care constitute additional barriers to appropriate mental health services for Hispanics. When Uebelacker and colleagues (2012) asked Hispanic patients at a medical health center to report barriers to engagement with medical providers, they indicated short allotments of time in appointments, lack of timely access to appointments, disregard for mental health problems, and being treated in a "dehumanizing" manner by medical health professionals. These patients reported they would be more engaged if medical providers were to make eye contact, ask about family members, ask directly about problems, and form a social partnership with them in addressing their medical and mental health problems; although these preferences likely generalize to members of other ethnic groups, they may be particularly important for Hispanic patients in consideration of cultural values (e.g., *personalismo*).

Hispanics tend to show a pattern of having a crisis orientation by seeking services during a crisis and terminating them abruptly when the crisis passes (Antshel, 2002). It may be due to the numerous barriers faced by Hispanics that the benefits of seeking traditional therapy services may only outweigh the cost in the case of an emergency. Culturally adapted therapies have been found to reduce some of these barriers to treatment engagement for Hispanics and integrated behavioral health care shows promise for reducing many internal and external barriers as well (Benish et al., 2011; Bridges et al., 2014).

Recommendations to Increase Engagement in Health Services Treatment

Systemic considerations. Before ever stepping foot into a medical examination room, or even into the building, primary care clinics already communicate their cultural responsivity to the patients they serve. Advertisements, websites, promotional materials, and outreach efforts all provide a public face of the clinic to the community. The use of bilingual and bicultural clinic representatives for community outreach, for example, can help make clinic services more accessible to the Hispanic community, especially recent immigrants (Musser-Granski & Carrillo, 1997). Having website and promotional resources available in Spanish as well as English can also assist in increasing engagement (Glasgow et al., 2011; Matthews, Darbisi, Sandmann, Galen, & Rubin, 2009). Even considering carefully the location of the clinic is important. For example, locating satellite sites in or near Hispanic communities and ensuring clinics are near major public transportation routes can reduce disparities associated with transportation (Bridges & Lindly, 2008).

Once patients arrive at the clinic, signage and other visual indicators can promote engagement by conveying to the patient that the clinic is aware of and responsive to their cultural and linguistic needs. For example, Community Clinic has artwork that reflects the diverse patients served by the clinic (professional photographers took portraits of patients and, with patient consent, these enlarged black and white photographs pepper the halls of the clinic). They also display maps and other artwork reflective of the Hispanic and Marshallese communities served by the clinic. This is consistent with Bathje and Shelton (2012), whose checklist for cultural competence in traditional mental health care clinics emphasizes the display of artwork and other visual cues indicating cultural responsivity.

Clinics should provide materials and have staff members who can speak the preferred language of patients. Having front office staff and telephone receptionists who speak Spanish will reduce the linguistic barriers often associated with lack of treatment engagement in Hispanics, especially recent immigrants (Bridges et al., 2012). Clinic forms, patient consent forms, notices of privacy, prescription information, pamphlets and brochures, and other paper products should be easy to read and understand. This requires clinics to invest in good interpreter services to ensure that the language of all forms is conceptually equivalent (and appropriate for the specific subgroups of Hispanics the clinic serves).

Relatedly, clinics where Hispanics represent a sizeable portion of patients served should strongly consider hiring trained interpreters (Jacobs et al., 2001). Research has consistently documented the beneficial effects of trained interpreters on treatment engagement in Hispanics; often, the therapeutic alliance between behavioral health specialists and patients is just as strong when a trained interpreter is present as when the patient and provider are able to communicate directly, and treatment outcomes are comparable (Brune, Eiroá-Orosa, Fischer-Ortman, Delijaj, & Haasen, 2011; Schulz, Resick, Huber, & Griffin, 2006; Villalobos et al., 2016). Increasingly, technology is assisting with linguistic barriers patients often face. For instance, telehealth allows for consultation with interpreter services that are provided at a distance and translation applications on the computer or on smart devices are increasingly sophisticated and helpful.

Other clinic policies and procedures, aside from artwork and linguistic services, can promote treatment engagement in Hispanic patients. For instance, having extended hours for services allows patients who may experience difficulties attending appointments because of relatively inflexible work schedules additional opportunities to engage in treatment (Bridges & Lindly, 2008). Having options for child care, or providing concurrent child—and parent—appointments or behavioral health education groups, can increase willingness to engage in treatment (Snell-Johns, Mendez, & Smith, 2004).

At the level of individual interactions with clinic staff and providers, it is helpful to consider the following. First, as reviewed above, many Hispanics approach physical and behavioral health problems from a crisis orientation; that is, they tend to seek services during periods of crisis and may end treatment abruptly, as soon as the crisis subsides (Rosado & Elias, 1993). Integrated care is especially responsive to this cultural style of help-seeking during crisis; the lack of a significant waiting period between when a need is identified and when the patient can receive services may be seen as particularly helpful. The crisis orientation approach, however, means expectations providers have for how long patients should remain in treatment should be adjusted, with behavioral health specialists recognizing that a decision not to return for a planned follow-up does not mean the services were perceived as unhelpful, or that the patient was disengaged. Instead, the flexibility of the integrated care model and the benefit of having patients return to their primary care medical home frequently for myriad services can help behavioral health specialists "check in" on clients after a critical incident to ensure the situation was adequately resolved. This flexible approach to services may significantly increase treatment adherence in Hispanic patients, compared to more traditional mental health services that require weekly 1-h appointments for many months (Antshel, 2002; Snell-Johns et al., 2004).

Second, clinic staff and providers may want to engage in small talk and some degree of self-disclosure with their Hispanic patients. This behavior is consistent with the Hispanic value of *personalismo*, a communication style that encompasses warm and friendly exchanges and a relationship between people, rather than between a person and an institution (Añez, Silva, Paris, & Bedregal, 2008). When interactions are perceived as warm and friendly, Hispanic patients may see the clinic and its personnel more positively and this, in turn, can enhance treatment engagement.

Finally, directors of primary care clinics that seek to enhance the cultural competence of their services should make it their mission to train *all* clinic staff, from the executive team on down, in multiculturalism and cultural sensitivity (Bathje & Shelton, 2012). This training can also include information about the diverse clientele served by the clinic, important historical facts or events that may shape the experiences of clinic patients, and even how culture impacts health behaviors and expressions of behavioral health concerns.

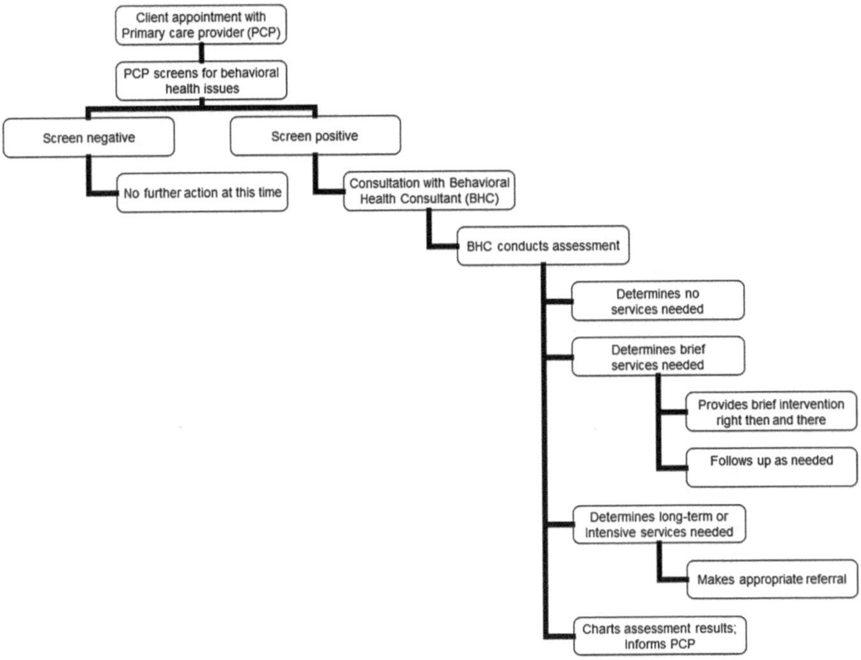

Fig. 8.1 Steps for integrated care patients' screening, treatment, and referral

We turn next to increasing treatment engagement at the various steps of integrated behavioral health care services. We have developed a brief flow chart to illustrate the various steps of patient screening, treatment, and referral that are commonly utilized in integrated care programs (Fig. 8.1). We organize our set of recommendations by these steps, beginning with screening, followed by warm hand-offs, intervention activities, and making outside referrals.

Screening. Aside from receiving referrals directly from primary care providers, behavioral health specialists working in integrated care settings may want to use behavioral health screening tools with all or a subset of patients. Screening instruments may also be used at initial sessions and follow up encounters to track patient progress on key behavioral health indicators. In general, screening instruments appropriate for primary care will be brief (typically no more than 5–20 questions), appropriate for a wide audience (e.g., adolescents, young adults, older adults), easy to read, and easy to score. Ideally, screening instruments will be normed with Hispanic patients and already translated into Spanish, so that they may be readily incorporated into practices with diverse patients.

Numerous Internet resources are available that provide integrated care clinics with free screening instruments. For example, the U.S. Substance Abuse and Mental Health Services Administration (SAMHSA) website has a list of screening tools appropriate for primary care (http://www.integration.samhsa.gov/clinical-practice/screening-tools#sample screening forms). The screening instruments cover a range of behavioral health topics, including depression, anxiety, trauma, drug and alcohol use, suicide, and general health/functional impairment. Most are freely available on the website and many contain scoring information, but many of the instruments are not available in Spanish. The Integrated Behavioral Health Project also lists many brief screening instruments available in English and Spanish that are appropriate for primary care (http://www.ibhp.org/uploads/file/IBHScreeningToolsRevFinal 100313.pdf). This large portable digital file also includes pictorial symptom checklists appropriate for use with pediatric and low-literacy populations.

One concern that may arise for behavioral health care providers working with Hispanic patients is that many Hispanic patients report somatic symptoms of distress, rather than mood or anxiety concerns (Escobar et al., 1987). As such, screening instruments that assess behavioral and health concerns broadly, and that include items assessing somatic concerns, may be more beneficial that more focused screening instruments. For example, the Kessler Psychological Distress Scale (K10; Kessler et al., 2002) is a ten-item screening instrument that assesses depression and anxiety, but includes items such as feeling "tired out for no good reason," "restless or fidgety," and "that everything was an effort." In addition, the Kessler 10 asks a few questions assessing the functional impairment patients experience because of their symptoms, including number of days in the past month the patient was unable to work or carry out normal daily activities and degree to which physical health problems caused the symptoms.

A second concern, one not well addressed by existing screening instruments, is that many Hispanic patients will see problems from a family or multisystemic perspective. Indeed, this more systemic approach to treatment is considered culturally responsive and even recommended by some scholars and clinicians (e.g., Añez, Paris, Bedregal, Davidson, & Grilo, 2005; Chowdhary et al., 2014). In our own practice, we often give screening instruments to patients and to a family member, such as a spouse, in order to gather multiple perspectives on the patient's functioning. While we cannot use these data in a normative fashion, the results are descriptive and can help inform treatment, particularly if the behavioral health specialist opts to include family members in the session.

A third concern in using screening instruments with Hispanic primary care patients is that the psychometric properties of these instruments are often unknown, particularly when one considers that country of origin, years living in the U.S., and literacy rates are all likely important factors that would affect screening norms. The literature is mixed with regard to the appropriateness of norms developed on primarily White nonminority patients for Hispanic patients. For example, Novy, Stanley, Averill, and Daza (2001) found comparability across many measures of anxiety disorders in English and Spanish with bilingual and literate adults. Similarly, Ruggero, Johnson, and Cuellar (2004) reviewed Spanish language measures of depression and mania and evaluated them with bilingual college students, finding psychometric equivalence across English and Spanish versions. However, both of these studies were conducted with people of high English and Spanish fluency and of high educational attainment. It is not certain that similar comparability would be obtained in low-literacy Spanish-speaking patients or in monolingual Spanish-speaking populations.

Dawes and colleagues (2010) found scores on the Beck Depression Inventory (BDI) had to be adjusted for formal education and gender in Spanish speakers near the U.S.-Mexico border. Specifically, women and respondents with lower formal education tended to endorse greater symptoms of depression than men or people with higher educational attainment. The authors recommend clinical cut-off scores of screening instruments be adjusted for these demographic variables, although they recognize their study was unable to determine whether differences in BDI scores were because of true differences in the base rates of depression, artifacts of measurement, or due to something else, such as level of acculturation or socioeconomic stress.

Other scholars have suggested cut-off scores of screening instruments may need to be modified for Hispanic populations, especially those with little formal education and limited literacy (in both English and Spanish). For instance, Reyes de Beaman and colleagues (2004) examined scores on a revised and translated Mini-Mental State Exam (MMSE) in a sample of 203 Mexican older adults (age 60 years or greater). In order to achieve good sensitivity and specificity associated with detection of true cognitive impairment, the authors had to adjust MMSE cut-off scores by level of formal education; otherwise, persons with low educational attainment were more likely to be incorrectly identified as having cognitive impairment.

Technology is likely to revolutionize the way behavioral health specialists conduct screenings in integrated care. In our own clinical work, we have begun using iPads and electronic medical records in order to help expedite screening and assessment in a culturally responsive manner. For example, given the relative low literacy rates among our patients, especially our Hispanic patients, we have created an application to be used with our iPads that allows us to input freely available behavioral health screening instruments. The application also permits us to record audio files of us reading the questions (and answer options) aloud. These audio files are automatically played for participants when they highlight questions and response options, allowing them to complete screenings in private. The application automatically scores the screener and provides the behavioral health specialist with the score and interpretation, so the information can be used in real time, during the behavioral health encounter. One need not hire computer programmers to take advantage of this technology: similar applications are now available and providers can create customized screenings for patients using commercial survey software such as Qualtrics offline (http://www.qualtrics.com/research-suite/mobile-surveys/).

Warm hand-offs. After a provider identifies a behavioral health concern in a patient or a patient screens positive on a behavioral health instrument, such as those described above, the next step is for the provider to introduce the behavioral health specialist in what has been called a warm hand-off (Strosahl, 1998). The hand-off allows the provider to introduce the behavioral health specialist as a member of the health care team and is thought to facilitate the development of rapport with patients. This facet of integrated services is particularly well suited for many Hispanic patients, as it naturally incorporates aspects of Hispanic culture that are important for treatment engagement. First, a warm hand-off by the primary care medical provider to the behavioral health specialist is highly personal—typically the medical provider explains to the patient why the behavioral health specialist is being included in the patient's care (therefore it corresponds with the value of *personalismo*). Second, the chance for the behavioral health specialist to talk briefly with the patient about the patient's presenting concerns also allows the behavioral health specialist to solicit information from the patient about *why* patients believe that they are experiencing these symptoms. This solicitation from the patient about their own illness myth (or explanation for the symptoms), and the incorporation of the patient's beliefs about the causes of their symptoms into the rationale for treatment, is a critical moderator of the effectiveness of cultural adaptations of psychotherapy on therapy outcomes (Benish et al., 2011). Third, following the solicitation from the patient about their explanation for their symptoms, behavioral health specialists are able to provide brief education to the patient about the rationale for integrated services and set expectations for the behavioral health session, including expectations for any potential follow-up visits. In so doing, the behavioral health specialist avoids using stigmatizing terms and opts instead for culturally responsive phrasing, such as describing behavior as "unhelpful" rather than "maladaptive." Such orientation to services and avoidance of stigma may be especially helpful at increasing treatment engagement and reducing premature drop-out in minority patients (Hays, 2009; Swift, Greenberg, Whipple, & Kominiak, 2012), who may not have the same cultural expectations about therapy as nonminority Whites (Kouyoumdjian et al., 2003).

Interventions. After conducting a warm hand-off and introducing behavioral health services to patients, behavioral health specialists are ready to begin their interventions. As reviewed above, often we meet with patients only one or two times for a particular presenting concern (Bridges et al., 2014; Corso et al., 2012), although we may meet with them multiple times over the years for different concerns, as the need arises. In each episode of care we provide, we approach interventions in a stepped care fashion (Bower & Gilbody, 2005; O'Donohue & Draper, 2011). Stepped care models begin by providing minimal treatment (or low treatment intensity) to patients. These "minimal treatments" must have some degree of efficacy, of course, so that it is likely many people will benefit. If a patient does not respond positively to this minimal treatment, then the patient receives more intensive treatment. For example, minimal treatment in integrated care may involve the provision of psychoeducation about panic disorder in someone who recently experienced a first panic attack. The hope is that with some education about the nature of panic, panic attacks, and why panic disorder develops in some people, the patient is able to use the information to avoid catastrophic evaluation of future fear responses and therefore will not develop full-blown panic disorder. Indeed, we have had such successes in our own clinical practice. However, for some patients this small dose of intervention is insufficient to ward off symptom development or ameliorate existing symptoms; for these patients, follow-up behavioral health sessions may include exposure to interoceptive panic cues and assignment of homework that involves approaching feared situations. If the patient's symptoms worsen or seem to require more than 4–6 sessions, typically we would make a referral to a traditional mental health care provider for continued treatment (see next section).

In general, research has shown that if Hispanics are able to initiate and remain in treatment, they receive comparable benefits as their non-Hispanic White counterparts. For instance, Bridges and colleagues (2014) demonstrate outcomes of integrated behavioral health care services are comparable between Hispanic and non-Hispanic White primary care patients (both pediatric and adult). Voss Horrell (2008) reviews the literature on the efficacy of traditional cognitive-behavioral therapy for ethnic minority patients; while the author notes the literature is quite sparse, the bulk of studies suggest it is effective for diverse patient groups.

On the other hand, there is increasing evidence that interventions are enhanced when cultural modifications are made (Benish et al., 2011). For example, Kanter, Santiago-Rivera, Rusch, Busch, and West (2010) show evidence that culturally adapted behavioral activation is effective for reducing depression in Latinos at a community mental health center. Adaptations included simplification of treatment rationale and case conceptualization, addition of structure, including the family and community into intervention, and patient-therapist linguistic and ethnic match. As mentioned above in the section on screenings, López et al. (2009) and Chowdhary et al. (2014) discuss the importance of including family members and other key people into treatment as a culturally-congruent way to intervene. Fortunately, in primary care settings we oftentimes have the option of easily including key family members into treatment. We have taken advantage of this and often include spouses, grandparents, nephews, or other important persons into the treatment of our patients. When doing so, however, additional concerns emerge and the behavioral health specialists must take care to explain carefully to patients and others the extent of and limits to confidentiality.

Hays (2009) has a list of several recommendations for doing brief, action-oriented interventions in a culturally sensitive manner, including things like framing certain beliefs as being "unhelpful" rather than "irrational," recognizing, assessing, and valuing the patients' experiences of discrimination and oppression, and clarifying what aspects of the problems are primarily external (environmental) or internal (part of the patient's belief system). All of these modifications can easily be incorporated into brief behavioral health interventions delivered to Hispanic primary care patients.

Outside referrals. One challenge we face in providing culturally responsive services to our Hispanic patients is coordinating care with outside providers and other community partners. Whether it is because the scope of services the patient requires is outside that which we can provide in our integrated care clinics, or because the patient prefers seeking more traditional therapy, we have a difficult time finding bilingual service providers who are able to accept our referrals. Many of the external barriers we articulated above as challenges to engaging Hispanics in treatment resurface when we need to make an outside referral: lack of insurance and low income serve as critical barriers for many of our patients. We have partnered with our local university's Psychological Clinic to accept referrals for traditional therapy.

While this significantly reduces cost barriers, the clinic is located at some distance from the primary care clinics transportation can be difficult. In addition, oftentimes the bilingual student clinicians have full caseloads; therefore wait times for services may extend to many months. Nevertheless, we have continued to forge relationships with other providers. In our experience, two significant efforts on our part help reduce frustration for our patients. First, we are likely to pick up the telephone and make a first contact with a new referral source. We ask questions about the scope of their services, wait times, eligibility requirements, payments accepted, availability of Spanish-speaking providers, locations, and other factors relevant for our patients. Second, we employ behavioral health case managers who can assist our patients with ensuring the outside referrals we make are utilized by our patients. Our behavioral health case managers will call patients to ensure they were able to make appointments, or will even call referrals on our patients' behalf (with proper consent). If patients do not follow through with outside referrals, our case managers can work with our patients to problem-solve barriers and, if need be, schedule them to return to us for additional services within the primary care clinic.

A Public Health Perspective

The integrated care model promises to reduce the large health disparities experienced by many minority groups in the United States, including Hispanics. Integrated care operates from a public health perspective, meaning the emphasis of interventions is on their *impact* rather than efficacy. The impact of an intervention is a function of the efficacy of the intervention and the rate of participation, or percentage of the population that is able to access the intervention (Impact = Participation Rate × Efficacy; Whitlock, Orleans, Pender, & Allan, 2002). For instance, an intervention for depression that is 80 % efficacious but can only be delivered to 5 % of patients will have an impact that is five times lower (impact = 0.8 × 0.05 = 0.04) than a depression intervention that is only 50 % efficacious but reaches 40 % of patients (impact = 0.5 × 0.4 = 0.20). Brief interventions delivered "just in time" in primary care settings to patients are responsive, efficacious, and can reach a great deal more patients than more intensive interventions delivered over many months. In addition, these interventions can be delivered before or shortly after behavioral health symptoms emerge, possibly preventing the onset of more serious illness. López and colleagues (2009) discuss the importance of increasing mental health literacy in Hispanic family members of people suffering from schizophrenia—the recognition of symptoms of psychotic disorders can help people seek services early on, before symptoms worsen or full relapse occurs.

Conclusions

The growing emphasis on integrating behavioral health services into primary care coincides with an increasingly diverse population in the U.S. This coinciding of events is quite fortunate, since the integrated approach to whole-person care is in fact quite amenable to culturally responsive behavioral health care service provision, especially for Hispanic patients. Integrated services reduce many of the intrinsic and external barriers Hispanics face when seeking care, from reducing stigma and responding to somatic expressions of distress to reducing cost barriers and delivering care in a brief, personal manner. Clinics that move towards embracing the growing diversity of their patients, and who opt to integrate behavioral health services into their medical homes, have the potential to make a significant impact on the health and well-being of their patients.

References

Alegría, M., Canino, G., Shrout, P. E., Woo, M., Duan, N., Vila, D., … Meng, X. -L. (2008). Prevalence of mental illness in immigrant and non-immigrant U.S. Latino groups. *American Journal of Psychiatry, 165*, 359–369. doi:10.1176/appi.ajp.2007.07040704.

Andrés-Hyman, R. C., Ortiz, J., Añez, L. M., Paris, M., & Davidson, L. (2006). Culture and clinical practice: Recommendations for working with Puerto Ricans and other Latinas(os) in the United States. *Professional Psychology: Research and Practice, 37*, 694–701. doi:10.1037/0735-7028.37.6.694.

Añez, L. M., Paris, M. R., Bedregal, L. E., Davidson, L., & Grilo, C. M. (2005). Application of cultural constructs in the care of first generation Latino clients in a community mental health setting. *Journal of Psychiatric Practice, 11*, 221–230. doi:10.1097/00131746200507000-00002.

Añez, L. M., Silva, M. A., Paris, M., Jr., & Bedregal, L. E. (2008). Engaging Latinos through the integration of cultural values and motivational interviewing principles. *Professional Psychology: Research and Practice, 39*, 153–159. doi:10.1037/0735-7028.39.2.153.

Antshel, K. M. (2002). Integrating culture as a means of improving treatment adherence in the Latino population. *Psychology, Health & Medicine, 7*, 435–449. doi:10.1080/1354850021000015258.

Arkansas Center for Health Improvement [ACHI]. (2015). *The impact of expanded coverage on Arkansas's health care safety net services.* Retrieved from http://www.achi.net/Docs/285/.

Bathje, G. J., & Shelton, K. (August, 2012). *Multicultural competence checklist for college and university counseling centers.* Poster presented at the annual meeting of the American Psychological Association, Orlando, FL.

Benish, S. G., Quintana, S., & Wampold, B. E. (2011). Culturally adapted psychotherapy and the legitimacy of myth: A direct-comparison meta-analysis. *Journal of Counseling Psychology, 58*, 279–289. doi:10.1037/a0023626.

Blount, A. (1998). *Integrated primary care: The future of medical and mental health collaboration.* New York, NY: Norton.

Bower, P., & Gilbody, S. (2005). Stepped care in psychological therapies: Access, effectiveness and efficiency. *British Journal of Psychiatry, 186*, 11–17. doi:10.1192/bjp.186.1.11.

Bridges, A. J., Andrews, A. I., Villalobos, B. T., Pastrana, F. A., Cavell, T. A., & Gomez, D. (2014). Does integrated behavioral health care reduce mental health disparities for Latinos? Initial findings. *Journal of Latina/o Psychology, 2*, 37–53. doi:10.1037/lat0000009.

Bridges, A. J., Andrews, A. I., & Deen, T. L. (2012). Mental health needs and service utilization by Hispanic immigrants residing in Mid-southern United States. *Journal of Transcultural Nursing, 23*, 359–368. doi:10.1177/1043659612451259.

Bridges, A. J., & Lindly, E. (2008). Service utilization and case management. In *Workgroup on adapting Latino services, Adaptation guidelines for serving Latino children and families affected by trauma* (1st ed.). San Diego, CA: Chadwick Center for Children and Families.

Brune, M. M., Eiroá-Orosa, F. J., Fischer-Ortman, J. J., Delijaj, B. B., & Haasen, C. C. (2011). Intermediated communication by interpreters in psychotherapy with traumatized refugees. *International Journal of Culture and Mental Health, 4*, 144–151. doi:10.1080/17542863.2010.537821.

Bryan, C. J., Corso, M. L., Corso, K. A., Morrow, C. E., Kanzler, K. E., & Ray-Sannerud, B. (2012). Severity of mental health impairment and trajectories of improvement in an integrated primary care clinic. *Journal of Consulting and Clinical Psychology, 80*, 396–403. doi:10.1037/a0027726.

Cabassa, L. J., Lester, R., & Zayas, L. H. (2007). 'It's like being in a labyrinth': Hispanic immigrants' perceptions of depression and attitudes toward treatments. *Journal of Immigrant and Minority Health, 9*, 1–16. doi:10.1007/s10903-006-9010-1.

Chang, J., Natsuaki, M. N., & Chen, C. (2013). The importance of family factors and generation status: Mental health service use among Latino and Asian Americans. *Cultural Diversity and Ethnic Minority Psychology, 19*, 236–247. doi:10.1037/a0032901.

Chowdhary, N., Jotheeswaran, A. T., Nadkarni, A., Hollon, S. D., King, M., ... Patel, V. (2014). The methods and outcomes of cultural adaptations of psychological treatments for depressive disorders: A systematic review. *Psychological Medicine, 44*, 1131–1146. doi: 10.1017/S0033291713001785.

Corso, K. A., Bryan, C. J., Corso, M. L., Kanzler, K. E., Houghton, D. C., Ray-Sannerud, B., & Morrow, C. E. (2012). Therapeutic alliance and treatment outcome in the primary care behavioral health model. *Families, Systems, & Health, 30*, 87–100. doi:10.1037/a0028632.

Davis, J. M., & Liang, C. H. (2015). A test of the mediating role of gender role conflict: Latino masculinities and help-seeking attitudes. *Psychology of Men & Masculinity, 16*, 23–32. doi:10.1037/a0035320.

Dawes, S. E., Suarez, P., Vaida, F., Marcotte, T. D., Atkinson, J. H., Grant, I., ... HNRC group. (2010). Demographic influences and suggested cut-scores for the Beck Depression Inventory in a non-clinical Spanish speaking population from the US-Mexico border region. *International Journal of Culture and Mental Health, 3*, 34–42. doi: 10.1080/17542860903533640.

Reyes de Beaman, S., Beaman, P. E., Garcia-Peña, C., Villa, M. A., Heres, J., Córdova, A., & Jagger, C. (2004). Validation of a modified version of the Mini-Mental State Examination (MMSE) in Spanish. *Aging Neuropsychology and Cognition, 11*, 1–11. doi: 10.1076/anec.11.1.1.29366.

Escobar, J. I., Goldring, J. M., Hough, R. L., Karno, M., Burnam, M. A., & Wells, K. B. (1987). Somatization in the community: Relationship to disability and use of services. *American Journal of Public Health, 77*, 837–840. doi:10.2105/AJPH.77.7.837.

Gary, F. A. (2005). Stigma: Barrier to mental health care among ethnic minorities. *Issues in Mental Health Nursing, 26*, 979–999. doi:10.1080/01612840500280638.

Glasgow, R. E., Christiansen, S. M., Kurz, D., King, D. K., Woolley, T., Faber, A. J., ... Dickman, J. (2011). Engagement in a diabetes self-management website: Usage patterns and generalizability of program use. *Journal of Medical Internet Research, 13*, 73–87. doi:10.2196/jmir.1391.

Gonzalez, J. M., Alegría, M., & Prihoda, T. J. (2005). How do attitudes toward mental health treatment vary by age, gender, and ethnicity/race in young adults? *Journal of Community Psychology, 33*, 611–629. doi:10.1002/jcop.20071.

Hays, P. A. (2009). Integrating evidence-based practice, cognitive-behavior therapy, and multicultural therapy: Ten steps for culturally competent practice. *Professional Psychology: Research and Practice, 40*, 354–360. doi:10.1037/a0016250.

Hirai, M., Vernon, L. L., Popan, J. R., & Clum, G. A. (2015). Acculturation and enculturation, stigma toward psychological disorders, and treatment preferences in a Mexican American sample: The role of education in reducing stigma. *Journal of Latina/o Psychology, 3*, 88–102. doi:10.1037/lat0000035.

Hunter, C. L., Goodie, J. L., Oordt, M. S., & Dobmeyer, A. C. (2009). *Integrated behavioral health in primary care: Step-by-step guidance for assessment and intervention*. Washington, DC: American Psychological Association.

Interian, A., Martinez, I. E., Guarnaccia, P. J., Vega, W. A., & Escobar, J. I. (2007). A qualitative analysis of the perception of stigma among Latinos receiving antidepressants. *Psychiatric Services, 58*, 1591–1594. doi:10.1176/appi.ps.58.12.1591.

Jacobs, E. A., Lauderdale, D. S., Meltzer, D., Shorey, J. M., Levinson, W., & Thisted, R. A. (2001). Impact of interpreter services on delivery of health care to limited-English-proficient patients. *JournalofGeneralInternalMedicine, 16*,468–474.doi:10.1046/j.1525-1497.2001.016007468.x.

Jang, Y., Chiriboga, D. A., Herrera, J. R., Martinez Tyson, D., & Schonfeld, L. (2011). Attitudes toward mental health services in Hispanic older adults: The role of misconceptions and personal beliefs. *Community Mental Health Journal, 47*, 164–170. doi:10.1007/s10597-009-9274-8.

Kanter, J. W., Santiago-Rivera, A. L., Rusch, L. C., Busch, A. M., & West, P. (2010). Initial outcomes of a culturally adapted behavioral activation for Latinas diagnosed with depression at a community clinic. *Behavior Modification, 34*, 120–144. doi:10.1177/0145445509359682.

Kessler, R. C., Andrews, G., Colpe, L. J., Hiripi, E., Mroczek, D. K., … Zaslavsky, A. M. (2002) Short screening scales to monitor population prevalences and trends in non-specific psychological distress. *Psychological Medicine, 32*, 959–956. doi: 10.1017/S0033291702006074.

Kim, G., Loi, C. A., Chiriboga, D. A., Jang, Y., Parmelee, P., & Allen, R. S. (2011). Limited English proficiency as a barrier to mental health service use: A study of Latino and Asian immigrants with psychiatric disorders. *Journal of Psychiatric Research, 45*, 104–110. doi:10.1016/j.psychires.2010.04.031.

Kinoshita, L. M., Sorocco, K. H., & Gallagher-Thompson, D. (2008). Mental health and aging: Current trends and future directions. In J. E. Maddux & B. A. Winstead (Eds.), *Psychopathology: Foundations for a contemporary understanding* (2nd ed., pp. 417–443). New York, NY: Routledge/Taylor and Francis Group.

Kouyoumdjian, H., Zamboanga, B. L., & Hansen, D. J. (2003). Barriers to community mental health services for Latinos: Treatment considerations. *Clinical Psychology: Science and Practice, 10*, 394–422. doi:10.1093/clipsy/bpg041.

López, S. R. (2002). A research agenda to improve the accessibility and quality of mental health care for Latinos. Psychiatric Services, 53, 1569–1573. doi: 10.1176/appi.ps.53.12.1569.

López, S. R., Lara, M. C., Kopelowicz, A., Solano, S., Foncerrada, H., & Aguilera, A. (2009). La CLAve to increase psychosis literacy of Spanish-speaking community residents and family caregivers. *Journal of Consulting and Clinical Psychology, 77*, 763–774. doi:10.1037/a0016031.

Matthews, P. H., Darbisi, C., Sandmann, L., Galen, R., & Rubin, D. (2009). Disseminating health information and diabetes care for Latinos via electronic information kiosks. *Journal of Immigrant and Minority Health, 11*, 520–526. doi:10.1007/s10903-008-9134-6.

McCabe, K. M. (2002). Factors that predict premature termination among Mexican-American children in outpatient psychotherapy. *Journal of Child and Family Studies, 11*, 347–359. doi:10.1023/A:1016876224388.

Miranda, J., Bernal, G., Lau, A., Kohn, L., Hwang, W. C., & La Fromboise, T. (2005). State of the science on psychosocial interventions for ethnic minorities. *Annual Review of Clinical Psychology, 1*, 113–142. doi:10.1146/annurev.clinpsy.1.102803.143822.

Musser-Granski, J., & Carrillo, D. F. (1997). The use of bilingual, bicultural paraprofessionals in mental health services: Issues for hiring, training, and supervision. *Community Mental Health Journal, 33*, 51–60. doi:10.1023/A:1022417211254.

Novy, D. M., Stanley, M. A., Averill, P., & Daza, P. (2001). Psychometric comparability of English- and Spanish-language measures of anxiety and related affective symptoms. *Psychological Assessment, 13*, 347–355. doi:10.1037/1040-3590.13.3.347.

O'Donohue, W. T., & Draper, C. (2011). *Stepped care and e-health: Practical applications to behavioral disorders*. New York, NY: Springer.

Olfson, M., Moitabai, R., Sampson, N. A., Hwang, I., Druss, B., Wang, P. S., … Kessler, R. C. (2009). Dropout from outpatient mental health care in the United States. *Psychiatric Services, 60*, 898–907. doi: 10.1176/appi.ps.60.7.898.

Rastogi, M., Massey-Hastings, N., & Wieling, E. (2012). Barriers to seeking mental health services in the Latino/a community: A qualitative analysis. *Journal of Systemic Therapies, 31*, 1–17. doi:10.1521/jsyt.2012.31.4.1.

Ray-Sannerud, B. N., Dolan, D. C., Morrow, C. E., Corso, K. A., Kanzler, K. E., Corso, M. L., & Bryan, C. J. (2012). Longitudinal outcomes after brief behavioral health intervention in an integrated primary care clinic. *Families, Systems, & Health, 30*, 60–71. doi:10.1037/a0027029.

Robinson, P., & Reiter, J. (2007). *Behavioral consultation and primary care: A guide to integrating services*. New York, NY: Springer Science and Business Media.

Rosado, J. W., & Elias, M. J. (1993). Ecological and psychocultural mediators in the delivery of services for urban, culturally diverse Hispanic clients. *Professional Psychology: Research and Practice, 24*, 450. doi:10.1037/0735-7028.24.4.450.

Ruggero, C. J., Johnson, S. L., & Cuellar, A. K. (2004). Spanish-language measures of mania and depression. *Psychological Assessment, 16*, 381–385. doi:10.1037/1040-3590.16.4.381.

Ryan, C. (2013). *Language use in the United States, 2011*. American Community Survey Reports, ACS-22. U. S. Census Bureau, Washington, DC: US Government Printing Office. Retrieved from https://www.census.gov/prod/2013pubs/acs-22.pdf.

Sanchez, K., Chapa, T., Ybarra, R., & Martinez, O. N. (2012). *Eliminating disparities through the integration of behavioral health and primary care services for racial and ethnic minority populations, including individuals with limited English proficiency: A literature review report*. Washington, DC: United States Department of Health and Human Services. Office of Minority Health.

Schulz, P. M., Resick, P. A., Huber, L., & Griffin, M. G. (2006). The effectiveness of cognitive processing therapy for PTSD with refugees in a community setting. *Cognitive and Behavioral Practice, 13*, 322–331. doi:10.1016/j.cbpra.2006.04.011.

Sentell, T., Shumway, M., & Snowden, L. (2007). Access to mental health treatment by English language proficiency and race/ethnicity. *Journal of General Internal Medicine, 22*, 289–293. doi:10.1007/s11606-007-0345-7.

Shattell, M. M., Hamilton, D., Starr, S. S., Jenkins, C. J., & Henderliter, N. A. (2008). Mental health service needs of a Latino population: A community-based participatory research project. *Issues in Mental Health Nursing, 29*, 351–370. doi:10.1080/01612840801904316.

Snell-Johns, J., Mendez, J. L., & Smith, B. H. (2004). Evidence-based solutions for overcoming access barriers, decreasing attrition, and promoting change with underserved families. *Journal of Family Psychology, 18*, 19–35. doi:10.1037/0893-3200.18.1.19.

Strosahl, K. (1998). Integrating behavioral health and primary care services: The primary mental health care model. In A. Blount & A. Blount (Eds.), *Integrated primary care: The future of medical and mental health collaboration* (pp. 139–166). New York, NY: W.W. Norton & Co.

Sue, S. (1988). Psychotherapeutic services for ethnic minorities: Two decades of research findings. *American Psychologist, 43*, 301. doi:10.1037/0003-066X.43.4.301.

Swift, J. K., Greenberg, R. P., Whipple, J. L., & Kominiak, N. (2012). Practice recommendations for reducing premature termination in therapy. *Professional Psychology: Research and Practice, 43*, 379–387. doi:10.1037/a0028291.

Tonigan, J. S. (2003). Project Match treatment participation and outcome by self-reported ethnicity. *Alcoholism, Clinical and Experimental Research, 27*, 1340–1344. doi:10.1097/01.ALC.0000080673.83739.F3.

U.S. Department of Health and Human Services. (2001). *Mental health: Culture, race, and ethnicity—A supplement to mental health: A report of the surgeon general*. Rockville, MD: Author.

Uebelacker, L. A., Marootian, B. A., Pirraglia, P. A., Primack, J., Tigue, P. M., Haggarty, R., & Miller, I. W. (2012). Barriers and facilitators of treatment for depression in a Latino community: A focus group study. *Community Mental Health Journal, 48*, 114–126. doi:10.1007/s10597-011-9388-7.

Varela, R., Vernberg, E. M., Sanchez-Sosa, J., Riveros, A., Mitchell, M., & Mashunkashey, J. (2004). Anxiety reporting and culturally associated interpretation biases and cognitive schemas: A comparison of Mexican, Mexican American, and European American families. *Journal of Clinical Child and Adolescent Psychology, 33*, 237–247. doi:10.1207/s15374424jccp3302_4.

Vega, W. A., Kolody, B., Aguilar-Gaxiola, S., & Catalano, R. (1999). Gaps in service utilization by Mexican Americans with mental health problems. *American Journal of Psychiatry, 156*, 928–934. doi:10.1176/ajp.156.6.928.

Villalobos, B. T., Bridges, A. J., Anastasia, E. A., Ojeda, C. A., Hernandez Rodriguez, J., & Gomez, D. (2016). Effects of language concordance and interpreter use on therapeutic alliance in Spanish-speaking integrated behavioral health care patients. *Psychological Services, 13*, 49.

Villatoro, A. P., Morales, E. S., & Mays, V. M. (2014). Family culture in mental health help-seeking and utilization in a nationally representative sample of Latinos in the United States: The NLAAS. *American Journal of Orthopsychiatry, 84*, 353–363. doi:10.1037/h0099844.

Voss Horrell, S. C. (2008). Effectiveness of cognitive-behavioral therapy with adult ethnic minority clients: A review. *Professional Psychology: Research and Practice, 39*, 160–168. doi:10.1037/0735-7028.39.2.160.

Wang, P. S., Lane, M., Olfson, M., Pincus, H. A., Wells, K. B., & Kessler, R. C. (2005). Twelve-month use of mental health services in the United States: Results from the National Comorbidity Survey Replication. Archives of General Psychiatry, 62, 629–640. doi: 10.1001/archpsyc.62.6.629.

Wells, A., Lagomasino, I. T., Palinkas, L. A., Green, J. M., & Gonzalez, D. (2013). Barriers to depression treatment among low-income, Latino emergency department patients. *Community Mental Health Journal, 49*, 412–418. doi:10.1007/s10597-012-9547-5.

Whitlock, E. P., Orleans, T., Pender, N., & Allan, J. (2002). Evaluating primary care behavioral counseling interventions: An evidence-based approach. *American Journal of Preventive Medicine, 22*, 267–284. doi:10.1016/S0749-3797(02)00415-4.

Young, A. S., Klap, R., Sherbourne, C. D., & Wells, K. B. (2001). The quality of care for depressive and anxiety disorders in the United States. *Archives of General Psychiatry, 58*, 55–61. doi:10.1001/archpsyc.58.1.55.

Chapter 9
Hispanic Children and Integrated Care

Jessica Urgelles, Michelle Pitts, and Lauren Gorog

Introduction

More than 20 % of US children meet criteria for a mental health diagnosis (Van Landeghem & Hess, 2005). The age of onset of major mental illness can be as young as 7 years of age, and predictors of mental health problems are sometimes seen in preschoolers (National Center for Children in Poverty, 2006). The consequences of childhood mental illness can be devastating. Half of high school-aged youth with a mental illness drop out of school and 70 % of juvenile justice-involved youth have a mental illness (National Institute of Mental Health, 2006). Furthermore, suicide is the third leading cause of death among youth aged 10–24 (Pearson, Stanley, King, & Fisher, 2001).

Unfortunately, 75–80 % of children who need mental health services do not receive them (Van Landeghem & Hess, 2005). Parents often seem willing to follow through with referrals to meet with a psychologist/behavioral health provider (BHP) during pediatric visits but frequently fail to follow through. Integrated pediatric primary care may be a solution to this problem, as most parents report a preference to meet with BHPs at their primary care office over an outside agency (Kolko, Campo, Kilbourne, & Kelleher, 2012).

Compared to other ethnic groups, Hispanic youth are the least likely to receive needed mental health care (Kataoka, Zhang, & Wells, 2002). This is particularly

J. Urgelles (✉)
Division of Clinical Psychology, Brown University Alpert Medical School,
Providence, RI 02912, USA
e-mail: jurgelles@msn.com

M. Pitts
Department of Psychology, University of Nevada, Las Vegas, Las Vegas, NV 89154, USA

L. Gorog
School of Graduate Psychology, Pacific University, Hillsboro, OR 97123, USA

© Springer International Publishing Switzerland 2016

L.T. Benuto, W. O'Donohue (eds.), *Enhancing Behavioral Health in Latino Populations*, DOI 10.1007/978-3-319-42533-7_9

concerning given national estimates that suggest Hispanic adolescents may be one of the most vulnerable groups with higher rates of suicidal thoughts, suicide attempts, and symptoms of depression and anxiety (Kataoka et al., 2002). They also tend to have higher rates of dropping out of high school, substance use, driving when drinking alcohol, unsafe sex, overweight and obesity, and unhealthy eating habits (Chapman, Laird, Ifill, & KewalRamani, 2011; Eaton et al., 2012). Integrated primary care may be part of the solution in creating healthcare equality. Comparable utilization rates and clinical outcomes have been demonstrated between Hispanics and non-Hispanic White patients in adult integrated care settings (Bridges et al., 2014), suggesting that integrated care may reduce some of the barriers to quality healthcare for Hispanic youth.

Barriers to Quality Healthcare

Knowledge and Training

Many symptoms presented to pediatric primary care providers (PPCPs), such as sleep difficulties, toileting problems, tantrums, abdominal pain, and mealtime struggles do not have a biological cause. Approximately 50 % of pediatric primary care visits are associated with emotional, behavioral, and educational problems (Pidano, 2007). Routine behavioral health screening in primary care is necessary, but is not common practice. This is a missed opportunity to address mental health problems early, before they become chronic and debilitating conditions.

Simply making behavioral health screens a routine procedure of well-child visits is not the solution. PPCPs are inaccurate at identifying developmental and mental health problems, with sensitivities below 54 % (Sheldrick, Merchant, & Perrin, 2011). In addition, PPCPs may be attempting to address mental health concerns without adequate training. The majority of PPCPs report not having enough knowledge and training to recognize and treat mental health problems in children (Nasir, Watanabe-Galloway, & DiRenzo-Coffey, 2014; Pidano, Kimmelblatt, & Nease, 2011). In a survey of PPCPs, more than 90 % of respondents reported seeing at least one patient per month with a diagnosed mental health problem, but only 10 % felt they were well-prepared to diagnose and treat these problems (Davis et al., 2012). Many PPCPs identified lack of communication and consultation with mental health providers as a barrier to quality care.

PPCP's lack of expertise may be noticeable to parents. Some parents have reported that their PPCPs initially normalized their concerns when they first presented them to their PPCPs (Brown, Girio-Herrera, Sherman, Kahn, & Copeland, 2014). Others report receiving little feedback from their PPCPs about how to address behavioral health problems in their children. Instead, caregivers are routinely given referrals to go elsewhere, but may not have a clear understanding of why there are being referred or what to expect from the referral services.

Financial Cost and Logistical Issues

Healthcare is costly for families and could present a significant barrier to following through with referrals and interventions. This may be a particularly salient barrier for Hispanic families. With the signing of the Patient Protection and Affordable Care Act in 2010, more Americans have access to health insurance. However, Hispanic children continue to be disproportionately uninsured. In 2013, 12.1 % of Hispanic children were uninsured compared to 5.4 % non-Hispanic White children, 7.5 % of Black children, and 8.4 % of Asian children (Smith & Medalia, 2014). Hispanic households also have one of the lowest median incomes and highest rates of poverty. In 2013, the poverty rate for Hispanics in the US was 23.5 %, compared to only 9.6 % for non-Hispanic Whites (DeNavas-Walt & Proctor, 2014). Mental disorders were the most costly condition ($13.9 billion) for youth in 2012 (Center for Financing, Access, & Cost Trends, 2012) and the average annual cost per child is highest for mental disorders ($2195). In addition, families with Medicaid typically have limited options for mental health services.

In traditional pediatric primary care, parents report spending 11–20 min with their PPCP (Halfon, Stevens, Larson, & Olson, 2011). This may not provide parents with enough time to adequately get their needs met. Longer visits are associated with more anticipatory guidance, and more psychosocial risk and developmental assessment. Parents are also more likely to report feeling respected and understood during longer appointments. This is evidence that pediatric well-child visits are not structured in a way to adequately meet the needs of families. This may be particularly relevant for Hispanic families who already have cultural barriers to feeling respected and understood.

There are several logistical barriers that are particularly salient for low-income families. The cost of transportation, lack of transportation options, inability to take time off work, lack of time, lack of childcare, and a higher incidence of day-to-day stress have all been identified as barriers to accessing healthcare for children from low-income households (Bringewatt & Gershoff, 2010; Santiago, Kaltman, & Miranda, 2013).

Cultural

A caregiver's culture will shape their perception of their child's emotional and behavioral problems. Hispanics tend to respond to psychological distress with somatic complaints. As a result, they are more likely to present to primary care for mental health problems (Bridges et al., 2014). Some Hispanic groups may have different views about when to seek professional assistance or feel unsure about when their children are in need of services.

Some parents feel uncomfortable discussing emotional issues because they view them as private family matters. A fragmented health care system makes this barrier even more prominent, as parents will prefer to speak with a provider with whom they have already established trust. Indeed, the quality of the therapist–family relationship is one of the most important factors associated with premature drop-out in community mental health centers (Stevens, Kelleher, Ward-Estes, & Hayes, 2006). The perceived relevance of treatment is another major factor associated with treatment attrition rates. Low expectations of the usefulness of referrals may make it less likely caregivers will follow through with treatment recommendations.

The use of home remedies is common among some Hispanic groups (Risser & Mazur, 1995). Some Hispanic caregivers report using a combination of pharmaceutical and herbal remedies to treat illnesses such as asthma, fever, and infections. Curanderos, or folk healers, are highly respected in some Hispanic cultures. Parents' beliefs about folk remedies and healers will affect how much faith they put into medical explanations and interventions. Culturally competent clinicians will be better able to effectively explain treatment rationales in a way that takes the family's cultural beliefs into consideration and makes it relevant to the family's perceived needs.

Miscommunication between caregivers and providers is a common reason for treatment nonadherence. Miscommunications are likely if providers cannot speak with families in a language they can understand. Parents may rely on a limited understanding of English, creating another barrier for quality healthcare. While most Hispanic children speak English very well, more than half of Hispanic children who live with both parents have at least one parent who does not speak English well (Murphey, Guzman, & Torres, 2014). Unfortunately, bilingual and ethnic minority providers are lacking. Approximately 25 % of the US population under the age of 18 is of Hispanic origin (Colby & Ortman, 2014). In contrast, only 2.8 % of US physicians identified as Hispanic in 2004 (Castillo-Page, 2006). Fortunately, physicians are becoming more diverse, as 8.5 % of medical matriculants identified as Hispanic in 2011 (Castillo-Page, 2012). There is also a lack of diversity among BHPs. It has been estimated that approximately 90 % of behavioral health professionals are non-Hispanic White (Annapolis Coalition, 2007).

When providers lack cultural competence in working with Hispanic families, their biases can act as a barrier to treatment. If providers and support staff lack cultural sensitivity to specific values, common stressors, and potential barriers to treatment for a family's specific Hispanic culture, inaccurate assumptions and misinterpretations are possible. Providers may be quick to label patients as "difficult" and make assumptions about their attitudes about treatment, possibly making fewer attempts to reach a family for follow-up after a missed appointment.

There are also limited options for culturally sensitive assessment and treatment. Families from some Hispanic cultures may want to include other family members, spiritual healers, or teachers in their child's treatment team. The Latino value of *familismo* suggests some Hispanic families will expect family members to take an active role in treatment and family-based interventions may be preferred.

Stigma and Fear

Many Hispanic individuals have experienced discrimination, making them feel uncomfortable in unfamiliar settings. Hispanic individuals living in the US often report feeling misunderstood, or even maltreated (Santiago et al., 2013). These experiences can lead to distrust of other ethnic groups. In addition, Hispanic immigrant families without proper documentation may experience fear associated with their immigration status and fear of deportation, making them reluctant to access care for their children.

There are several potential fears that may prevent caregivers from utilizing services. Hispanics and other low-income groups have reported a fear of losing custody of their children if they admit to having difficulty caring for their children or managing behavioral problems. An alarming number of minority children have been relinquished to child welfare agencies so that they can receive needed mental health services (Children's Defense Fund, 2009). Fear associated with not being able to afford services and what might happen if they cannot afford services may keep some caregivers from following through with referrals.

Further, there continues to be a stigma associated with needing mental health services. Some Hispanic families may fear disapproval from relatives and community members, or that others and providers will blame them for their problems with their child. They may also receive feedback that discourages them from following through with mental health referrals. Some families may prefer to seek help through informal sources over traditional mental health settings.

Integrated Care

Traditional healthcare has failed to address the many barriers to quality healthcare faced by many Hispanic families and integrated care may be the solution. There is no clear definition of integrated care but there are models of collaborative care with varying levels of integration. Often the terms coordinated care, co-located care, and integrated care are used interchangeably, making it difficult to interpret the existing literature. In coordinated care, medical and mental health services occur in different settings. There is a referral relationship between PPCPs and BHPs, as well as other community resources. There is limited integration in this model and the majority of the aforementioned barriers still exist. In a co-located model, medical and behavioral health services are located in the same facility, but there is still a referral process for medical cases to be seen by BHPs. Co-located practices are rare and do not guarantee enhanced communication between providers (Guevara, Greenbaum, Shera, Bauer, & Schwarz, 2009).

In integrated care, there is one treatment plan for both medical and behavioral health components of care. Primary care and behavioral health are usually co-located. The treatment plan is delivered by staff that closely work together. Teams usually consist of a physician and some combination of physician's assistants, nurse practitioners, nurses, social workers, case managers, family advocates, psychologists, or behavioral health therapists. Ideally, there would be more than one BHP for each PPCP, so that while one is performing treatment the other is available for "warm handoffs." Evidence suggests that the ideal ratio of PPCP to BHP is 1:6 (Cummings, O'Donohue, & Cummings, 2009).

In a fully integrated pediatric primary care practice, behavioral health is part of routine medical care which includes direct patient care, as well as screening and prevention services. There is a holistic approach to healthcare that appreciates all aspects of an individual's health, including culture. Integrated pediatric primary care programs typically offer psychoeducation, medication, psychotherapy, and care management strategies. Pharmacological interventions are monitored collaboratively by all team members. BHPs in primary care tend to have larger caseloads and more flexible session time limits than in traditional outpatient mental health settings (Stancin, Perrin, & Ramirez, 2009). They also tend to use briefer, short-term interventions, use less-extensive documentation, and have flexible treatment plans. Interventions tend to be skills-based and patients may be taught self-management strategies to increase health knowledge and self-efficacy. Informal "curbside" consultations are common. The role of a BHP may extend beyond psychotherapy, and include patient education, physician education, case management, telephone monitoring, and skill coaching. BHPs may provide training to physicians on improving cultural competence and communication with families.

Integrated care also provides an important opportunity for developmental screening, promotion of healthy parent–child interactions, and detection of parental mental health problems and child maltreatment (Stancin et al., 2009). Assistance from other team members will help ensure that children who need additional services are not missed and allow PPCPs to focus their time on procedures for which they are better trained. Barriers to care are openly addressed and some programs may provide additional resources, such as transportation assistance, childcare, or meeting with children while they are at school.

Integrated care is associated with improved access to mental health services, greater patient satisfaction, higher quality care, improved patient compliance to treatment, greater provider satisfaction and perceived skill, better clinical outcomes and follow-ups, and a reduction in medical costs (Blount, 2003; Cummings et al., 2009; Hwang, Chang, LaClair, & Paz, 2013). The "warm handoff" in integrated models results in up to 90 % of patients entering mental health treatment, compared to 10 % through a traditional referral system (Cummings et al., 2009). These findings provide convincing evidence that integrated care is the way to eliminate the aforementioned barriers to quality healthcare that are often experienced by Hispanic families.

Implementation Challenges

The more integrated a program, the more likely it will be successful. However, there are several challenges when it comes to integrating care. It would likely take time to develop the infrastructure to support this system. There is also a lack of adequate payment options and many complex coding and billing issues (Stancin & Perrin, 2014). In integrated care, families will often attend joint or sequential appointments with pediatricians and BHPs. Unfortunately, some payers will not pay for more than one service per day for the same diagnosis and there is no mechanism available to pay BHPs to facilitate parent education groups in a pediatric practice. Therefore, integrated models will not be sustainable without changes in policy, and the management of billing and repayments. A crucial component of the future of integrated care is education. Many training programs are training psychologists and other mental health professionals to work in this fast-paced setting.

Special Topics in Treating Hispanic Youth

Integrated care provides opportunities for regular assessment and early intervention of childhood mental health disorders while reducing barriers for Hispanic families. It is also the ideal setting to coordinate care for children with chronic physical and mental health problems. Mental health is interconnected with physical health and both should be addressed concurrently. Below are examples special topics relevant to the health of Hispanic youth and examples of how integrated care can help reduce disparities in these areas.

Attention-Deficit/Hyperactivity Disorder

The prevalence and heritability of attention-deficit/hyperactivity disorder (ADHD) is similar across different cultural groups (e.g., Rohde et al., 2005). However, Hispanic youth are less likely to receive an ADHD diagnosis compared to White youth, even when they present with the same symptoms (Morgan, Staff, Hillemeier, Farkas, & Maczuga, 2014). This is especially the case in non-English-speaking families. This means that many Hispanic children are not being properly assessed and diagnosed, and not receiving needed treatment. Likely, a result of the many barriers to treatment described above. ADHD is highly comorbid with other mental health disorders, such as depression, anxiety, and substance-use disorders. It is also associated with an increase in risk taking behaviors and poor school performance. A recent study found that there is a high prevalence of ADHD symptoms among Hispanic prison inmates (González, Vélez-Pastrana, Ruiz Varcárcel, Levin, & Albizu-García, 2015).

Evidence-based interventions for ADHD include pharmacological management and behavioral treatment (Daly, Cohen, Carpenter, & Brown, 2009). In traditional pediatric settings, children are prescribed psychostimulant medications by their PPCP and given a referral for behavioral treatment through a BHP. The aforementioned barriers often keep families from following through with needed behavior modification interventions and parent training. An integrated care model is ideal for treating ADHD because collaboration between PPCPs, BHPs, and school personnel is the gold standard. Collaborative care is an effective model for treating Hispanic youth with ADHD (Myers, Vander Stoep, Thompson, Zhou, & Unützer, 2010).

Violence

Hispanic adolescents are involved in physical altercations more often than White adolescents, with approximately one-quarter engaged in fighting (Shetgiri, Kataoka, Ponce, Flores, & Chung, 2010). Homicide is the second leading cause of death for Hispanics adolescents (Center for Disease Control and Prevention, 2010). Oppositional defiant disorder and conduct disorder are often risk factors for later violence. Early identification and intervention of these problems is crucial for reducing risk for later violence. Being a bully and being a victim of bullying are both associated with physical altercation injuries (Glew, Fan, Katon, & Rivara, 2008). Involvement in bullying is linked to negative psychological outcomes such as anger, depression, and suicidal ideation (van der Wal, de Wit, & Hirasing, 2003), and to a higher likelihood for criminality by early adulthood (Renda, Vassallo, & Edwards, 2011).

PPCPs are well positioned to take preventative action for youth at-risk for violence involvement. However, children are infrequently screened about current involvement in violence, or risk of future violence perpetration at routine visits. In fact, one study demonstrated that 76 % of practitioners never or rarely asked adolescents about involvement in physical fighting (Borowsky & Ireland, 2004). In general, pediatricians are not comfortable addressing issues of violence with their patients (Chaffee, Bridges, & Boyer, 2000; Finch, Weiley, Ip, & Barkin, 2008).

Violence-prevention strategies can be integrated into pediatric practice. Both the American Medical Association (AMA) and the AAP have strongly encouraged PCPs to screen youth for violence-related involvement and link at-risk youth to necessary intervention and follow-up services (AAP, 2009; Knox, Lomonaco, & Elster, 2005). This process would include appropriate screening for a history of injuries associated with violence and risk of retaliatory violence (Whiteside & Cunningham, 2009). Some key questions to assist in determining risk of future violence include school attendance and achievement, witnessing of violence, previous physical fights, bullying, substance use, and access to firearms (Borowsky & Ireland, 2004).

Many effective violence-prevention strategies and interventions are available that can easily be implemented by BHPs in primary care. Connected Kids (AAP, 2006) is a freely available strength-based prevention program designed for use in primary care that has demonstrated reductions in both fighting and related injuries in a randomized controlled trial (Borowsky, Mozayeny, Stuenkel, & Ireland, 2004). Parent–child Interaction Therapy (PCIT; Zisser & Eyberg, 2010) is a parent training intervention for children between the ages of 2 and 7 with disruptive behavior disorders. Abbreviated versions that have been adapted for primary care have shown improvements in child behavior through increased effectiveness of parenting strategies for child behavior management (Berkovits, O'Brien, Carter, & Eyberg, 2010).

Substance Abuse

Hispanic adolescents are disproportionately affected by substance use (Chen & Jacobson, 2012). Identification and treatment of substance use in Hispanic adolescents is inadequate and inconsistent (Saloner, Carson, & Lê Cook, 2014). Hispanics experience higher severity substance use and more severe consequences later in life as a result of early onset substance use (Hingson & Zha, 2009), and an increased likelihood of experiencing co-occurring mental health disorders (Chisolm, Mulatu, & Brown, 2009). Untreated substance use in Hispanic youths is also associated with problem behaviors such as unsafe sexual behavior (Prado et al., 2006), conduct problems, and delinquency (Barnes, Hoffman, Welte, Farrell, & Dintcheff, 2006).

Routine substance use screening of adolescents is recommended by the AAP (Levy, Kokotailo, & Committee on Substance Abuse, 2011). Screening, Brief Intervention, and Referral to Treatment (SBIRT; Babor et al., 2007) is a research-supported approach for this purpose that has been effective in adult populations. SBIRT is intended to identify current substance use along a spectrum and implement appropriate intervention at every health care visit in primary care (see Levy et al., 2011 for intervention goals based on level of substance use). Those in need of extensive substance abuse treatment are typically referred to outside providers, but within an integrated model this would be unnecessary. An exception would be if the adolescent was in need of inpatient or detoxification services. A number of outpatient evidence-based treatments exist for adolescent substance abuse, including ecological family therapy, multidimensional family therapy, brief motivational interventions, and cognitive behavioral therapy (Hogue, Henderson, Ozechowski, & Robbins, 2014). Family-based interventions are the gold standard and can be incorporated into primary care.

Overweight and Obesity

Childhood obesity is linked to serious medical conditions such as type 2 diabetes and cardiovascular disease (Weiss et al., 2004). Diabetes diagnosed before the age of 20 can reduce life expectancy by up to 27 % (Mayer-Davis et al., 2009). Childhood obesity places children at risk to a number of psychosocial consequences including depression, anxiety, impulsivity, and ADHD (Kalarchian & Marcus, 2012). Obese youth often have low self-esteem and negative body image, and face social discrimination and bullying (Puder & Munsch, 2010).

Although being overweight is directly related to the imbalance of caloric intake and physical activity, the current obesity epidemic proves to be more complex. Hispanic youth have higher rates of overweight and obesity than children of other ethnicities (Ogden, Carroll, Kit, & Flegal, 2014). Although there is a strong genetic component disproportionally predisposing certain racial and ethnic groups to diabetes, complex cultural and socioeconomic barriers place Hispanic youth at greater risk. Factors such as parental obesity, lack of time for meal preparation, higher cost of healthy foods, lack of access to healthy foods, meals traditionally higher in fat and carbohydrates, and caregivers using sugary foods as rewards have all been implicated in the high rate of obesity in Hispanic youth (He et al., 2013; Snethen, Hewitt, & Petering, 2007). Factors associated with decreased physical activity in the Hispanic community include limited time, lack of transportation, sedentary activities (e.g., watching television, playing video games), lack of safe options for recreational activities, racism from other ethnic groups or police, and the cost of organized athletic activities. Lack of parental health knowledge may also be an important contributing factor and a reasonable target for intervention.

The provision of educational materials is a common obesity intervention in pediatric primary care; however, this often leaves Hispanic families with more questions than answers., Hispanic parents were more likely than White parents to rate the quality of advice received regarding nutrition and physical activity at their most recent primary care visits as poor or fair (Taveras, Gortmaker, Mitchell, & Gillman, 2008). Many primary care offices now have educational information in Spanish about metabolism, nutrition, healthy snacks, portion size, and fitness (Stacia et al., 2010). However, there is a strong need for skilled health educators to provide culturally competent nutritional education that respects Hispanic heritage and beliefs about diet and potential barriers to regular physical activity. Family-based interventions are likely to be the most effective and acceptable method for working with Hispanic families.

Rather than relying on visual appearance, which is only noticeable when children are already obese, all children should be screened for overweight and obesity and risk factors. This can be accomplished by calculating the Body Mass Index (BMI) of each child at every well child visit (Barlow & Expert Committee, 2007). Regardless of BMI percentile, all children should receive a medical and behavioral assessment of risk factors for obesity, as well as an assessment of attitudes that affect lifestyle and habits. Children with a BMI below the 85th percentile and no evidence of health risk should get continued screening, prevention messages, and reinforcement for maintaining a healthy lifestyle. Those with a BMI at the 85th percentile or higher should get different stages of intervention depending on their level of risk. For some, prevention counseling will be sufficient, while others will require more active forms of treatment. In most cases, a multidisciplinary team consisting of social workers, psychologists, other BHPs, registered dietitians, exercise specialists (e.g., physical therapist), and community resources are only utilized in more severe cases. BHPs' expertise in behavioral change makes them well-suited to assess behavior and attitudes, teach behavioral-change strategies, as well as address the psychosocial consequences of overweight and obesity. In integrated primary care, BHPs can be involved in the prevention stage, possibly mitigating the need more intensive interventions.

Obesity interventions may be more effective when they extend beyond the primary care setting. Interventions that incorporate both primary care and community resources may help combat risk factors unique to Hispanic and low-income families. For example, *Healthy Living Today*! is a family-centered, culturally sensitive intervention that focuses on nutrition, physical activity, and stress management. It is effective and well tolerated by Hispanic families (Arauz Boudreau, Kurowski, Gonzalez, Dimond, & Oreskovic, 2013).

Asthma

Asthma is the most common chronic illness among children in the US. It is a chronic inflammatory disorder of the airways that is characterized by variable and recurring airflow obstruction and bronchial hyperresponsiveness (National Institutes of Health [NIH], 2007). Physical symptoms include difficulty breathing, wheezing, coughing, and mucus secretions. The severity of asthma exacerbations can vary from mild to fatal.

Asthma is currently conceptualized as a disorder with genetic, environmental, and psychological factors. Asthma disproportionately affects low-income and urban communities, likely due to various environmental factors, such as higher exposure to indoor and outdoor pollutants, as well as psychosocial stressors (Canino et al., 2006). While Hispanic children as a whole tend to have lower rates of asthma compared to other ethnic groups, a large disparity exists between different Hispanic subgroups. Puerto Rican youth have the highest prevalence of asthma than any other US racial or ethnic group, even after controlling for known risk factors (Lara, Akinbami, Flores, & Morgenstern, 2006). US born Hispanic youth tend to have higher rates of asthma compared to foreign-born Hispanic youth, with higher prevalence of asthma in later generations (Balcazar, Grineski, & Collins, 2015).

Maternal distress during pregnancy may disrupt fetal lung development and immunomodulation (Wright et al., 2010). Continued exposure to maternal distress and parenting difficulties into infancy and early childhood may negatively impact immune functioning and contribute to how infants learn to regulate physiological and emotional stress (Klinnert et al., 2001; Kozyrskyj et al., 2008). Stress and emotions are common triggers for many children with asthma, especially when exposed to stressful life events (McQuaid & Abramson, 2009).

Hispanic children have very poor adherence to prescribed asthma regimens, with less than half of Hispanic families adhering to the treatment recommendations described by the NIH (Acevedo-Nieves, 2008). Failing to fill prescriptions, incorrect dosage, inaccurate dosing intervals, and premature discontinuation of asthma medications are all common, especially if medications are expensive, have unpleasant side effects, are difficult to take, or if the benefits are not seen immediately. A major contributor to noncompliance with prescribed regimens among Hispanic families may be lack of asthma awareness. Hispanic caregivers are less likely to receive adequate training on how to control their child's asthma than non-Hispanic White caregivers (Inkelas, Garro, McQuaid, & Ortega, 2008). Hispanic parents report that they need more help understanding asthma and how to use medications to control it, which may contribute to a reliance on folk remedies (Mosnaim et al., 2006).

There are several ways an integrated approach can reduce barriers to adequate asthma care for Hispanic families. Several asthma educational programs for patients and families have been developed (McQuaid & Abramson, 2009). The most successful programs provide information about asthma and incorporate behavioral-change strategies. BHPs can also assist with physician training programs. The Physician Asthma Education program consists of teaching communication techniques and reviewing asthma guidelines with physicians (Cabana et al., 2014). It has been associated with higher adherence to guidelines by physicians, improved communication with patients, and better patient outcomes.

BHPs can identify psychosocial barriers to asthma management and provide interventions to address these barriers. One purpose of psychosocial interventions is to improve the family's autonomy in the self-management of asthma. Interventions may include self-management training, problem-solving techniques, family-based interventions, motivational interviewing, relaxation training, and biofeedback (McQuaid & Abramson, 2009). As the patient ages into adolescence, the focus of self-management training shifts from the caregivers to the child. Patients are taught to appropriately take medications and may be taught stress-management strategies to reduce autonomic arousal and emotional distress during an asthma exacerbation. A culturally adapted, family-based, asthma educational program called CALMA was found to improve patient outcomes and caregiver confidence in treating asthma in island and mainland Puerto Rican families (Canino et al., 2008).

School-Readiness and Literacy

Hispanic youth have lower levels of educational attainment and academic achievement than non-Hispanic White youth (Garcia & Miller, 2008). Children who attend high-quality preschool programs evidence greater school readiness; however, the long-term benefits are unclear. Hispanic families often do not have access to affordable, high-quality programs, which puts the pressure solely on parents to prepare children for school. Unfortunately, Hispanic caregivers are less likely than White caregivers to read daily to their young children (Murphey et al., 2014). The AAP recommendations that PPCPs promote early literacy with caregivers beginning when children are in infancy (High, Klass, & Council on Early Childhood, 2014). National programs, such as Reach Out and Read (ROR) are designed for PPCPs to teach the caregivers of preschoolers about the importance of reading aloud, teach book-reading strategies, and provide caregivers with developmentally appropriate books for their children during each well-child visit. Caregivers in ROR are more likely to read regularly with their children and children in the program evidence significantly improved language development at 24 months of age (High et al., 2014). This program has demonstrated to be efficacious with Hispanic populations (Sanders, Gershon, Huffman, & Mendoza, 2000).

Including other providers into primary care may enhance these outcomes. Programs such as Healthy Steps (Zuckerman, Parker, Kaplan-Sanoff, Augustyn,

& Barth, 2004) and the Video Interaction Project (VIP; Mendelsohn et al., 2007) utilize child development specialists to teach caregivers about child development, assess caregiver emotional health, reframe negative parental attributions about their child, and model positive interactions during well-child visits. Healthy Steps has been associated with greater adherence to well-child visits and better parenting. Caregivers in VIP meet with child develop specialists to discuss caregiver expectations and concerns about the child's development. They are videotaped while playing together with their child for several minutes. The video is watched and the specialist reinforces parenting strengths and teaches caregivers how to engage children and navigate disruptive behavior. VIP is associated with lower levels of parenting stress, greater likelihood of normal cognitive development, and lower likelihood of developmental delays in children. It has been implemented with both English- and Spanish-speaking families.

Conclusion

Mental health problems are prevalent in children, but the majority of these children do not receive needed services. Hispanic children are less likely to receive these services than children of other ethnic groups, likely due to barriers associated with physician training and knowledge, financial cost and logistical issues, culture, and stigma and fear. Integrated care has been shown to reduce these barriers and provide a setting for a higher quality, culturally competent, and holistic approach to healthcare.

References

Acevedo-Nieves, R. M. (2008). Exposing barriers to asthma care in Hispanic children. *The Nurse Practitioner, 33*, 37–42. doi:10.1097/01.NPR.0000314756.03293.ca.

American Academy of Pediatrics. (2006). *Connected kids: Safe, strong, secure clinical guide.* Retrieved from http://www2.aap.org/connectedkids/ClinicalGuide.pdf.

American Academy of Pediatrics. (2009). Policy statement – Role of the pediatrician in youth violence prevention. *Pediatrics, 124*, 393–402. doi:10.1542/peds.2009-0943.

Annapolis Coalition. (2007). *An action plan for behavioral health workforce development: A framework for discussion.* Substance Abuse and Mental Health Administration. Shortage Designation: HPSAs, MUAs, & MUPs. Retrieved from http://annapoliscoalition.org/wp-content/uploads/2013/11/action-plan-full-report.pdf.

Arauz Boudreau, A. D., Kurowski, D. S., Gonzalez, W. I., Dimond, M. A., & Oreskovic, N. M. (2013). Latino families, primary care, and childhood obesity: A randomized controlled trial. *American Journal of Preventative Medicine, 44*, S247–S257. doi:10.1016/j.amepre.2012.11.026.

Babor, T. F., McRee, B. G., Kassebaum, P. A., Grimaldi, P. L., Ahmed, K., & Bray, J. (2007). Screening, brief intervention, and referral to treatment (SBIRT): Toward a public health approach to the management of substance abuse. *Substance Abuse, 28*, 7–30. doi:10.1300/J465v28n03_03.

Balcazar, A. J., Grineski, S. E., & Collins, T. W. (2015). The Hispanic health paradox across generations: The relationship of child generational status and citizenship with health outcomes. *Public Health, 129*, 691–697. http://dx.doi.org/10.1016/j.puhe.2015.04.007.

Barlow, S. E., & Expert Committee. (2007). Expert committee recommendations regarding the prevention, assessment, and treatment of child and adolescent overweight and obesity: Summary report. *Pediatrics, 120*, S164–S192. doi:10.1542/peds.2007-2329C.

Barnes, G. M., Hoffman, J. H., Welte, J. W., Farrell, M. P., & Dintcheff, B. A. (2006). Effects of parental monitoring and peer deviance on substance use and delinquency. *Journal of Marriage and Family, 68*, 1084–1104. doi:10.1111/j.1741-3737.2006.00315.x.

Berkovits, M. D., O'Brien, K. A., Carter, C. G., & Eyberg, S. M. (2010). Early identification and intervention for behavior problems in primary care: A comparison of two abbreviated versions of parent-child interaction therapy. *Behavior Therapy, 41*, 375–387. doi:10.1016/j.beth.2009.11.002.

Blount, A. (2003). Integrated primary care: Organizing the evidence. *Family, Systems, & Health, 21*, 121–133. doi:10.1037/1091-7527.21.2.121.

Borowsky, I. W., & Ireland, M. (2004). Predictors of future fight-related injury among adolescents. *Pediatrics, 113*, 530–536.

Borowsky, I. W., Mozayeny, S., Stuenkel, K., & Ireland, M. (2004). Effects of a primary care-based intervention on violent behavior and injury in children. *Pediatrics, 114*(4), e392–e399. doi:10.1542/peds.2004-0693.

Bridges, A. J., Andrews, A. R., Villalobos, B. T., Pastrana, F. A., Cavell, T. A., & Gomez, D. (2014). Does integrated behavioral health care reduce mental health disparities for Latinos? Initial findings. *Journal of Latina/o Psychology, 2*, 37–53. doi:10.1037/lat0000009.

Bringewatt, E. H., & Gershoff, E. T. (2010). Falling through the cracks: Gaps and barriers in the mental health system for America's disadvantaged children. *Children and Youth Services Review, 32*, 1291–1299. doi:10.1016/j.childyouth.2010.04.021.

Brown, C. M., Girio-Herrera, E. L., Sherman, S. N., Kahn, R. S., & Copeland, K. A. (2014). Pediatricians may address barriers inadequately when referring low- income preschool- aged children to behavioral health services. *Journal of Health Care for the Poor and Underserved, 25*, 406–424. doi:10.1353/hpu.2014.0018.

Cabana, M. D., Slish, K. K., Evans, E., Mellins, R. B., Brown, R. W., Lin, X., … Clark, N. M. (2014). Impact of physician asthma care education on patient outcomes. Health Education & Behavior, 41, 509–517. doi:10.1177/1090198114547510.

Canino, G., Koinis-Mitchell, D., Ortega, A. N., McQuaid, E. L., Fritz, G. K., & Alegría, M. (2006). Asthma disparities in the prevalence, morbidity, and treatment of Latino children. *Social Science & Medicine, 63*, 2926–2937. doi:10.1016/j.socscimed.2006.07.017.

Canino, G., Vila, D., Normand, S. -L. T., Acosta-Pérez, E., Ramírez, R., García, P., & Rand, C. (2008). Reducing asthma health disparities in poor Puerto Rican children: The effectiveness of a culturally tailored family intervention. *Journal of Allergy & Clinical Immunology, 121*, 665–670. doi:10.1016/j.jaci.2007.10.022.

Castillo-Page, L. (2006). *Diversity in the physician workforce: Facts and figures 2006*. Washington, DC: American Association of Medical Colleges. Retrieved from https://www.aamc.org/download/386176/data/diversityinthephysicianworkforce-factsandfigures2006.pdf.

Castillo-Page, L. (2012). *Diversity in medical education: Facts & figures 2012*. Washington, DC: American Association of Medical Colleges. Retrieved from https://members.aamc.org/eweb/upload/Diversity%20in%20Medical%20Education%20Facts%20and%20Figures%202012.pdf.

Center for Financing, Access, and Cost Trends, AHRQ. (2012). *Household component of the medical expenditure panel survey.* Retrieved from http://meps.ahrq.gov/mepsweb/data_files/publications/st472/stat472.shtml.

Centers for Disease Control and Prevention, National Center for Injury Prevention Control. (2010). *Web-based injury statistics query and reporting system* [Data file]. Retrieved from www.cdc.gov/injury.

Chaffee, T. A., Bridges, M., & Boyer, C. B. (2000). Adolescent violence prevention practices among California pediatricians. *Archives of Pediatrics & Adolescent Medicine, 154*, 1034–1041. doi:10.1001/archpedi.154.10.1034.

Chapman, C., Laird, J., Ifill, N., & KewalRamani, A. (2011). *Trends in high school dropout and completion rates in the United States: 1972–2009.* (NCES 2012-006). U.S. Department of Education. Washington, DC: National Center for Education Statistics. Retrieved from http://nces.ed.gov/pubs2012/2012006.pdf.

Chen, P., & Jacobson, K. C. (2012). Developmental trajectories of substance use from early adolescence to young adulthood: Gender and racial/ethnic differences. *Journal of Adolescent Health, 50*, 154–163. doi:10.1016/j.jadohealth.2011.05.013.

Children's Defense Fund. (2009). *The barriers: Why is it so difficult for children to get mental health screens and assessments*? Retrieved from http://www.childrensdefense.org/library/data/barriers-children-mental-health-screens-assesments.pdf.

Chisolm, D. J., Mulatu, M. S., & Brown, J. R. (2009). Racial/ethnic disparities in the patterns of co-occurring mental health problems in adolescents in substance abuse treatment. *Journal of Substance Abuse Treatment, 37*, 203–210. http://dx.doi.org/10.1016/j.jsat.2008.11.005.

Colby, S. L., & Ortman, J. M. (2014). *Projections of the size and composition of the U.S. population: 2014 to 2060*, Current Population Reports, P25-1143, U.S. Census Bureau: Washington, DC. Retrieved from https://www.census.gov/content/dam/Census/library/publications/2015/demo/p25-1143.pdf.

Cummings, N. A., O'Donohue, W. T., & Cummings, J. L. (2009). The financial dimension of integrated behavioral/primary care. *Journal of Clinical Psychology in Medical Settings, 16*, 31–39. doi:10.1007/s10880-008-9139-2.

Daly, B. P., Cohen, J. S., Carpenter, J. L., & Brown, R. T. (2009). Attention-deficit/hyperactivity disorder in pediatric context. In M. C. Roberts & R. G. Steele (Eds.), *Handbook of pediatric psychology* (4th ed., pp. 540–555). New York, NY: The Guilford Press.

Davis, D. W., Honaker, S. M., Jones, V. F., Williams, P. G., Stocker, F., & Martin, E. (2012). Identification and management of behavioral/mental health problems in primary care pediatrics: Perceived strengths, challenges, and new delivery models. *Clinical Pediatrics, 51*, 978–982. doi:10.1177/0009922812441667.

DeNavas-Walt, C., & Proctor, B. D. (2014). *Income and poverty in the United States: 2013. U.S. Census Bureau*, Current Population Reports, P60-249. U.S. Government Printing Office: Washington, DC. Retrieved from http://www.census.gov/content/dam/Census/library/publications/2014/demo/p60-249.pdf?eml=gd&utm_medium=email&utm_source=govdelivery.

Eaton, D. K., Kann, L., Kinchen, S., Shanklin, S., Flint, K. H., Hawkins, J., … Wechsler, H. (2012). Youth risk behavior surveillance—United States, 2011, *Morbidity and Mortality Weekly Report, 61*, 1–162. Retrieved from http://www.cdc.gov/mmwr/pdf/ss/ss6104.pdf.

Finch, S. A., Weiley, V., Ip, E. H., & Barkin, S. (2008). Impact of pediatricians' perceived self-efficacy and confidence on violence prevention counseling: A national study. *Maternal and Child Health Journal, 12*, 75–82. doi:10.1007/s10995-007-0223-2.

Garcia, E. E., & Miller, L. S. (2008). Findings and recommendations of the national task force on early childhood education for Hispanics. *Child Development Perspectives, 2*, 53–58. doi:10.1111/j.1750-8606.2008.00042.x.

Glew, G. M., Fan, M. Y., Katon, W., & Rivara, F. P. (2008). Bullying and school safety. *The Journal of Pediatrics, 152*, 123–128. doi:10.1016/j.jpeds.2007.05.045.

González, R. A., Vélez-Pastrana, M. C., Ruiz Varcárcel, J. J., Levin, F. R., & Albizu-García, C. E. (2015). Childhood ADHD symptoms are associated with lifetime and current illicit substance-use disorders and in-site health risk behaviors in a representative sample of Latino prison inmates. *Journal of Attention Disorders, 19*, 301–312. doi:10.1177/1087054712461690.

Guevara, J. P., Greenbaum, P. E., Shera, D., Bauer, L., & Schwarz, D. F. (2009). Survey of mental health consultation and referral among primary care pediatricians. *Academic Pediatrics, 9*, 123–127. doi:10.1016/j.acap.2008.12.008.

Halfon, N., Stevens, G. D., Larson, K., & Olson, L. M. (2011). Duration of a well-child visit: Association with content, family-centeredness, and satisfaction. *Pediatrics, 128*, 657–664. doi:10.1542/peds.2011-05860.

He, M., Wilmoth, S., Bustos, D., Jones, T., Leeds, J., & Yin, Z. (2013). Latino church leaders' perspectives on childhood obesity prevention. *American Journal of Preventive Medicine, 44*, S232–S239. doi:10.1016/j.amepre.2012.11.014.

High, P. C., Klass, P., & Council on Early Childhood. (2014). American Academy of Pediatrics policy statement: Literacy Promotion: An essential component of primary care pediatric practice. *Pediatrics, 134*, 404–409. doi:10.1542/peds.2014.1384.

Hingson, R. W., & Zha, W. (2009). Age of drinking onset, alcohol use disorders, frequent heavy drinking, and unintentionally injuring oneself and others after drinking. *Pediatrics, 123*, 1477–1484. doi:10.1542/peds.2008-2176.

Hogue, A., Henderson, C. E., Ozechowski, T. J., & Robbins, M. S. (2014). Evidence base on outpatient behavioral treatments for adolescent substance use: Updates and recommendations 2007–2013. *Journal of Clinical Child & Adolescent Psychology, 43*, 695–720. doi:10.1080/15374416.2014.915550.

Hwang, W., Chang, J., LaClair, M., & Paz, H. (2013). Effects of integrated delivery system on cost and quality. *American Journal of Managed Care, 19*, e175–e184.

Inkelas, M., Garro, N., McQuaid, E. L., & Ortega, A. N. (2008). Race/ethnicity, language, and asthma care: Findings from a 4-state survey. *Annals of Allergy, Asthma & Immunology, 100*, 120–127. doi:10.1016/S1081-1206(10)60420-6.

Kalarchian, M. A., & Marcus, M. D. (2012). Psychiatric comorbidity of childhood obesity. *International Review of Psychiatry, 24*, 241–246. doi:10.3109/09540261.2012.678818.

Kataoka, S. H., Zhang, L., & Wells, K. B. (2002). Unmet need for mental health care among U.S. children: Variation by ethnicity and insurance status. *American Journal of Psychiatry, 159*, 1548–1555. doi:10.1176/appi.ajp.159.9.1548.

Klinnert, M. D., Nelson, H. S., Price, M. R., Adinoff, A. D., Leung, D. Y. M., & Mrazek, D. A. (2001). Onset and persistence of childhood asthma: Predictors from infancy. *Pediatrics, 108*, e69. doi:10.1542/peds.108.4.e69.

Knox, L. M., Lomonaco, C., & Elster, A. (2005). American Medical Association's youth violence prevention training and outreach guide. *American Journal of Preventive Medicine, 29*, 226–229. http://dx.doi.org/10.1016/j.amepre.2005.08.029.

Kolko, D. J., Campo, J. V., Kilbourne, A. M., & Kelleher, K. (2012). Doctor-office collaborative care for pediatric behavioral problems: A preliminary clinical trial. *Archives of Pediatric & Adolescent Medicine, 166*, 224–231. doi:10.1001/archpediatrics.2011.201.

Kozyrskyj, A. L., Mai, X. M., McGrath, P., HayGlass, K. T., Becker, A. B., & MacNeil, B. (2008). Continued exposure to maternal distress in early life is associated with an increased risk of childhood asthma. *American Journal of Respiratory and Critical Care Medicine, 177*, 142–147. doi:10.1164/rccm.200703-381OC.

Lara, M., Akinbami, L., Flores, G., & Morgenstern, H. (2006). Heterogeneity of childhood asthma among Hispanic children: Puerto Rican children bear a disproportionate burden. *Pediatrics, 117*, 43–53. doi:10.1542/peds.2004-1714.

Levy, S. J., Kokotailo, P. K., & Committee on Substance Abuse. (2011). Substance use screening, brief intervention, and referral to treatment for pediatricians. *Pediatrics, 128*, e1330–e1340. doi:10.1542/peds.2011-1754.

Mayer-Davis, E. J., Bell, R. A., Dabelea, D., D'Agostino Jr., R., Imperatore, G., Lawrence, J. M., … Marcovina, S. (2009). The many faces of diabetes in American youth: Type 1 and type 2 diabetes in five race and ethnic populations: The SEARCH for diabetes in youth study. *Diabetes Care, 32*, S99–S101. doi:10.2337/dc09-S201.

McQuaid, E. L., & Abramson, N. W. (2009). Pediatric asthma. In M. C. Roberts & R. G. Steele (Eds.), *Handbook of pediatric psychology* (4th ed., pp. 254–270). New York, NY: The Guilford Press.

Mendelsohn, A. L., Valdez, P. T., Flynn, V., Foley, G. M., Berkule, S. B., Tomopoulos, S., … Dreyer, B. P. (2007). Use of videotaped interactions during pediatric well-child care: Impact at 33 months on parenting and on child development. *Journal of Developmental & Behavioral Pediatrics, 28*, 206–212. doi:10.1097/DBP.0b013e3180324d87.

Morgan, P. L., Staff, J., Hillemeier, M. M., Farkas, G., & Maczuga, S. (2014). Racial and ethnic disparities in ADHD diagnosis from kindergarten to eighth grade. *Pediatrics, 132*, 85–93. doi:10.1542/peds.2012-2390.

Mosnaim, G., Kohrman, C., Sharp, L. K., Wolf, M. E., Sadowski, L. S., Ramos, L., & Grammer, L. C. (2006). Coping with asthma in immigrant Hispanic families: A focus group study. *Annals of Allergy, Asthma & Immunology, 97*, 477–483. doi: 10.1016/S1081-1206(10)60938-6.

Murphey, D., Guzman, L., & Torres, A. (2014). America's Hispanic children: Gaining ground, looking forward. *Child Trends*. Retrieved from http://www.childtrends.org/wp-content/uploads/2014/09/2014-38AmericaHispanicChildren.pdf.

Myers, K., Vander Stoep, A., Thompson, K., Zhou, C., & Unützer, J. (2010). Collaborative care for the treatment of Hispanic children diagnosed with attention-deficit hyperactivity disorder. *General Hospital Psychiatry, 32*, 612–614. doi:10.1016/j.genhosppsych.2010.08.004.

Nasir, A., Watanabe-Galloway, S., & DiRenzo-Coffey, G. (2014). Health services for behavioral problems in pediatric primary care. *Journal of Behavioral Health Services & Research*. Advance online publication. doi: 10.1007/s11414-014-9450-7.

National Center for Children in Poverty. (2006). *Children's mental health: Facts for policymakers*. Retrieved from http://www.nccp.org/publications/pdf/text_687.pdf.

National Institute of Mental Health. (2006). *Mental illness exacts heavy toll, beginning in youth*. Retrieved from http://www.nimh.nih.gov/news/science-news/2005/mental-illness-exacts-heavy-toll-beginning-in-youth.shtml.

National Institutes of Health. (2007). *Expert panel report 3: Guidelines for the diagnosis and management of asthma—Full report 2007*. Bethesda, MD: Author. Retrieved from http://www.nhlbi.nih.gov/files/docs/guidelines/asthgdln.pdf.

Ogden, C. L., Carroll, M. D., Kit, B. K., & Flegal, K. M. (2014). Prevalence of childhood and adult obesity in the United States, 2011-2012. *JAMA, 311*, 806–814. doi:10.1001/jama.2014.732.

Pearson, J. L., Stanley, B., King, C., & Fisher, C. (2001). *Issues to consider in intervention research with persons at high risk for suicidality*. Retrieved from http://www.nimh.nih.gov/health/topics/suicide-prevention/issues-to-consider-in-intervention-research-with-persons-at-high-risk--for-suicidality.shtml.

Pidano, A. E. (2007). How primary care providers respond to children's mental health needs: Strategies and barriers. In *Impact*. Farmington, CT: Child Health and Development Institute of Connecticut, Inc.. Retrieved from http://www.chdi.org/files/5614/1203/7734/impact_how_primary_care_providers_respond_to_children_with_mental_health_needs.pdf.

Pidano, A. E., Kimmelblatt, C. A., & Nease, W. P. (2011). Behavioral health in the pediatric primary care setting: Needs, barriers, and implications for psychologists. *Psychological Services, 8*, 151–165. doi:10.1037/a0019535.

Prado, G., Schwartz, S. J., Pattatucci-Aragon, A., Clatts, M., Pantin, H., Fernandez, M. I., … Szapocznik, J. (2006). The prevention of HIV transmission in Hispanic adolescents. *Drug Alcohol Dependence, 84(S1)*, S43–S53. doi: 10.1016/j.drugalcdep.2006.05.006.

Puder, J. J., & Munsch, S. (2010). Psychological correlates of childhood obesity. *International Journal of Obesity, 34*, S37–S43. doi:10.1038/ijo.2010.238.

Renda, J., Vassallo, S., & Edwards, B. (2011). Bullying in early adolescence and its association with anti-social behaviour, criminality and violence 6 and 10 years later. *Criminal Behaviour and Mental Health, 21*, 117–127. doi:10.1002/cbm.805.

Risser, A. L., & Mazur, L. J. (1995). Use of folk remedies in a Hispanic population. *Archives of Pediatric & Adolescent Medicine, 149*, 978–981. doi:10.1001/archpedi.1995.02170220044006.

Rohde, L. A., Szobot, C., Polanczyk, G., Schmitz, M., Martins, S., & Tramontina, S. (2005). Attention-deficit/hyperactivity disorder in a diverse culture: Do research and clinical findings support the notion of a cultural construct for the disorder? *Biological Psychiatry, 57*, 1436–1441. doi:10.1016/j.biopsych.2005.

Saloner, B., Carson, N., & Lê Cook, B. (2014). Explaining racial/ethnic differences in adolescent substance abuse treatment completion in the United States: A decomposition analysis. *Journal of Adolescent Health, 54*, 646–653. doi:10.1016/j.jadohealth.2014.01.002.

Sanders, L. M., Gershon, T. D., Huffman, L. C., & Mendoza, F. S. (2000). Prescribing books for immigrant children: A pilot study to promote emergent literacy among the children of Hispanic immigrants. *Archives of Pediatric & Adolescent Medicine, 154*, 771–777. doi:10.1001/archpedi.154.8.771.

Santiago, C. D., Kaltman, S., & Miranda, J. (2013). Poverty and mental health: How do low-income adults and children fare in psychotherapy? *Journal of Clinical Psychology: In Session, 69*, 115–126. doi:10.1002/jclp.21951.

Sheldrick, R. C., Merchant, S., & Perrin, E. C. (2011). Identification of developmental-behavioral problems in primary care: A systematic review. *Pediatrics, 128*, 356–363. doi:10.1542/peds.2010-3261.

Shetgiri, R., Kataoka, S., Ponce, N., Flores, G., & Chung, P. J. (2010). Adolescent fighting: Racial/ethnic disparities and the importance of families and schools. *Academic Pediatrics, 10*, 323–329. doi:10.1016/j.acap.2010.06.004.

Smith, J. C., & Medalia, C. (2014). *Health insurance coverage in the United States: 2013. U.S. Census Bureau*, Current Population Reports, P60-250, U.S. Government Printing Office: Washington, DC. Retrieved from https://www.census.gov/content/dam/Census/library/publications/2014/demo/p60-250.pdf.

Snethen, J. A., Hewitt, J. B., & Petering, D. H. (2007). Addressing childhood overweight: Strategies learned from one Latino community. *Journal of Transcultural Nursing, 18*, 366–372. doi:10.1177/1043659607305197.

Stacia, M., Patricia, L., Diane, M. M., Darwin, D., Alice, F., Jason, F., Arthur, B. (2010). Evaluation of health educator consults in primary care. *Health Education, 110*, 209–224. http://dx.doi.org/10.1108/09654281011038877.

Stancin, T., & Perrin, E. C. (2014). Psychologists and pediatricians: Opportunities for collaboration in primary care. *American Psychologist, 69*, 332–343. doi:10.1037/a0036046.

Stancin, T., Perrin, E. C., & Ramirez, L. (2009). Pediatric psychology and primary care. In M. C. Roberts, R. G. Steele, M. C. Roberts, & R. G. Steele (Eds.), *Handbook of pediatric psychology* (4th ed., pp. 630–646). New York, NY: Guilford Press.

Stevens, J., Kelleher, K. J., Ward-Estes, J., & Hayes, J. (2006). Perceived barriers to treatment and psychotherapy attendance in child community mental health centers. *Community Mental Health Journal, 42*, 449–458. doi:10.1007/s10597-006-9048-5.

Taveras, E. M., Gortmaker, S. L., Mitchell, K. F., & Gillman, M. W. (2008). Parental perceptions of overweight counseling in primary care: The roles of race/ethnicity and parent overweight. *Obesity, 16*, 1794–1801. doi:10.1038/oby.2008.264.

van der Wal, M. F., de Wit, C. A., & Hirasing, R. A. (2003). Psychosocial health among young victims and offenders of direct and indirect bullying. *Pediatrics, 111*, 1312–1317.

Van Landeghem, K., & Hess, C. A. (2005). Children's mental health: An overview and key considerations for health system stakeholders. *Children's Mental Health.* Retrieved from http://www.nihcm.org/pdf/CMHReport-FINAL.pdf.

Weiss, R., Dziura, J., Burgert, T. S., Tamborlane, W. V., Taksali, S. E., Yeckel, C. W., … Caprio, S. (2004). Obesity and the metabolic syndrome in children and adolescents. *New England Journal of Medicine, 350*, 2362–2374. doi:10.1056/NEJMoa031049.

Whiteside, L. K., & Cunningham, R. M. (2009). Youth violence: Effective screening and prevention. *Virtual Mentor, 11*, 117–123.

Wright, R. J., Visness, C. M., Calatroni, A., Grayson, M. H., Gold, D. R., Sandel, M. T., Gern, J. E. (2010). Prenatal maternal stress and cord blood innate and adaptive cytokine responses in an inner-city cohort. *American Journal of Respiratory and Critical Care Medicine, 182*, 25–33. doi:10.1164/rccm.200904-0637OC.

Zisser, A., & Eyberg, S. M. (2010). Treating oppositional behavior in children using parent-child interaction therapy. In A. E. Kazdin & J. R. Weisz (Eds.), *Evidence-based psychotherapies for children and adolescents* (2nd ed., pp. 179–193). New York, NY: Guilford.

Zuckerman, B., Parker, S., Kaplan-Sanoff, M., Augustyn, M., & Barth, M. C. (2004). Healthy steps: A case study of innovation in pediatric practice. *Pediatrics, 114*, 820–826. doi:10.1542/peds.2003-0999-L.

Chapter 10
Integrated Depression Care Among Latinos

Susan Caplan and Frances Munet-Vilaró

Introduction

When asked to write this chapter on integrated depression care in primary care, I thought about my own experiences as a primary care provider two decades ago. At that time, there was no mental health parity and minimal or no insurance coverage of mental health conditions, and if there was coverage, there was no place to send my monolingual Spanish speaking patients, a problem that in the subsequent 20 years, remains a persistent barrier to health care access (Bridges, Andrews, & Deen, 2012). Thus, integrated care consisted of dispensing the SSRI du jour that the pharmaceutical rep had recently deposited. Yet it was also more than that. As we now know, it's the relationship with the provider that influences outcomes more than whatever technique is used and as a primary care provider who sees patients on a regular basis, one may be able to experience the privilege of being confided in and trusted by our patients. I heard from a Puerto Rican woman whose son committed suicide several years prior, upon return from Desert Storm and a Dominican woman whose children had become "too American" and no longer shared her values. There was a Mexican man, a former teacher who was experiencing a profound sense of grief due to his wife's infertility. A well-educated Ecuadorian woman quietly and tearfully spoke of having to leave her children behind while fleeing from a physically abusive husband. There was the Dominican woman who came every week with a new ailment, headaches, stomach aches, chest pain whom I prodded with the gentle question, "is there something going on in your life?" I quietly listened to the tearful Colombian woman who was grieving the loss of her 21-year-old son. "How did he die?" I asked. She responded that he was fleeing the military juntas and guerillas in Colombia, and boarded a boat that landed in Brazil. The ship's cargo of

S. Caplan (✉) • F. Munet-Vilaró
School of Nursing, Rutgers University, The State University of New Jersey,
180 University Avenue, Newark, NJ 07102, USA
e-mail: sc1140@sn.nursing.edu

© Springer International Publishing Switzerland 2016

L.T. Benuto, W. O'Donohue (eds.), *Enhancing Behavioral Health in Latino Populations*, DOI 10.1007/978-3-319-42533-7_10

illegal immigrants was detained in prison and the son mysteriously was found dead the next morning. When my patient, his mother, was finally able to arrange with the Consulate to send his body back to Colombia, an autopsy was performed to determine the cause of death. It was impossible to determine the cause of death because her son's body had been disemboweled. It is in these intimate interactions that we begin to understand some of the underlying factors contributing to depression in our patients.

Depression is the leading cause of disability in the United States (Lopez, Mathers, Ezzati, Jamison, & Murray, 2001). In spite of successful treatment options for depression, 75 % of Americans do not receive adequate care (Shim, Baltrus, Ye, & Rust, 2011). Treatment rates among low-acculturated Hispanics, also referred to as Latinos and Latinos with limited English proficiency, are significantly lower (Alegría, Polo, et al., 2008; Bauer, Chen, & Alegría, 2010). People of Hispanic origin (Latinos) are the largest minority group in the United States, representing 17 % of the population (United States Census Bureau, 2013a). By 2060, it is predicted that Latinos will make up 31 % of the United States population, or approximately one in three residents (United States Census Bureau, 2012). Although, past year mental illness and depression rates for Latinos are similar or slightly less than the population as a whole, 15.3 vs. 19 (any mental illness) and 6.9 % vs. 7 % respectively for depression, this differs by ethnic background, nativity, and generational status (Alegría, Mulvaney-Day, Torres, Polo, et al., 2007; SAMSHA, 2015). Puerto Ricans have higher rates of depression than non-Hispanic Whites (Alegría, Mulvaney-Day, Torres, Polo, et al., 2007). Moreover, many Latinos have demographic characteristics that increase their vulnerability to depression: unemployment, poverty, chronic illness, exposure to violence and chronic stress, and less than a high school education (Bromet et al., 2011; March et al., 2014). Latinos are among the most impoverished of all ethnic and racial groups in the United States, with one quarter of Latinos living in poverty compared to 11.6 % of non-Hispanic Whites (Taylor, Kochhar, Fry, Velasco, & Motel, 2011; United States Census Bureau, 2013b). Among primary care populations, refugees, and monolingual Spanish-speaking populations, there is a high prevalence of affective disorders, estimated at 20–45 % due to the above-mentioned factors associated with depression (Cardemil et al., 2007; March et al., 2014; Tarricone et al., 2012). In addition, for Latino immigrants, experiences of loss of previously existing social support systems, changes in cultural values, and social roles are stressors that have been associated with depression, as well as perceived discrimination, and neighborhood safety (Alegría, Shrout, Woo, Guarnaccia, et al., 2007).

Latinos suffer from large health disparities when compared to non-Hispanic Whites (Alegría, Mulvaney-Day, Torres, Polo, et al., 2007; Alegría, Mulvaney-Day, Woo, Torres, et al., 2007; SAMSHA, 2015). Only half of Latino immigrants with severe mental health disorders receive any type of mental health treatment (SAMSHA, 2015). The rates of mental health service use from 2008 to 2012 for any mental illness were 27.3 % for Hispanics compared to 46.3 % for non-Hispanic Whites (SAMSHA, 2015). These mental health disparities also include decreased access to care and lower rates of care that conform to evidenced-based guidelines in terms of referrals for specialty mental health care, psychopharmacology, and duration of treatment compared to non-Hispanic Whites (Alegría, Mulvaney-Day, Woo, Torres, et al., 2007; Alegría, Polo, et al., 2008; Shim et al., 2011).

Factors Contributing to Health Care Disparities

Disparities in mental health care for Latinos may be due to systemic barriers to obtaining treatment, including an insufficient supply of Medicaid specialty services in Latino neighborhoods creating long waits for treatment, lack of bilingual providers and language barriers, and lack of adequate insurance (Alegría, Polo, et al., 2008; González, Tarraf, Whitfield, & Vega, 2010; González, Vega, et al., 2010; SAMSHA, 2015). However, when taking into account many of these factors, Latino mental health care utilization is still half that of Hispanics (SAMSHA, 2015). Thus, provider and patient level factors strongly influence decisions to seek help, particularly in undiagnosed conditions when cultural factors and level of acculturation become particularly salient (Keyes et al., 2012). When Latinos do seek mental health care services, it is most often in the primary care sector (Alegría, Mulvaney-Day, Woo, Torres, et al., 2007). Although research consistently indicates that Latinos prefer therapy to medication (Dwight-Johnson et al., 2010; Interian, Lewis-Fernandez, Gara, & Escobar, 2013; Vargas et al., 2015), preferences do not determine actual uptake of treatment. In one sample of Latinos in the Northeast, there was a greater likelihood that patients would follow recommendations for pharmacological treatment, rather than psychotherapy, most likely due to the fact that medication is a much more accessible form of treatment (Ishikawa et al., 2014).

There are numerous patient-level factors contributing to low treatment rates for mental disorders among Latinos. Language barriers or educational level contributing to low mental health literacy, and stigma are significant barriers to care (Alegría, Shrout, Woo, Guarnaccia, et al., 2007; Tarricone et al., 2012). Language barriers make it difficult for the Latino patient to understand the options available to treat depression. Results of some research indicate that patients have better outcomes when they are culturally and linguistically matched with their mental health provider (Sue, 1988). However, Latino primary care providers and mental health providers, in particular, are underrepresented in the health care workforce (Jackson & Gracia, 2014).

Cultural values and beliefs, including the reluctance to share personal problems outside of the family and disclose personal problems, a value on self-sufficiency, and stigma about mental illness create barriers to treatment engagement (Cabassa, Lester, & Zayas, 2007; Caplan et al., 2013; Interian, Martinez, Guarnaccia, Vega, & Escobar, 2007; Nadeem et al., 2007; Vega, Rodriguez, & Ang, 2010). Thus, it becomes essential to understand the barriers to treatment engagement and develop a roadmap to facilitate effective and quality care for Latino patients with depression. In this chapter we will walk you through the steps of effective care from: (1) recognition of and screening for depression; (2) understanding cultural barriers to treatment engagement; (3) strategies to improve treatment engagement; (4) providing evidenced-based treatment; and (5) situating depression care within the appropriate social, economic, and political context.

Recognition of and Screening for Depression

Depression is far more frequently diagnosed and treated in the primary care setting than in specialty mental health care (Harman, Veazie, & Lyness, 2006; Uebelacker, Wang, Berglund, & Kessler, 2006). Primary care providers (PCPs) are responsible for providing up to 80 % of all prescriptions for antidepressants (Mojtabai & Olfson, 2008). Nevertheless, access to treatment is hindered by lack of recognition in primary care in as many as 30–60 % of patients (Borowsky et al., 2000; Kamphuis et al., 2012; Mitchell, Vaze, & Rao, 2009; Schmaling & Hernandez, 2005). Primary care providers' recognition of depression is increased the more often a patient is seen (Menchetti, Belvederi-Murri, Bertakis, Bortolotti, & Berardi, 2009). However, many Latinos and individuals with limited English proficiency do not have a usual source of health care (Agency for Healthcare Research and Quality [AHRQ], 2010).

Although the United States Preventive Services Task Force (USPSTF) (USPSTF) (2009) has recommended screening of all patients for depression in the primary care setting when systems are in place to provide appropriate treatment and follow-up, most patients do not receive screening. Instead primary care providers rely on their own clinical judgment, which is much less effective in detecting depression than the use of formal screening instruments (AHRQ, 2013). The Patient Health Questionnaire (PHQ-9) (Kroenke, Spitzer, & Williams, 2001) is the most commonly used depression screener in primary care. It is a 9-item scale with a sensitivity of 88 % and a specificity of 88 % for major depression at a score of greater than or equal to 10 (Kroenke et al., 2001). When the PHQ-9 is used to screen it aids in the initiation of treatment (Moore et al., 2012); however, it has not been shown to be consistently used in primary care (Fuchs et al., 2015; Gilbody, Richards, Brealey, & Hewitt, 2007). A shorter version of the PHQ-9, the PHQ-2 just uses the first two questions of the PHQ-9:

"To what extent have you been bothered by the following:

(1) Little interest or pleasure in doing things and
(2) Feeling down, depressed, or hopeless?" (Kroenke, Spitzer, & Williams, 2003).

The PHQ-2 is highly sensitive as a first step in the screening process when followed by the PHQ-9 and can be self-administered in the waiting room.

For patients who may not be literate in Spanish or English there is a bilingual computerized voice recognition screener that is as reliable as paper and pencil administration Muñoz, McQuaid, González, Dimas, and Rosales (1999)(or an Interactive Voice Response System which can be used via phone screening, Kim et al., 2012).

While the PHQ-9 has been shown to be reliable in Spanish-speaking populations (Diez-Quevedo, Rangil, Sanchez-Planell, Kroenke, & Spitzer, 2001; Wulsin, Somoza, & Heck, 2002), there are instances where the validity may be questionable for Latino immigrants (Caplan et al., 2010). In a study of 177 predominantly Colombian, Ecuadorian, and Dominican immigrants in primary care, 21 participants perceived that they had a mental health problem, but did not meet criteria for depression on the PHQ-9 (subjective depression). Participants' descriptions of symptoms had a predominantly somatic component. The most common complaints were *ánimo bajo* (low energy) and *decaimiento* (weakness). Participants with "subjective" depression had mean scores of somatic symptoms and depression severity that were significantly lower than the participants with "objective" depression and significantly higher than the group with no depression ($P < 0.0001$). Therefore, it is possible that some Latinos with depression may be missed by traditional depression screeners. These patients still have significant distress and impairment. To avoid having these patients "fall through the cracks," it is important to take into account culturally accepted idiomatic and behavioral expressions of distress and the meaning of illness for the individual and develop alternative ways of screening for depression (Sentell & Braun, 2012).

Self-Rated Health. One of the often cited reasons that primary care providers do not formally screen is lack of time. Many providers prefer a targeted approach of screening people they believe to be at high risk. If this approach seems more feasible in one's particular setting, certainly all patients with chronic illness should be screened given the high comorbidities of depression and chronic illness (Ducat, Philipson, & Anderson, 2014; Houts, Lipinski, Olsen, Baldwin, & Hasan, 2010; Scott et al., 2007). Given the time constraints in primary care, one very important question to ask about is self-rated health. How would you rate your health?

Self-rated health has been defined as the intersection of biology and culture since it relies upon lay meanings of symptoms (Jylha, 2009). Self-rated health has consistently been a predictor of mortality, primarily because it encompasses more than a biomedical definition of health, and includes functional abilities, social relationships, mental health, and spirituality. In one study of Puerto Ricans in the Northeast, depressive symptoms, functional problems, allostatic load (an indicator of the biological stress response), and physical comorbidities strongly predicted self-rated health (Todorova et al., 2013). Thus, one simple, fast, and potentially effective screening method would be to add in an open-ended question on self-rated health: "How would you rate your health? Responses range from 1 to 5: 1—Excellent (Excelente), 2—Very Good (Muy Buena), 3—Good, (Buena), 4—Fair (Regular), 5—Poor (Mala)" ***in addition to using the PHQ-2 as described above***.

Once you are satisfied that your patient has depression that cannot be managed with watchful waiting, the next question is how do you effectively convey that information to your patient, in a manner that is acceptable to the patient? Many Latinos will not follow-up on a recommendation to seek treatment in the specialty mental health care sector (De Figueiredo, Boerstler, & Doros, 2009) or even within an integrated primary care behavioral health care system (Caplan & Whittemore, 2013).

Understanding Cultural Barriers to Treatment Engagement

Treatment engagement is a concept that encompasses identification of a mental health problem, the decision to seek professional care, maintaining engagement throughout the course of care, adherence to treatment, and minimization of drop-out (Interian et al., 2013). For Latinos, the low cultural congruence of behavioral health treatment is a strong contributing factor to lower rates of treatment engagement (Vargas et al., 2015). The level of a Primary Care Provider's (PCP) cultural competence can determine the uptake of a recommendation to seek care for depression (Ishikawa et al., 2014). For example, Latinos use Spanish idioms to refer to affective feelings that don't necessarily translate well into English. In addition, the use of somatic symptoms to express emotional distress is also very common (Cheng, Chen, & Cunningham, 2007; Elder, Ayala, Parra-Medina, & Talavera, 2009; Katon, 1982; Rogler, Cortes, & Malgady, 1994). Providers not familiar with these types of behaviors might have difficulty making an accurate diagnosis and providing the appropriate referrals to treatment (Vargas et al., 2015).

What are Latino cultural values and how might they influence care? Latino values differ by ethnic group, class, level of acculturation, and geographic area. However, there are a few values that transcend between group differences. One particular cultural value among Latinos, *Familismo*, or the belief in strong family connections and unity, is believed to have a major influence, both positive and negative, upon help-seeking (Villatoro, Morales, & Mays, 2014). The value of *Familismo* may influence help-seeking either due to stigma or reluctance to disclose personal problems to outsiders, or fear of burdening one's family or guilt about being depressed (Dunn & O'Brien, 2009).

In Latino culture, *Machismo* (male gender roles) may be evidenced in behaviors that include honor, pride, and responsibility (Arciniega, Anderson, Tovar Blank, & Tracey, 2008) but may also include traits such as high alcohol consumption and a sense of entitlement and control within the family (Edelson, Hokoda, & Ramos-Lira, 2007). *Marianismo*, derived from beliefs about the Virgin Mary is an ideal female role that exalts endurance of suffering, submission, and self-sacrifice and the responsibility for mothers to create peaceful family relationships (Andres-Hyman, Ortiz, Paris, Davidson, & Añez, 2006). Acculturation can result in changing gender roles, that increase women's power, but also can increase familial stress. Latino culture emphasizes that men should be the breadwinners and women, the homemakers. Thus, traditional male and female roles in Latino culture may inhibit help-seeking.

The cultural value of *Personalismo*, or the importance of individual relationships and social interactions, rather than institutional loyalties, has strong implications for quality of care. Research has shown that the quality of the PCP relationship with the patient in terms of trustworthiness, genuineness, and openness in communication style will positively affect the outcomes of treatment recommendations (Kravitz et al., 2011). Moreover, the cultural value of *Respeto* (respect) for people in positions of authority will make it less likely that Latinos will voice disagreement or a reluctance to follow treatment recommendations.

Cultural and religious values are also apparent in many Latinos' attitudes towards coping with depression. For many Latinos, depression signifies weakness of character, lack of faith in God, an inability to confront life's challenges (Caplan & Cordero, 2015). Many Latinos believe that depression can be overcome by willpower (*fuerza de voluntad*), not paying attention to it, (*no darle mente*) or controlling oneself (*controlarse*) (Vargas et al., 2015). Latinos tend to have higher endorsement of cognitive escape/avoidance and distancing as a way of coping with physical and emotional health issues (Munet-Vilaró, Gregorich, & Folkman, 2002). Although some types of escapist coping are related to negative mental health outcomes (Folkman & Moskowitz, 2004), in some instances, the use of such strategies (wishful thinking, daydreaming) may actually reflect hope and are thus, not necessarily negative.

Strategies to Improve Treatment Engagement

There are a number of important tools to enable the PCP to most effectively overcome barriers to treatment engagement and effectively increase the likelihood that the patient will agree to a recommendation for treatment of depression. These strategies may include: (a) ethnographic interviewing, (b) the warm hand-off, increasing health literacy, (c) minimizing stigma, and (d) creating a working alliance.

Ethnographic Interviewing

Ethnographic interviewing is a means to understanding of the patient's perceptions of illness. Attention to cultural aspects of care is a critical component in engaging patients in care (Balan, Moyers, & Lewis-Fernandez, 2013; Benish, Quintana, & Wampold, 2011). There are specific assessment questions designed to understand the sociocultural contexts of people's health care needs (Kleinman, 1980) the noted medical anthropologist, recommends the following eight questions:

1. "What do you call the problem?
2. What do you think has caused the problem?
3. Why do you think it started when it did?
4. What do you think the sickness does? How does it work?
5. How severe is the sickness? Will it have a long or a short course?
6. What kind of treatment do you think the patient should receive?
7. What are the chief problems the sickness has caused?
8. What do you fear most about the sickness?"

Beginning a conversation about depression treatment with some version of the above questions will help to clarify treatment expectations for both the provider and patient (Fernandez et al., 2011).

The Warm Hand-Off

Due to the cultural value of *Personalismo* it is recommended that the referral to the mental health provider who is situated in the primary care setting be accomplished by personally introducing the patient to the mental health provider (Manoleas, 2008). This is believed to reduce stigma and aid in uptake of the referral. However, a recent study examining that hypothesis showed the many nuances in context and implementation of the warm hand-off. The warm hand-off did not make a difference in uptake for referrals among Spanish-speaking primary care patients and actually diminished the likelihood of seeing a specialist among English-speaking participants (Horevitz, Organista, & Arean, 2015). Details of the precise manner the hand-off was implemented in this study are lacking and in some instances, a warm-hand off conducted by a Medical Assistant rather than personally by the PCP may have been off-putting for patients. Nevertheless, these data indicate that it may be premature to endorse the concept of the warm hand-off.

Increasing Health Literacy

Health literacy and the understanding of depression as a treatable illness may also affect help seeking behaviors (Horner-Johnson, Dobbertin, Lee, & Andresen, 2014; Koskan, Friedman, & Messias, 2010; US Department of Health and Human Services, 2015). Although unique culture-specific life experiences are shared by many Latino groups, their understanding, responses to distress and depression, and the seriousness they place on the expression of distress may differ (Myers et al., 2015). Among some Latinos, there is the belief that succumbing to depression will eventually lead to craziness (Vargas et al., 2015). Latinos may label their illness as "stress," rather than depression (Caplan et al., 2010; Vargas et al., 2015). Major stressors that impact the mental health in the lives of Latino cultural groups living in the U.S. include health, family, and intergenerational conflict, discrimination, underemployment and exploitive employment, financial issues, and unsafe living environments (Falcon, Todorova, & Tucker, 2009; Greenberg, 2006). Trying to adapt to a new lifestyle and the impact of dissimilar cultural norms can generate anxiety and emotional dissonance that contributes to or creates other major sources of emotional distress (McIntyre, Korn, & Matsuo, 2008; Nicklett & Burgard, 2009; Torres & Rollock, 2007). While stressful events are experienced by many, Latinos tend to disregard the effect daily stressful events have on their mood and well-being (Munet-Vilaró, Folkman, & Gregorich, 1999; Winkelman, Chaney, & Bethel, 2013).

Minimizing Stigma

Mental health diagnoses often result in experiences of stigma and shame for the person bearing the diagnosis. Indeed, labeling a person is one of the underlying mechanisms in the process of stigmatizing and individual (Link, Yang, Phelan, &

Collins, 2004). Labeled people can be negatively categorized by the dominant society as "us and them," resulting in separation, status loss, and discrimination. Thus, other words that convey emotional distress might be more acceptable to the patient and result in greater acceptance of the need for treatment. "Stress," "family problems," are much less laden with negative connotations and are something people can understand.

Working Alliance

The PCP's working alliance is a key factor in a patient's decision to follow-up on treatment recommendations, although stated intention is not necessarily correlated with actual behavior (Ishikawa et al., 2014). Creating trusting bonds that leads to shared decision-making and understanding patients' views about treatment, their expectations of the kind of care they should be receiving are the most important ways to enhance patients' satisfaction with care (Julius, Novitsky, & Dubin, 2009; Lin & Fagerlin, 2014). The RESPECT framework for cultural assessment, based on the series of eight questions developed by Kleinman (listed above), provides a model for culturally competent assessment in the medical setting (Mostow et al., 2010). RESPECT is an acronym for Respect, Explanatory model, Sociocultural context, Power, Empathy, Concerns and fears, and Therapeutic alliance/trust.

Respect and *empathy* are attitudes that demonstrate to the patient that his/her concerns are valued and he/she is understood. The patient's *explanatory model* is his/her understanding of what is the cause of his/her illness. The *sociocultural context* denotes factors in a person's life that may contribute to the current state of health and expectations for treatment, such as poverty, stress, and social support. *Power* refers to the importance of acknowledging that the patient is in a vulnerable position and that there is a difference between patients and health care providers in terms of access to resources, knowledge level, and control over outcomes. The loss of power and control that a patient faces can contribute to *concerns and fears* about treatment, illness outcomes, and the future. These concepts can enhance communication and assessment skills and create a working alliance characterized by trust.

Providing Evidenced-Based Behavioral Interventions in Primary Care

The most comprehensive type of integrated behavioral healthcare (IBH) occurs when the mental health professional is embedded within the primary care team. Preliminary outcomes of this model indicates that it reduces depression, disparities in treatment engagement, increases satisfaction, and may reduce stigma and other barriers to care (Bridges et al., 2014). IBH has the potential to decrease disparities in quality of treatment.

Although evidenced-based psychotherapeutic treatment is equally effective in minorities and non-Hispanic Whites, they are less frequently utilized for Latino patients. Latinos are much less likely than non-Hispanic Whites to receive minimally adequate care, defined as four or more visits with a provider while taking antidepressant medication or eight or more visits with a specialty mental health provider (Alegría, Canino, et al., 2008). Between one half and two thirds of the population are likely to drop out of treatment, a statistic that is much worse among Latinos (Corrigan, 2004). Latinos are three times more likely than non-Hispanic Whites to stop going to therapy prematurely (Olfson, Moitabai, Sampson, Hwang, & Kessler, 2009).

Integrated mental health care requires innovative models of care delivery that address provider, systems-level barriers, and patient level barriers. These include the use of culturally modified interventions; technological innovations to mental health care delivery, and the use of community health workers and peer counselors.

Culturally Modified Interventions

Culturally modified psychotherapeutic and psychoeducational interventions can be used in primary care and have been shown to reduce health care disparities (Interian, Allen, Gara, & Escobar, 2008). The interventions with the strongest evidence base for use in Latinos with depression include Cognitive Behavioral Therapy (CBT), Behavioral Activation (BA), Mindfulness and Motivational Interviewing.

1. *CBT*. CBT is a widely recognized evidenced-based treatment for depression that is as effective in Latinos as in non-Hispanic Whites (Alegría, Ludman, et al., 2014; Miranda et al., 2003). Interian et al. (2008) have developed a culturally modified (Cognitive Behavioral Therapy) CBT intervention that was effectively piloted in the primary care setting. This intervention used the methods of CBT which include cognitive interventions that help patients recognize and identify patterns of thinking that contribute to negative self-evaluations. CBT also focuses on behaviors strategies that will counteract the effects of depression such as assertiveness training, relaxation, and increasing pleasurable activities (Beck et al., 1979). Cultural modification was employed by using a case-conceptualization approach that acknowledged the specific stressors that are predominant among low-income Hispanics. It was also employed in specific recommendations for behavioral strategies. For example, assertiveness training was adapted to include the cultural value of respect (*respeto*) so that assertiveness could be employed while maintaining respect. Similarly, cultural values were used to illustrate the value of changing cognitions such as (*poniendo de su parte*) or putting in effort.
2. *Behavioral activation*. Studies indicate that the application of behavioral activation therapy is effective in depression. Behavioral activation treatment (BAT) for

depression addresses problems a patient is experiencing in life that are not considered rewarding. Inaction is the most common depressive reaction to life situations that are not considered rewarding. Basic behavioral activation strategies are usually used in combination with cognitive behavioral therapy and initially target the inertia that occurs in depression. In BAT, emphasis is given to engaging the patient in activities that are considered rewarding and can be mastered; less emphasis is given to problems related to thoughts and biological processes (Lejuez, Hopko, Acierno, Daughters, & Pagoto, 2011). The patient is coached by the therapist to take an active participation in decision-making by establishing goals and begin to take steps to re-engage in life despite the lack of motivation or the negative feelings (Barry & Edgman-Levitan, 2012). Collaboration in the decision-making process is important when applying BA (Alegría, Carson, et al., 2014; Dimidjian, Barrera, Martell, Munoz, & Lewinsohn, 2011) and requires that both the client and clinician share information and that BA activities take into account the patients' cultural values and preferences (Barry, 2012; Comas-Diaz, 2006).

3. *Mindfulness-meditation.* Another approach is mindfulness-meditation which is a method that has been used for more than two decades to treat psychiatric disorders including depression (Chiesa & Serretti, 2011). It has been successfully culturally modified and can be used in the primary care setting as a brief intervention to improve symptoms in people with chronic illness (Gucht, Takano, Broeck, & Raes, 2015; Keyworth et al., 2014). This approach emphasizes focused, nonjudgmental awareness of experiences happening in the present moment as an alternative to worrying about future situations. Some studies have found that this therapy can help patients improve their quality of life and particularly with bilingual patients, help them manage their stress and anxiety (Roth & Robbins, 2004). Mindfulness-based stress reduction (MBSR) is a series of techniques that an individual or group of individuals can use such as informal mindfulness, yoga, and mindful breathing, that teaches directed attention to reduce anxiety (Keng, Smoski, & Robins, 2011) and depression (Deyo, Wilson, Ong, & Koopman, 2009; Godfrin & Van Heeringen, 2010).
4. *Motivational interviewing.* The use of motivational interviewing (MI), that is, the process of talking to a person in an empathetic and nonconfrontational way is an approach that can create confidence in the patient to actively participate in treatment decisions and facilitate interaction between the provider and the patient (Balan et al., 2013; Lewis-Fernandez et al., 2013). This approach can be effective when providers use cultural terms and idioms patients are familiar with to explain symptoms, distinguish medically unexplained symptoms, and differentiate them from significant clinical signs (Añez, Paris, Bedregal, Davidson, & Grilo, 2005; Britigan, Murnan, & Rojas-Guyler, 2009; McCaffery, Smith, & Wolf, 2010; Sentell & Braun, 2012).

Many Latinos have the misconception that medications used in the treatment of depression are addictive (Interian et al., 2007; Vargas et al., 2015) and are not aware that depression has a genetic component (Caplan et al., 2013). This misconception can result in patients not accepting or adhering to their medication treatment. The use of motivational interviewing when integrated to psychopharmacotherapy sessions is reported to effectively facilitate interaction between the provider and the patient and improve adherence to medication for depression (Balan et al., 2013; Lewis-Fernandez et al., 2013). Motivational pharmacotherapy offers the provider and patient the opportunity to use their respective expertise when deciding medication treatment, encourages self-efficacy in patients so they can overcome barriers and can incorporate language and relevant cultural aspects that help the patient become engage in their pharmacotherapy. A motivational interviewing study on anti-depressive medication adherence that was adapted for Latinos found that the intervention was effective in helping patients change their conceptual and emotional viewpoint of adhering to medication treatment from a perceived mandated therapy to a personal and motivational way to fight (l*ucha*r) for improving their mental health (Interian, Martinez, Rios, Krejci, & Guarnaccia, 2010).

Technology

Technological innovations to mental health care delivery include the use of mobile apps, computer-based applications of psychotherapy and psychoeducation, and telephone-based therapy. Telephone-based psychotherapy has shown to be effective in reducing levels of depression and improving mood (Ludman, Simon, Tutty, & Von Korff, 2007). A Spanish language culturally modified telephone CBT was more effective and cost saving than face-to-face CBT among Latino patients (Kafali, Cook, Canino, & Alegría, 2014).

Case Management and Community Health Workers

Many Latino immigrants in the U.S. might not have the social links or intercultural competence needed to learn how to access and utilize mental health care services that can assist them to cope with depression (Torres, 2010; Torres & Rollock, 2007). Community health workers (*promotoras*) are widely used in public health interventions and chronic disease prevention, because of their knowledge of the cultural and communities from which they are from and their ability to provide support, advocacy, and education.

1. *Peer to Peer Communication.* Similar to the support provided by Community Health Workers, peers can provide advocacy and increase access to care for people experiencing stigmatizing conditions, such as mental illness (Deering et al., 2009). Peer counseling programs have been successfully used to prevent depression among low income, minority families at high risk for depression (Acri, Olin, Burton, Herman, & Hoagwood, 2014; Boyd, Diamond, & Bourjolly, 2006). Among Latino populations, peers have also been used to implement depression screening and treatment engagement interventions through messages of

empowerment and patient activation or psychoeducation to train patients to ask questions and interact in a collaborative manner with their PCPs (Alegría, Polo, et al., 2008).

Situating Depression Care Within the Appropriate Social, Economic, and Political Context

The concept of integrated care is a misnomer if it solely refers to the incorporation of behavioral health care in the primary care setting. There is no such thing as "integrated behavioral health care is one fails to address the underlying social determinants of health that are among the primary root causes of depression: economic inequalities, discrimination, poverty, interpersonal violence (IPV), and lifelong exposure to adverse events" (Myers et al., 2015) and societal stigma that is a barrier to help-seeking for many people with depression (Corrigan, Morris, Michaels, Rafacz, & Rusch, 2012).

All ethnic and racial minority groups have poverty rates exceeding the national average for non-Hispanic Whites of 11.6 %. Among racial groups, the highest national poverty rates were for American Indians and Alaska Natives (27.0 %) followed by Blacks or African Americans (25.8 %) and Native Hawaiians and Other Pacific Islanders (17.6 %). By country of origin among Asians, poverty rates were highest for Vietnamese (14.7 %) and Koreans (15.0 %). Among Hispanics, poverty rates are highest for Dominicans, exceeding Blacks at 26.3 %, followed by, Puerto Ricans (25.6 %), Guatemalans, and Mexicans (24.9 %) and Salvadoreans (18/9 %) (Macartney, Bishaw, & Fontenot, 2013). Contributing to the high rates of poverty and psychosocial stressors among Dominicans and Puerto Ricans and African Americans are the two and three times higher than average rates of single parent homes with children under 18 when compared to non-Hispanic whites (Vespa, Lewis, & Kreider, 2013).

As a primary care provider, you may feel that it would be impossible to address societal factors that contribute to ill health. Thinking in this manner will ultimately lead to burn-out as you recognize that your treatment is essentially bandaging wounds. One of the most important ways to address the needs of our patients is to partner with communities and become informed of the community's health needs. Is the neighborhood too unsafe for children and parents to walk outside for exercise? Do the local corner groceries provide low fat products and fresh fruits? Is there are bus depot emitting fumes which contribute to high rates of asthma? Are there green spaces in the community? Working with Community Boards to identify and address health issues within the community is an effective way to ensure the long-term health of your patients.

A very high risk population that is often overlooked in primary care are patients with current or past histories of domestic violence, child abuse, and gender-based violence. Due to societal and economic stressors and cultural norms, racial and ethnic minorities, particularly immigrants in the United States may be at even greater risk for adverse psychiatric consequences of IPV. Lifetime prevalence of IPV, including rape, physical violence, and stalking among ethnic and racial minorities are significantly higher than among White women (Black et al., 2010).

Legal status in the United States is a societal aspect that creates barriers to care that affects many immigrant families. Immigration status impedes help-seeking behavior and provides a readily available mechanism by which women can be coerced. Women may silently endure domestic violence because of fears of being deported and losing their children. Some may fear that their partners will be jailed or deported leaving them without any financial support. Most immigrant women are not aware of the legal protections available to them (Bhuyan & Senturia, 2005) such as the U.S. Violence against Women Act (VAWA) which allows battered women living in the United States to petition for permanent resident status even if they leave their American partner.

Many immigrant and minority women will not disclose intimate details of their personal lives (Hamdy, 2004; Nicolaidis et al., 2011).

Internalized or self-perceived stigma inhibits help-seeking for depression, as well as IPV. Stigma also operates at the structural institutional level. Less funding is given to mental health research compared to other disorders and residential treatment facilities for psychiatric patients are often located in undesirable neighborhoods. Therefore, it is important to advocate for societal changes in mental health care and recommend that our patients join advocacy organizations such as the National Alliance for Mental Illness (NAMI) which has extensive programming and learning materials in Spanish.

Screening and Prevention of Domestic Violence. The United States Preventive Services Task Force has recently provided new guidelines recommending routine screening for IPV among women of childbearing age 18–46 (Moyer & U.S. Preventive Services, 2013). There is ample evidence of the benefits of screening as the health care risks of unaddressed IPV are great, including the chronic health conditions mentioned above; poor birth outcomes in pregnant women experiencing IPV (El-Mohandes, Kiely, Gantz, & El-Khorazaty, 2011; Shah, Shah, & Knowledge Synthesis Group on Determinants of Preterm/LBW Births, 2010); and chronic and persistent mental illnesses. Screening can be accomplished with the simple four question HITS which has strong validity in English- and Spanish-speaking populations.

As a provider, you may be thinking that you don't want to open that can of worms; however, women who experience IPV have greater psychological problems than women who have not experienced IPV, including PTSD, depression, low self-esteem, substance abuse, anxiety, eating disorders, and suicide attempts (Black et al., 2010; Coker et al., 2002; Edelson et al., 2007). Treating depression without addressing the underlying domestic violence that carries with it a high risk of injury or death is tantamount to malpractice. Effective interventions exist such as home visits, counseling, referrals to community service agencies and creating safety plans that have served to prevent these adverse outcomes, such as IPV in pregnancy; assaults and risk for homicide and prematurity in neonates (McFarlane, Groff, O'Brien, & Watson, 2005).

Truly integrated depression care for Latinos requires a multifaceted, interdisciplinary approach starting with community-based efforts at prevention, culturally sensitive screening, appropriate referrals, strategies to improve adherence and minimize drop-out, and effective behavioral interventions within the health care setting.

References

Acri, M., Olin, S. S., Burton, G., Herman, R. J., & Hoagwood, K. E. (2014). Innovations in the identification and referral of mothers at risk for depression: Development of a peer-to-peer model. *Journal of Child and Family Studies, 23*, 837–843. doi:10.1007/s10826-013-9736-z.

Agency for Healthcare Research and Quality (AHRQ). (2010). *National healthcare disparities report, 2010*, Rockville, MD. Retrieved May 22, 2015, from http://www.ahrq.gov/research/findings/nhqrdr/nhqrdr10/minority.html.

Agency for Healthcare Research and Quality, Rockville, MD. (April 2013). *Screening for depression in adults*. Retrieved May 20, 2015, from http://www.ahrq.gov/professionals/clinicians-providers/resources/depression/depsum1.html.

Alegría, M., Canino, G., Shrout, P. E., Woo, M., Duan, N., Vila, D., … Meng, X. -L. (2008). Prevalence of mental illness in immigrant and nonimmigrant U.S. Latino groups. *American Journal of Psychiatry, 165,* 359–369. doi:10.1176/appi.ajp.2007.07040704.

Alegría, M., Carson, N., Flores, M., Li, X., Shi, P., Lessios, A. S., … Shrout, P. E. (2014). Activation, self-management, engagement, and retention in behavioral health care: A randomized clinical trial of the DECIDE intervention. *JAMA Psychiatry, 71*(*5*), 557–565. doi:10.1001/jamapsychiatry.2013.4519.

Alegría, M., Ludman, E., Kafali, E. N., Lapatin, S., Ramirez, R., Vila, D., … Canino, G. (2014). Effectiveness of the engagement and counseling for Latinos (ECLA) intervention in low-income Latinos. *Medical Care*, *52*(*11*), 989–97.

Alegría, M., Mulvaney-Day, N., Torres, M., Polo, A., Cao, Z., & Canino, G. (2007). Prevalence of psychiatric disorders across Latino subgroups in the United States. *American Journal of Public Health, 97*(1), 68–75. PMCID: PMC1716243.

Alegría, M., Mulvaney-Day, N., Woo, M., Torres, M., Gao, S., & Oddo, V. (2007). Correlates of past-year mental health service use among Latinos: Results from the National Latino and Asian American study. *American Journal of Public Health, 97*, 76–83.

Alegría, M., Polo, A., Gao, S., Santana, L., Rothstein, D., Jimenez, A., … Normand, S. L. (2008). Evaluation of a patient activation and empowerment intervention in mental health care. *Medical Care*, *46*, 247–256.

Alegría, M., Shrout, P. E., Woo, M., Guarnaccia, P., Sribney, W., Vila, D., … Canino, G. (2007). Understanding differences in past year psychiatric disorders for Latinos living in the US. *Social Science & Medicine*, *65*, 214–226.

Andres-Hyman, R. C., Ortiz, J., Paris, M., Davidson, L., & Añez, L. M. (2006). Culture and clinical practice: Recommendations for working with Puerto Ricans and other Latinas(os) in the United States. *Professional Psychology: Research and Practice, 6*, 694–701.

Añez, L. M., Paris, M., Jr., Bedregal, L. E., Davidson, L., & Grilo, C. M. (2005). Application of cultural constructs in the care of first generation Latino clients in a community mental health setting. *Journal of Psychiatric Practice, 11*(4), 221–230.

Arciniega, G. M., Anderson, T. C., Tovar Blank, Z. G., & Tracey, T. J. G. (2008). Toward a fuller conception of machismo: Development of a traditional *Machismo* and *Caballerismo* scale. *Journal of Counseling Psychology, 55*(1), 19–33. Retrieved from http://dx.doi.org/10.1037/0022-0167.55.1.19.

Balan, I. C., Moyers, T. B., & Lewis-Fernandez, R. (2013). Motivational pharmacotherapy: Combining motivational interviewing and antidepressant therapy to improve treatment adherence. *Psychiatry, 76*(3), 203–209. http://dx.doi.org/10.1521/psyc.2013.76.3.203.

Barry, M. J. (2012). Shared decision making: Informing and involving patients to do the right thing in health care. *The Journal of Ambulatory Care Management, 35*(2), 90–98. doi:10.1097/JAC.0b013e318249482f.

Barry, M. J., & Edgman-Levitan, S. (2012). Shared decision making--Pinnacle of patient-centered care. *The New England Journal of Medicine, 366*(9), 780–781. doi:10.1056/NEJMp1109283.

Bauer, A. M., Chen, C. N., & Alegría, M. (2010). English language proficiency and mental health service use among Latino and Asian Americans with mental disorders. *Medical Care, 48*(12), 1097–1104.

Benish, S. G., Quintana, S., & Wampold, B. E. (2011). Culturally adapted psychotherapy and the legitimacy of myth: A direct-comparison meta-analysis. *Journal of Counseling Psychology, 58*(3), 279–289. doi:10.1037/a0023626.

Bhuyan, R., & Senturia, K. (2005). Understanding domestic violence resource utilization and survivor solutions among immigrant and refugee women: Introduction to the special issue. *Journal of Interpersonal Violence, 20*(8), 895–901.

Black, M. C., Basile, K. C., Breiding, M. J., Smith, S. G., Latlers, M. L., Merrick, M. T., … Stevens, M. R. (2010). *National Intimate Partner and Sexual Violence Survey (NISVS) 2010 Summary Report.*

Borowsky, S. J., Rubenstein, L. V., Meredith, L. S., Camp, P., Jackson-Triche, M., & Wells, K. B. (2000). Who is at risk of nondetection of mental health problems in primary care. *Journal of General Internal Medicine, 15*(6), 381–388.

Boyd, R. C., Diamond, G. S., & Bourjolly, J. N. (2006). Developing a family-based depression prevention program in urban community mental health clinics: A qualitative investigation. *Family Process, 45*, 187–203.

Bridges, A. J., Andrews, A. R., Villalobos, B. T., Pastrana, F. A., Cavell, T. A., & Gomez, D. (2014). Does integrated behavioral health care reduce mental health disparities for Latinos? Initial findings. *Journal of Latina/o Psychology, 2*(1), 37–53.

Bridges, A. J., Andrews, A. R. I., & Deen, T. L. (2012). Mental health needs and service utilization by Hispanic immigrants residing in mid-southern United States. *Journal of Transcultural Nursing, 23*, 359–368. doi:10.1177/1043659612451259.

Britigan, D. H., Murnan, J., & Rojas-Guyler, L. (2009). A qualitative study examining Latino functional health literacy levels and sources of health information. *Journal of Community Health, 34*(3), 222–230. doi:10.1007/s10900-008-9145-1.

Bromet, E., Andrade, L. H., Hwang, I., Sampson, N. A., Alonso, J., de Girolamo, G., … Kessler, R. C. (2011). Cross-national epidemiology of DSM-IV major depressive episode. *BMC Medicine, 9*, 90–94.

Cabassa, L. J., Lester, R., & Zayas, L. H. (2007). "It's like being in a labyrinth": Hispanic immigrants' perceptions of depression and attitudes toward treatments. *Journal of Immigrant and Minority Health, 9*(1), 1–16. Retrieved from http://dx.doi.org/10.1007/s10903-006-9010-1.

Caplan, S., Alvidrez, J., Paris, M., Escobar, J., Desai, M., Whittemore, R., … Scahill, L. (2010). Subjective versus objective: An exploratory analysis of Latino primary care patients who have self-perceived depression, but do not Fulfill PRIME-MD Patient Health Questionnaire (PHQ-9) Criteria for Depression. *The Primary Care Companion to the Journal of Clinical Psychiatry, 12(5)*, e1–e12. doi: 10.4088/PCC.099m00899blu.

Caplan, S., & Cordero, C. (2015). Development of a faith-based mental health literacy program to improve treatment engagement among Caribbean Latinos in the Northeastern United States of America. *International Quarterly of Community Health Education, 35*, 199–214.

Caplan, S., Escobar, J., Desai, M. M., Paris, M., Alvidrez, J., Scahill, L. D., … Whittemore, R. (2013). Cultural influences upon causal beliefs about depression among Latino immigrants: Faith and resilience. *Journal of Transcultural Nursing, 24*, 68–77.

Caplan, S., & Whittemore, R. (2013). Barriers to treatment engagement for depression among Latinas. *Issues in Mental Health Nursing, 34*(6), 412–424. doi:10.3109/01612840.2012.762958.

Cardemil, E. V., Adams, S. T., Calista, J. L., Connell, J., Encarnacion, J., Esparza, N., … Wang, E. (2007). The Latino mental health project: A local mental health needs assessment. *Administration and Policy in Mental Health and Mental Health Services Research, 34,* 331–341.

Cheng, E. M., Chen, A., & Cunningham, W. (2007). Primary language and receipt of recommended health care among Hispanics in the United States. *Journal of General Internal Medicine, 22*(Suppl 2), 283–288. doi:10.1007/s11606-007-0346-6.

Chiesa, A., & Serretti, A. (2011). Mindfulness based cognitive therapy for psychiatric disorders: A systematic review and meta-analysis. *Psychiatry Research, 187*(3), 441–453. doi:10.1016/j.psychres.2010.08.011.

Coker, A. L., Davis, K. E., Arias, I., Desai, S., Sanderson, M., Brandt, H. M., & Smith, P. H. (2002). Physical and mental health effects of intimate partner violence for men and women. *American Journal of Preventive Medicine, 2*, 260–268.

Comas-Diaz, L. (2006). Latino healing: The integration of ethnic psychology into psychotherapy. *Psychotherapy (Chicago, Ill.), 43*(4), 436–453. doi:10.1037/0033-3204.43.4.436.

Corrigan, P. W. (2004). How stigma interferes with mental health care. *American Psychologist, 59,* 614–625.

Corrigan, P. W., Morris, S. B., Michaels, P. J., Rafacz, J. D., & Rusch, N. (2012). Challenging the public stigma of mental illness: A meta-analysis of outcome studies. *Psychiatric Services, 63*(10), 963–973. doi:10.1176/appi.ps.201100529.

De Figueiredo, J. M., Boerstler, H., & Doros, G. (2009). Failure of high-risk minority patients to show up for outpatient psychiatric treatment. *International Journal of Mental Health, 38,* 91–105. 2009-08142-005.

Deering, K. N., Shannon, K., Sinclair, H., Parsad, D., Gilbert, E., & Tyndall, M. W. (2009). Piloting a peer-driven model to increase access and adherence to antiretroviral therapy and HIV care among street-entrenched HIV-positive women in Vancouver. *AIDS Patient Care and STDs, 23,* 603–609.

Deyo, M., Wilson, K. A., Ong, J., & Koopman, C. (2009). Mindfulness and rumination: Does mindfulness training lead to reductions in the ruminative thinking associated with depression? *Explore (NY), 5*(5), 265–271. doi:10.1016/j.explore.2009.06.005.

Diez-Quevedo, C., Rangil, T., Sanchez-Planell, L., Kroenke, K., & Spitzer, R. L. (2001). Validation and utility of the Patient Health Questionnaire in diagnosing mental disorders in 1003 general hospital Spanish inpatients. *Psychosomatic Medicine, 63*, 679–686.

Dimidjian, S., Barrera, M., Jr., Martell, C., Munoz, R. F., & Lewinsohn, P. M. (2011). The origins and current status of behavioral activation treatments for depression. *Annual Review of Clinical Psychology, 7,* 1–38. doi:10.1146/annurev-clinpsy-032210-104535.

Ducat, L., Philipson, L. H., & Anderson, B. J. (2014). The mental health comorbidities of diabetes. *JAMA, 312*(7), 691–692. doi:10.1001/jama.2014.8040.

Dunn, M. G., & O'Brien, K. M. (2009). Psychological health and meaning in life: Stress, social support, and religious coping in Latina/Latino immigrants. *Hispanic Journal of Behavioral Sciences, 31*, 204–227. doi:10.1177/0739986309334799.

Dwight-Johnson, M., Lagomasino, I., Hay, M. J., Zhang, P. L., Tang, M., Green, J. M., & Duan, N. (2010). Effectiveness of collaborative care in addressing depression treatment preferences among low-income Latinos. *Psychiatric Services, 61,* 1112–1118. doi:10.1176/appi.ps.61.11.1112.

Edelson, M. G., Hokoda, A., & Ramos-Lira, L. (2007). Differences in effects of domestic violence between Latina and non-Latina women. *Journal of Family Violence, 1*(22), 1–10.

Elder, J. P., Ayala, G. X., Parra-Medina, D., & Talavera, G. A. (2009). Health communication in the Latino community: Issues and approaches. *Annual Review of Public Health, 30*, 227–251. doi:10.1146/annurev.publhealth.031308.100300.

El-Mohandes, A. A., Kiely, M., Gantz, M. G., & El-Khorazaty, M. N. (2011). Very preterm birth is reduced in women receiving an integrated behavioral intervention: A randomized, controlled trial. *Maternal & Child Health Journal, 15*, 19–28.

Falcon, L. M., Todorova, I., & Tucker, K. (2009). Social support, life events, and psychological distress among the Puerto Rican population in the Boston area of the United States. *Aging & Mental Health, 13*(6), 863–873. doi:10.1080/13607860903046552. Pii 916452718.

Fernandez y Garcia, E., Franks, P., Jerant, A., Bell, R. A., & Kravitz, R. L. (2011). Depression treatment preferences of Hispanic individuals: Exploring the influence of ethnicity, language, and explanatory models. *Journal of the American Board of Family Medicine, 24*, 39–50. doi:10.3122/jabfm.2011.01.100118.

Folkman, S., & Moskowitz, J. T. (2004). Coping: Pitfalls and promise. *The Annual Review of Psychology, 55*, 745–774. http://dx.doi.org/10.1146/annurev.psych.55.090902.141456.

Fuchs, C. H., Haradhvala, N., Hubley, S., Nash, J. M., Keller, M. B., Ashley, D., … Uebelacker, L. A. (2015). Physician actions following a positive PHQ-2: Implications for the implementation of depression screening in family medicine practice. *Families, Systems, & Health, 33(1)*, 18–27. doi:10.1037/fsh0000089.

Gilbody, S., Richards, D., Brealey, S., & Hewitt, C. (2007). Screening for depression in medical settings with the patient health questionnaire (PHQ): A diagnostic meta-analysis. *Journal of General Internal Medicine, 22*(11), 1596–1602. doi:10.1007/s11606-007-0333-y.

Godfrin, K. A., & Van Heeringen, C. (2010). The effects of mindfulness-based cognitive therapy on recurrence of depressive episodes, mental health and quality of life: A randomized controlled study. *Behaviour Research and Therapy, 48*(8), 738–746. doi:10.1016/j.brat.2010.04.006.

González, H. M., Tarraf, W., Whitfield, K. E., & Vega, W. A. (2010). The epidemiology of major depression and ethnicity in the United States. *Journal of Psychiatric Research, 44*(15), 1043–1051. http://doi.org/10.1016/j.jpsychires.2010.03.017.

González, H. M., Vega, W. A., Williams, D. R., Tarraf, W., West, B. T., & Neighbors, H. W. (2010). Depression care in the United States: Too little for too few. *Archives of General Psychiatry, 67*, 37–46. doi:10.1001/archgenpsychiatry.2009.168.

Greenberg, A. B. J. (2006). *Stress and mind/body health: Hispanics*. Retrieved February 2, 2008, from http://www.greenbergresearch.com/articles/1800/2340_apa06_Hispanic_final.pdf.

Gucht, K., Takano, K., Broeck, N., & Raes, F. (2015). A mindfulness-based intervention for economically disadvantaged people: Effects on symptoms of stress, anxiety, and depression and on cognitive reactivity and overgeneralization. *Mindfulness, 6*, 1042. doi:10.1007/s12671-014-0353-8.

Hamdy, S. L. (2004). *Sexual victimization in Indian Country: Barriers and resources for native women seeking help*. Harrisburg, PA: VAWnet. Retrieved November 4, 2013, from http://www.vawnet.org.

Harman, J. S., Veazie, P. J., & Lyness, J. M. (2006). Primary care physician office visits for depression by older Americans. *Journal of General Internal Medicine, 21*, 926–930.

Horevitz, E., Organista, K. C., & Arean, P. A. (2015). Depression treatment uptake in integrated primary care: How a "Warm Handoff" and other factors affect decision making by Latinos. *Psychiatric Services, 66*, 824–830. doi:10.1176/appi.ps.201400085.

Horner-Johnson, W., Dobbertin, K., Lee, J. C., & Andresen, E. M. (2014). Disparities in health care access and receipt of preventive services by disability type: Analysis of the medical expenditure panel survey. *Health Services Research, 49*(6), 1980–1999. doi:10.1111/1475-6773.12195.

Houts, A. C., Lipinski, D., Olsen, J. P., Baldwin, S., & Hasan, M. (2010). Use of the patient care monitor to screen for depression in adult cancer patients interviewed with the structured clinical interview for DSM-IV. *Psycho-Oncology, 19*(4), 399–407.

Interian, A., Allen, L. A., Gara, M. A., & Escobar, J. I. (2008). A pilot study of culturally adapted cognitive behavior therapy for Hispanics with major depression. *Cognitive and Behavioral Practice, 15*(1), 67–75. doi:10.1016/j.cbpra.2006.12.002.

Interian, A., Lewis-Fernandez, R., Gara, M. A., & Escobar, J. I. (2013). A randomized-controlled trial of an intervention to improve antidepressant adherence among Latinos with depression. *Depression and Anxiety, 30*(7), 688–696. doi:10.1002/da.22052.

Interian, A., Martinez, I. E., Guarnaccia, P. J., Vega, W. A., & Escobar, J. I. (2007). A qualitative analysis of the perception of stigma among Latinos receiving antidepressants. *Psychiatric Services, 58*(12), 1591–1594. http://dx.doi.org/10.1037/a0012820.

Interian, A., Martinez, I., Rios, L. I., Krejci, J., & Guarnaccia, P. J. (2010). Adaptation of a motivational interviewing intervention to improve antidepressant adherence among Latinos. *Cultural Diversity & Ethnic Minority Psychology, 16*(2), 215–225.

Ishikawa, R. Z., Cardemil, E. V., Alegría, M., Schuman, C. C., Joseph, R. C., & Bauer, A. M. (2014). Uptake of depression treatment recommendations among Latino primary care patients. *Psychological Services, 11*(4), 421–432. doi:10.1037/a0035716.

Jackson, C. S., & Gracia, J. N. (2014). Addressing health and health-care disparities: The role of a diverse workforce and the social determinants of health. *Public Health Reports, 129*(Suppl 2), 57–61.

Julius, R. J., Novitsky, M. A., & Dubin, W. R. (2009). Medication adherence: A review of the literature and implications for clinical practice. *Journal of Psychiatric Practice, 15*, 34–44. doi:10.1097/01.pra.0000344917.43780.77.

Jylha, M. (2009). Self-rated health between psychology and biology. A response to Huisman and Deeg. *Social Science & Medicine, 70*, 655–657. doi:10.1016/j.socscimed.2009.11.004.

Kafali, N., Cook, B., Canino, G., & Alegría, M. (2014). Cost effectiveness of a randomized trial to treat depression among Latinos. *The Journal of Mental Health Policy and Economics, 17*, 41–50.

Kamphuis, M. H., Stegenga, B. T., Zuithoff, N. P. A., King, M., Nazareth, I., de Wit, N. J., & Geerlings, M. I. (2012). Does recognition of depression in primary care affect outcome? The PREDICT-NL study. *Family Practice, 29*, 16–23. doi: 10.1093/fampra/cmr049.

Katon, W. (1982). Depression - Somatic symptoms and medical disorders in primary care. *Comprehensive Psychiatry, 23*(3), 274–287. doi:10.1016/0010-440x(82)90076-1.

Keng, S. L., Smoski, M. J., & Robins, C. J. (2011). Effects of mindfulness on psychological health: A review of empirical studies. *Clinical Psychological Reviews, 31*(6), 1041–1056. doi:10.1016/j.cpr.2011.04.006.

Keyes, K. M., Martins, S. S., Hatzenbuehler, M. L., Blanco, C., Bates, L. M., & Hasin, D. S. (2012). Mental health service utilization for psychiatric disorders among Latinos living in the United States: The role of ethnic subgroup, ethnic identity, and language/social preferences. *Social Psychiatry and Psychiatric Epidemiology, 47*(3), 383–394. http://doi.org/10.1007/s00127-010-0323-y.

Keyworth, C., Knopp, J., Roughley, K., Dickens, C., Bold, S., & Coventry, P. (2014). A mixed-methods pilot study of the acceptability and effectiveness of a brief meditation and mindfulness intervention for people with diabetes and coronary heart disease. *Behavioral Medicine, 40*(2), 53–64. doi:10.1080/08964289.2013.834865.

Kim, H. G., Geppert, J., Quan, T., Bracha, Y., Lupo, V., & Cutts, D. B. (2012). Screening for postpartum depression among low-income mothers using an interactive voice response system. *Maternal and Child Health Journal, 16*, 921–928. doi:10.1007/s10995-011-0817-6.

Kleinman, A. (1980). *Patients and healers in the context of culture*. Berkeley, CA: University of California Press.

Koskan, A., Friedman, D. B., & Messias, D. K. H. (2010). Health literacy among Hispanics: A systematic research review (1992-2008). *Hispanic Health Care International, 8*(2), 65–76. doi:10.1891/1540-4153.8.2.65.

Kravitz, R. L., Paterniti, D. A., Epstein, R. M., Rochlen, A. B., Bell, R. A., Cipri, C., … Duberstein, P. (2011). Relational barriers to depression help-seeking in primary care. *Patient Education and Counseling, 82*, 207–213. doi:10.1016/j.pec.2010.05.007.

Kroenke, K., Spitzer, R. L., & Williams, J. B. (2001). The PHQ-9: Validity of a brief depression severity measure. *Journal of General Internal Medicine, 16*, 606–613.

Kroenke, K., Spitzer, R. L., & Williams, J. B. (2003). The Patient Health Questionnaire-2: Validity of a two-item depression screener. *Medical Care, 41*, 1284–1292. http://dx.doi.org/10.1097/01.MLR.0000093487.78664.3C.

Lejuez, C. W., Hopko, D. R., Acierno, R., Daughters, S. B., & Pagoto, S. L. (2011). Ten year revision of the brief behavioral activation treatment for depression: Revised treatment manual. *Behavior Modification, 35*(2), 111–161. doi:10.1177/0145445510390929.

Lewis-Fernandez, R., Balan, I. C., Patel, S. R., Sanchez-Lacay, J. A., Alfonso, C., Gorritz, M., … Moyers, T. B. (2013). Impact of motivational pharmacotherapy on treatment retention among depressed Latinos. *Psychiatry, 76(3)*, 210–222. doi: 10.1521/psyc.2013.76.3.210.

Lin, G. A., & Fagerlin, A. (2014). Shared decision making: State of the science. *Circulation: Cardiovascular and Quality Outcomes, 7*, 328–334. http://dx.doi.org/10.1161/CIRCOUTCOMES.113.000322.

Link, B., Yang, L. H., Phelan, J. C., & Collins, P. Y. (2004). Measuring mental illness stigma. *Schizophrenia Bulletin, 30*(3), 511–541.

Lopez, A. D., Mathers, C. D., Ezzati, M., Jamison, D. T., & Murray, C. J. L. (2001). Global burden of disease and risk factors. In *Systematic analysis of population health data*. London: J. Onwhyn.

Ludman, E. J., Simon, G. E., Tutty, S., & Von Korff, M. (2007). A randomized trial of telephone psychotherapy and pharmacotherapy for depression: Continuation and durability of effects. *Journal of Consulting and Clinical Psychology, 75*(2), 257–266. http://dx.doi.org/10.1037/0022-006X.75.2.257.

Macartney, S., Bishaw, A., & Fontenot, K. (2013). Poverty rates for selected detailed race and Hispanic groups by state and place: 2007–2011. *American Community Survey Briefs*. U.S. Census Bureau, 2007–2011 American Community Survey. ACSBR/11-17. Retrieved November 15, 2013, from http://www.census.gov/prod/2013pubs/acsbr11-17.pdf.

Manoleas, P. (2008). Integrated primary care and behavioral health services for Latinos: A blueprint and research agenda. *Social Work in Health Care, 47*, 438–454.

March, D., Luchsinger, J. A., Teresi, J. A., Eimicke, J. P., Findley, S. E., Carrasquillo, O., & Palmas, W. (2014). High rates of depressive symptoms in low-income urban Hispanics of Caribbean origin with poorly controlled diabetes: Correlates and risk factors. *Journal of Health Care for the Poor and Underserved, 25(1)*, 321–331. doi:10.1353/hpu.2014.0027.

McCaffery, K. J., Smith, S. K., & Wolf, M. (2010). The challenge of shared decision making among patients with lower literacy: A framework for research and development. *Medical Decision Making, 30*(1), 35–44. doi:10.1177/0272989x09342279.

McFarlane, J. M., Groff, J. Y., O'Brien, J. A., & Watson, K. (2005). Prevalence of partner violence against 7,443 African American, White, and Hispanic women receiving care at urban public primary care clinics. *Public Health Nursing, 22*, 98–107. doi:10.1111/j.0737-1209.2005.220203.x.

McIntyre, K. P., Korn, J. H., & Matsuo, H. (2008). Sweating the small stuff: How different types of hassle result in the experience of stress. *Stress and Health, 24*, 383. doi:10.1002/smi.1190. Retrieved from www.interscience.wiley.com.

Menchetti, M., Belvederi-Murri, M., Bertakis, K., Bortolotti, B., & Berardi, D. (2009). Recognition and treatment of depression in primary care: Effect of patients' presentation and frequency of consultation. *Journal of Psychosomatic Research, 66*, 335–341.

Substance Abuse and Mental Health Services Administration, (SAMSHA). (2015). *Racial/ethnic differences in mental health service use among adults*. HHS Publication No. SMA-15-4906. Rockville, MD: Substance Abuse and Mental Health Services Administration.

Miranda, J., Duan, N., Sherbourne, C., Schoenbaum, M., Lagomasino, I., Jackson-Triche, M., & Wells, K. B. (2003). Improving care for minorities: Can quality improvement interventions improve care and outcomes for depressed minorities? Results of a randomized, controlled trial. *Health Services Research, 38*, 613– 630. doi:10.1111/1475-6773.00136.

Mitchell, A. J., Vaze, A., & Rao, S. (2009). Clinical diagnosis of depression in primary care: A meta-analysis. *Lancet, 374*, 609–619. doi:10.1016/S0140-6736(09)60879-5.

Mojtabai, R., & Olfson, M. (2008). National patterns in antidepressant treatment by psychiatrists and general medical providers: Results from the national comorbidity survey replication. *Journal of Clinical Psychiatry, 69*, 1064–1074. http://dx.doi.org/10.4088/JCP.v69n0704.

Moore, M., Ali, S., Stuart, B., Leydon, G. M., Ovens, J., Goodall, C., & Kendrick, T. (2012). Depression management in primary care: An observational study of management changes related to PHQ-9 score for depression monitoring. *The British Journal of General Practice, 62(599)*, e451–e457. Retrieved from http://dx.doi.org/10.3399/bjgp12X649151.

Mostow, C., Crosson, J., Gordon, S., Chapman, S., Gonzalez, P., Hardt, E., … David M. (2010). Treating and precepting with RESPECT: A relational model addressing race, ethnicity, and culture in medical training, *Journal of General Internal Medicine 25(Suppl 2)*, 146–154.

Moyer, V. A., & U.S. Preventive Services Task Force. (2013). Screening for intimate partner violence and abuse of elderly and vulnerable adults: U.S. preventive services task force recommendation statement. *Annals of Internal Medicine, 158*(6), 478–486. doi:10.7326/0003-4819-158-6-201303190-00588.

Munet-Vilaró, F., Folkman, S., & Gregorich, S. (1999). Depressive symptomatology in three Latino groups. *Western Journal of Nursing Research, 21*(2), 209–224.

Munet-Vilaró, F., Gregorich, S., & Folkman, S. (2002). Factor analysis of the Spanish version of the ways of coping questionnaire. *Journal of Applied Social Psychology, 32*(9), 1938–1954.

Muñoz, R. F., McQuaid, J. R., González, G., Dimas, J., & Rosales, V. (1999). Depression screening in a women's clinic: Using automated Spanish- and English-language voice recognition. *Journal of Consulting & Clinical Psychology, 67*, 502–510.

Myers, H. F., Wyatt, G. E., Ullman, J. B., Loeb, T. B., Chin, D., Prause, N., … Liu, H. (2015). Cumulative burden of lifetime adversities: Trauma and mental health in low-SES African Americans and Latino/as. *Psychological Trauma: Theory, Research, Practice, and Policy, 7(3)*, 243–251. doi:10.1037/a0039077.

Nadeem, E., Lange, H. M., Edge, D., Fongwa, M., Berlin, T., & Miranda, J. (2007). Does stigma keep poor young immigrant and U.S.-born Black and Latina women from seeking mental health care? *Psychiatric Services, 58*, 1547–1554.

Nicklett, E. J., & Burgard, S. A. (2009). Downward social mobility and major depressive episodes among Latino and Asian-American immigrants to the United States. *American Journal of Epidemiology, 170*(6), 793–801. doi:10.1093/aje/kwp192.

Nicolaidis, C., Perez, M., Mejia, A., Alvarado, A., Celaya-Alston, R., Galian, H., & Hilde, A. (2011). 'Guardarse las cosas adentro' (keeping things inside): Latina violence survivors' perceptions of depression. *Journal of General Internal Medicine*, *26(10)*, 1131–1137. PMID: 21626052.

Olfson, M., Moitabai, R., Sampson, N. A., Hwang, I., & Kessler, R. C. (2009). Dropout from outpatient mental health care in the United States. *Psychiatric Services, 60*, 898–907. doi:10.1176/appi.ps.60.7.898.

Rogler, L. H., Cortes, D. E., & Malgady, R. G. (1994). The mental-health relevance of idioms of distress anger and perceptions of injustice among New-York Puerto-Ricans. *Journal of Nervous and Mental Disease, 182*(6), 327–330. doi:10.1097/00005053-199406000-00003.

Roth, B., & Robbins, D. (2004). Mindfulness-based stress reduction and health-related quality of life: Findings from a bilingual inner-city patient population. *Psychosomatic Medicine, 66(1)*, 113–123. Retrieved from http://www.ncbi.nlm.nih.gov/pubmed/14747645.

Schmaling, K. B., & Hernandez, D. V. (2005). Detection of depression among low-income Mexican Americans in primary care. *Journal of Health Care for the Poor and Underserved, 16*, 780–790.

Scott, K. M., Bruffaerts, R., Tsang, A., Ormel, J., Alonso, J., Angermeyer, M. C., … Von Korff, M. (2007). Depression-anxiety relationships with chronic physical conditions: Results from the world mental health surveys. *Journal of Affective Disorders, 103(1–3)*, 113–120. doi:10.1016/j.jad.2007.01.015.

Sentell, T., & Braun, K. L. (2012). Low health literacy, limited English proficiency, and health status in Asians, Latinos, and other racial/ethnic groups in California. *Journal of Health Communication, 17*(Suppl 3), 82–99. doi:10.1080/10810730.2012.712621.
Shah, P. S., Shah, J., & Knowledge Synthesis Group on Determinants of Preterm/LBW Births. (2010). Maternal exposure to domestic violence and pregnancy and birth outcomes: A systematic review and meta-analyses. *Journal of Women's Health, 19*, 2017–2031.
Shim, R. S., Baltrus, P., Ye, J., & Rust, G. (2011). Prevalence, treatment, and control of depressive symptoms in the United States: Results from the National Health and Nutrition Examination Survey (NHANES), 2005–2008. *Journal of the American Board of Family Medicine, 24*, 33–38.
Sue, S. (1988). Psychotherapeutic services for ethnic minorities: Two decades of research findings. *American Psychologist, 43*, 301–308. doi:10.1037/0003-066X.43.4.301.
Tarricone, I., Stivanello, E., Poggi, F., Castorini, V., Marseglia, M. V., Fantini, M. P., Berardi, D. (2012). Ethnic variation in the prevalence of depression and anxiety in primary care: A systematic review and meta-analysis. *Psychiatry Research, 195*, 91–106.
Taylor, P., Kochhar, R., Fry, R., Velasco, G., Motel, S. (2011). Twenty-to-one: Wealth gaps rise to record highs between Whites, Blacks, and Hispanics. Pew Research Center, *Social and Demographic Trends*. Retrieved from http://www.pewsocialtrends.org/files/2011/07/SDT-Wealth-Report_7-26-11_FINAL.pdf.
Todorova, I. L. G., Tucker, K. L., Pescador, M., Jimenez, A. K., Lincoln, S. A., & Falcón, L. M. (2013). Determinants of self-rated health and the role of acculturation: Implications for health inequalities. *Ethnicity & Health, 18*, 563–585.
Torres, L. (2010). Predicting levels of Latino depression: Acculturation, acculturative stress, and coping. *Cultural Diversity and Ethnic Minority Psychology, 16*(2), 256. doi:10.1037/a0017357.
Torres, L., & Rollock, D. (2007). Acculturation and depression among Hispanics: The moderating effect of intercultural competence. *Cultural Diversity & Ethnic Minority Psychology, 13*(1), 10–17. doi:10.1037/1099-9809.13.1.10.
Uebelacker, L. A., Wang, P. S., Berglund, P., & Kessler, R. C. (2006). Clinical differences among patients treated for mental health problems in general medical and specialty mental health settings in the National Comorbidity Survey Replication. *General Hospital Psychiatry, 28*, 387–395. http://dx.doi.org/10.1016/j.genhosppsych.2006.05.001.
United States Census Bureau. (2012). *U.S. Census Bureau projections show a slower growing, older, more diverse nation a half century from now*. Retrieved from http://www.census.gov/newsroom/releases/archives/population/cb12-243.html.
United States Census Bureau. (2013a). *ACS Demographic and housing estimates 2012 American Community Survey 1-Year Estimates*. Retrieved from http://factfinder2.census.gov/faces/tableservices/jsf/pages/productview.xhtml?pid=ACS_12_1YR_DP05&prodType=table.
United States Census Bureau. (2013b). Poverty rates for selected detailed race and Hispanic groups by state and place, 2007–2011. *American Community Survey Briefs*. Retrieved from http://www.census.gov/prod/2013pubs/acsbr11-17.pdf.
United States Preventive Services Task Force (USPSTF). (2009). *Screening for depression in adults*. Retrieved from http://uspreventiveservicestaskforce.org.
US Department of Health and Human Services. (2015). *Access to health services*. Washington, DC: DHHS. Retrieved from http://www.healthypeople.gov/2020/topics-objectives/topic/Access-to-Health-Services.
Vargas, S. M., Cabassa, L. J., Nicasio, A., De La Cruz, A. A., Jackson, E., Rosario, M., …. Lewis Fernandez, R. (2015). Toward a cultural adaptation of pharmacotherapy: Latino views of depression and antidepressant therapy. *Transcultural Psychiatry, 52*(2), 244–273. doi:10.1177/1363461515574159.
Vega, W. A., Rodriguez, M. A., & Ang, A. (2010). Addressing stigma of depression in Latino primary care patients. *General Hospital Psychiatry, 32*(2), 182–191. doi:10.1016/j.genhosppsych.2009.10.008.

Vespa, J., Lewis, J. M., & Kreider, R. M. (2013). America's families and living arrangements: 2012 Population characteristics P20-570. U. S. Census Bureau, *American Community Survey, 2011*. Retrieved November 15, 2013, from http://www.census.gov/prod/2013pubs/p20-570.pdf.

Villatoro, A. P., Morales, E. S., & Mays, V. M. (2014). Family culture in mental health help-seeking and utilization in a nationally representative sample of Latinos in the united states: The NLAAS. *American Journal of Orthopsychiatry, 84*(4), 353–363.

Winkelman, S. B., Chaney, E. H., & Bethel, J. W. (2013). Stress, depression and coping among Latino migrant and seasonal farmworkers. *International Journal of Environmental Research and Public Health, 10*(5), 1815–1830. doi:10.3390/ijerph10051815.

Wulsin, L., Somoza, E., & Heck, J. (2002). The feasibility of using the Spanish PHQ-9 to screen for depression in primary care in Honduras. *Primary Care Companion of the Journal of Clinical Psychiatry, 4*, 191–195.

Chapter 11
Using Integrated Care to Treat Anxiety Among Latino Populations

Velma Barrios, Michelle Blackmore, and Denise Chavira

Introduction: Addressing Disparities Through Integrated Behavioral and Primary Care

The growth of the nation's Latino group is estimated to nearly double over the next half century (from 13 to 24 %; U.S. Census Bureau, 2003). Most notably, while the total U.S. population increased 10 % from 2000 to 2010, the Latino population increased 43 % (U.S. Census Bureau, 2010). This growth has taken place at a time when many social service systems are not prepared to address the needs of the culturally pluralistic Latino population. For instance, a significant number of Latinos have relatively high levels of mental health problems and unmet mental health needs (Kessler et al., 1994), contributing to Latinos' overrepresentation among individuals at risk for poor mental health outcomes (e.g., groups with lower socioeconomic status, limited English proficiency) (Derose & Baker, 2000; Ku & Matani, 2001; Vega, Alderete, Kolody, & Aguilar-Gaxiola, 1998). A significant gap exists between the need for and availability of culturally competent mental health services for Latinos. With new health care reform legislation, a unique opportunity exists to enhance the accessibility and quality of mental health services that are available in primary care settings for this population.

Latinos in the U.S. experience substantial difficulties in obtaining adequate access to health care (Alegría et al., 2002) and mental health services (Blanco et al., 2007; Center for Mental Health Services, 2000), and overall are underrepresented

V. Barrios, Ph.D. (✉)
Los Altos, CA 94022, USA
e-mail: vbarrios@paloaltou.edu

M. Blackmore, Ph.D.
Yonkers, NY 10710, USA

D. Chavira, Ph.D.
Los Angeles, CA 90095, USA

© Springer International Publishing Switzerland 2016

L.T. Benuto, W. O'Donohue (eds.), *Enhancing Behavioral Health in Latino Populations*, DOI 10.1007/978-3-319-42533-7_11

in mental health settings (e.g., Vega, Kolody, Aguilar-Gaxiola, & Catalano, 1999). Many Latinos seeking services for psychological problems tend to do so from their primary care providers, highlighting the need for culturally appropriate integrated care in this setting. Developing culturally competent integrated care models has the potential to significantly decrease disparities in access to and quality of behavioral health services among the Latino population in the U.S. The chief goal of this chapter is to examine how cultural considerations can be applied to evidence-based interventions for anxiety in an integrated care setting.

Latinos as an at-Risk Population

Research suggests that Latinos in the U.S. tend to have high prevalence rates of anxiety disorders and comorbidity—primarily with depression (Kessler et al., 1994). Some evidence indicates that Latinos also have higher rates of anxiety disorders when compared to other ethnic groups (Minsky, Vega, Miskimen, Gara, & Escobar, 2003). Though not statistically different, epidemiological data show that compared to whites, Latinos have greater levels of symptom severity and greater 12-month prevalence rates of anxiety disorders (21.4 % vs. 18.9 %) (Kessler, Chiu, Demler, & Walters, 2005). In other studies, Latinos have lower rates of anxiety disorders than non-Latino whites but, among Latinos who became ill, the disorder was more likely to be chronic than in non-Latino whites (Breslau, Kendler, Su, Gaxiola-Aguilar, & Kessler, 2005). That is, Latinos may be at high risk for developing chronic anxiety disorders when left untreated.

In recent decades, the U.S. has seen the greatest influx of Latino immigrants compared to other countries (Kaiser Commission on Medicaid and the Uninsured, 2004). Like many other immigrant populations, immigration for Latinos can lead to considerable familial, social, and environmental hardships (Perez & Fortuna, 2005), including separation from family, loss of family support and social status, lack of community, poorer living conditions, discrimination, and language and communication difficulties (Finch, Kolody, & Vega, 2000; Finch & Vega, 2003; Hovey, 2000a, 2000b; Perez & Fortuna, 2005). Many Latinos immigrate to the U.S. due to economic adversities and violence resulting from political oppression or war-related violence in their country of origin (Leslie & Lietch, 1989); factors that also contribute to psychological issues related to trauma, loss, and poverty (Organista & Muñoz, 1996). Given such negative life events are frequently linked to poor psychological adjustment (Hiott, Grzywacz, Arcury, & Quandt, 2006; Perez & Fortuna, 2005; Portes & Rumbaut, 2006), Latinos may be at particularly high risk for developing psychiatric disorders—particularly anxiety and depression (Plante, Manuel, Menedez, & Marcotter, 1995).

Anxiety and Service Use in Primary Care Settings

Currently, anxiety disorders are the most prevalent mental health problems seen in primary care settings (Kessler et al., 2005). Latinos, like other groups, underutilize psychiatric services. However, unlike other groups, Latinos overutilize primary care health services and are twice as likely to seek treatment for psychiatric disorders in publicly funded primary care rather than mental health specialty settings (U.S. Surgeon General, 2001). Overutilization of services may be due, at least in part, to differences in beliefs about psychiatric disorders and treatment preferences. For instance, the tendency for Latinos to believe that psychiatric disorders are biologically based makes them more likely to seek and receive mental health treatment in primary health care settings (Givens, Houston, Van Voorhees, Ford, & Cooper, 2007). Further, given the stigmatizing attitudes associated with visiting a mental health professional (Azocar, Areán, Miranda, & Muñoz, 2001), Latinos may feel more comfortable seeking services from their medical providers (i.e., primary care providers and allied professionals) than mental health specialists in community mental health agencies or private practices (Vega, Kolody, & Aguilar-Gaxiola, 2001).

Disparities in Quality of Care for Latinos in Primary Care

Disparities exist in detection and treatment of depression and anxiety in primary care. In a study that examined ethnic/racial disparities over a 10-year period, Latinos with anxiety and depression who had visits to primary care had significantly lower odds of receiving a diagnosis than non-Latino whites. Additionally, Latinos had significantly lower odds (compared with whites) of receiving an antidepressant prescription, and of receiving any care at all. Despite the significant number of patients with diagnosable anxiety disorders that present in primary care, it appears that anxiety is infrequently detected among ethnic/racial minorities (Stockdale, Lagomasino, Siddique, McGuire, & Miranda, 2008). Further, when anxiety is recognized, evidence-based psychological interventions are rarely used, and are particularly unlikely to be used when treating Latinos (Stockdale et al., 2008; Young, Klap, Sherbourne, & Wells, 2001).

Evidence-Based Treatments for Anxiety

At present, there is an abundance of data suggesting that psychosocial (i.e., cognitive behavioral therapy [CBT]), pharmacologic treatments (i.e., psychotropic medications) or a combination of the two are efficacious for the treatment of anxiety disorders (Norton & Price, 2007; Roy-Byrne & Cowley, 2007). A growing body of literature also suggests that these evidence-based interventions are effective in real-world settings, including primary care (Roy-Byrne et al., 2005, 2010). Moreover, clinical outcomes appear similar for Latinos and non-Latino whites who receive pharmacological and psychosocial interventions in primary care settings (Chavira et al., 2014). Below, we briefly describe pharmacotherapy and CBT for anxiety disorders.

Pharmacotherapy

Antidepressants are the first-line medication treatments for anxiety disorders, particularly the selective serotonin reuptake inhibitors (SSRIs) and serotonin-norepinephrine reuptake inhibitors (SNRIs). Response rates are in the range of 50–70 % (Stein, 2005). These classes of medication include fluoxetine (Prozac), fluvoxamine (Luvox), citalopram (Celexa), escitalopram (Lexapro), paroxetine (Paxil), and sertraline (Zoloft) for the SSRIs, and venlafaxine (Effexor) and duloxetine (Cymbalta) for the SNRIs. Although there is a 3–4 week delay in response, the reduced potential for addiction makes these medications more desirable for long-term management of anxiety symptoms. For patients with major functional impairments requiring short-term symptom relief, benzodiazepines like clonazepam (Klonopin) or alprazolam (Xanax) may be indicated for faster response or until satisfactory symptom reduction has been achieved with an SSRI, SNRI, or other treatment. Benzodiazepines can also be used on an as-needed basis. However, continuous long-term use of benzodiazepines can lead to physiological tolerance, abuse, and dependence, while discontinuing their use can lead to symptom relapse and abrupt discontinuation can lead to withdrawal symptoms (e.g., seizures). Other widely used pharmacotherapies for anxiety include Buspirone (Buspar), an anxiolytic that is primarily used for the treatment of generalized anxiety disorder (GAD).

Clomipramine (Anafranil) is a tricyclic antidepressant used specifically for the treatment of obsessive-compulsive disorder (OCD) or for patients with anxiety that do not respond well to SSRIs and SNRIs. Adverse side effects for tricyclics include anticholinergic symptoms (jitterness, postural hypotension, dry mouth, constipation), which makes tricyclics a less desirable form of treatment for patients with anxiety disorders. Monoamine oxidase inhibitors (MAOIs), like phenelzine (Nardil) and tranylcypromine (Parnate), are sometimes used for the treatment of panic disorder or generalized social anxiety. Importantly, their use requires strict dietary restrictions (limit foods rich in tyramine); otherwise, MAOIs have the potential to increase the risk of a hypertensive crisis, stroke, or even death. Because of this side effects' profile, health professionals limit their use for the treatment of anxiety, as other efficacious pharmacotherapies with more benign side effects (e.g., SSRIs) are available. Finally, beta-blockers, such as propranolol (Inderal) and atenolol (Tenormin), reduce tachycardia, trembling, and blushing and can be helpful on an as-needed basis for the treatment of anxiety related to performance situations.

Psychosocial Intervention: Cognitive Behavioral Therapy

Cognitive behavioral therapy (CBT) is an empirically supported treatment and the gold standard psychosocial treatment for the anxiety disorders (Chambless & Ollendick, 2001; Hofmann & Smits, 2008). Briefly, CBT involves systematic exposure to feared stimuli in order to reverse patterns of avoidance, as well as cognitive restructuring to alter irrational thoughts and beliefs. More specifically, over the course of treatment, individuals learn through direct experience (i.e., exposure) that fear, anxiety, and the associated stimuli and contexts are not harmful and that they can cope with anxiety-producing situations; this learning is facilitated by discussion and verbal processing (i.e., cognitive restructuring; Craske, 1999).

Integrated Models of Care

Despite demonstrated effectiveness of evidence-based treatments (e.g., CBT) for anxiety disorders, the majority of patients do not have access to these interventions partially due to fragmentation of behavioral and primary health care and lack of coordinated care among providers. Health care reform legislation aims to reduce ineffective silo-based systems of care by creating integrated behavioral and medical health care systems. The more successful integrated care efforts do not solely rely on being co-located, but improve care quality and outcomes through integration of screening, assessment, and treatment of behavioral health conditions into the overall health care of patients entering the primary care setting. In this model, all primary care staff and providers are part of the collaborative effort, from the front desk and office personnel, to the nurses, the PCPs, the behavioral health team, and the administrators and site leadership. For example, the front desk staff is often the first point of contact for the patient and can be responsible for handing out the behavioral health screen and briefly explaining the primary care physician's interest in the patient's overall health care, both behavioral and medical. The nurses can then collect and review the screen while rooming the patient for the primary care physician. The primary care physician, typically operating as the center of the team overseeing all aspects of the patient's care, can then confirm any symptomatology, possibly make a preliminary mental health diagnosis, and then either provide a brief intervention (including prescribing an antidepressant), seek consultation, or introduce the services provided by the behavioral health team and make a referral.

The integrated care team can consist of one or more behavioral health care specialist(s) (BHS; e.g., care manager, psychologist, consulting psychiatrist, and/or social worker) and their roles will vary depending on the model, the patient's needs, and the resources available (Collins, Hewson, Munger, & Wade, 2010). In a partially integrated model, communication between the BHS and the primary care providers (PCPs) is routine and on-site counseling and concrete services are offered or referrals are made to specialty providers. In a fully integrated model, behavioral health care is often co-located in primary care and treatment plans integrate behavioral and medical aspects, with a high degree of shared treatment responsibility between the BHS and primary care provider. Behavioral health treatment options can consist of medication management, evidence-based psychotherapy (e.g., CBT, Problem-Solving Therapy, Behavioral Activation, Motivational Interviewing), and/or care and case management. A stepped-care approach is often utilized to deliver treatments that are effective but conserve behavioral health resources. Monitoring the patient's progress using treat-to-target measures ensure the patient is moved to the next level of stepped care when necessary.

Regardless of the level of integration, the goal is to have the BHS collaborate with the primary care physician to design, implement, and adjust, as necessary, a treatment plan for every patient. If the behavioral health team consists of a consulting psychiatrist, their role may vary from providing consultation and supervision to the medical care team to becoming the primary provider for a complex patient who needs specialty behavioral health treatment. Ultimately, the BHS will be essential in providing a comprehensive assessment, confirming diagnoses, and monitoring the patients' mental health symptoms and needs within the parameters of a primary care setting. Coordination and communication amongst the health care team (e.g. BHS, PCP), including regular team meetings, is crucial to best synchronize health care visits, share knowledge of the patient's care, and monitor the patient's progress using treat-to-target measures.

Integrated models of care for anxiety are relatively new but are supported by a substantial body of research on integrated care for depression, which demonstrates their effectiveness in improving early detection, treatment, and short- and long-term mental health and medical care outcomes when compared to standard care (Gilbody, Bower, Fletcher, Richards, & Sutton, 2006; Katon et al., 2012; Katon, Unützer, Wells, & Jones, 2010; Unützer et al., 2008), including those utilizing psychological interventions (Coventry et al., 2014). In the presence of minor sociocultural adjustments to the model, similar improvements in health care outcomes and patient satisfaction in minority populations have been demonstrated, including in predominantly low-income Latino groups (Ell et al., 2010; Miranda et al., 2003).

Integrated Models of Care for Anxiety

Integrated care models for anxiety disorders have also shown promise. One study combining pharmacotherapy and a cognitive behavioral intervention for the treatment of panic disorder in primary care settings demonstrated significantly greater improvements across all outcome measures compared to treatment as usual (i.e. typical pharmacotherapy) (Roy-Byrne et al., 2005; Roy-Byrne, Katon, Cowley, & Russo, 2001). The collaborative care intervention included up to 6 sessions, across 12 weeks, of CBT modified for the primary care setting and provided by the BHS. Pharmacotherapy in the collaborative condition was provided by the primary care physician with guidance from a psychiatrist.

A subsequent study which included more anxiety disorders within an integrated care model sought to provide treatment for panic disorder and GAD using a telephone-based collaborative care intervention (Rollman et al., 2005). In the intervention group, non-mental health professionals provided psychoeducation, assessed preferences for guideline-based care, monitored treatment responses, and informed physicians of their patients' care preferences and progress via an electronic medical record system. The intervention proved more effective at improving anxiety symptoms, health-related quality of life, and work-related outcomes compared to care as usual (Rollman et al., 2005). Additional trials of integrated treatment of GAD support findings that the model is generally superior to care as usual in reducing symptoms (Archer et al., 2012; Muntingh et al., 2013; Price, Beck, Nimmer, & Bensen, 2000), as well as improving patients' satisfaction with their health care (Price et al., 2000). An integrated anxiety care approach within the practice of cardiology further addressed the interplay between behavioral and medical health, and helped patients adapt a more healthy lifestyle to improve health care outcomes (Janeway, 2009). While results are promising, these studies have not included adequate representation of Latinos; additional research is necessary to examine these models in ethnic minority populations.

The largest trial of integrated anxiety care to date is the Coordinated Anxiety Learning and Management (CALM) model, based on the IMPACT intervention for depression. The CALM model used a computer-assisted CBT program with possible phamacotherapy to treat four of the major anxiety disorders seen in primary care (i.e., GAD, panic disorder with or without agoraphobia, social phobia, and post-traumatic stress disorder). Treatment included approximately eight sessions of CBT and/or medication management treatment over 10–12 weeks, with follow-up phone calls for up to 1 year (Sullivan et al., 2007). Outcomes for intervention patients were significantly better than control patients for all measures, except physical health and satisfaction, at all time points (6, 12, 18 months). The CALM study was highly flexible and effective for a wide range of patients and targeted multiple anxiety disorders, making this model's application feasible and applicable in primary care settings. The computer assisted-CBT was also acceptable to patients and improved effectiveness of care (Craske et al., 2009; Roy-Byrne et al., 2010).

To our knowledge, the CALM study is the largest clinical trial examining CBT for anxiety in Latino adults (Chavira et al., 2014). Rates of treatment preference for Latinos in this study were similar to non-Latino whites; 40 % of Hispanic patients preferred CBT only, 52 % preferred CBT and medication, and 9 % preferred medication only (Chavira et al., 2014). Findings from this study suggest that the CBT intervention was similarly effective for Hispanic and non-Hispanic Whites with anxiety disorders, although the study's sample was made up of a primarily acculturated Latino group (e.g., bilingual, higher income). Scores on engagement-related outcome measures (e.g., adherence, commitment, treatment completion) were also mostly similar among Latinos and non-Latino whites, other than a measure on understanding of CBT principles. Studies examining the effectiveness of CBT for other psychiatric conditions, such as depression, also demonstrate favorable outcomes for Latinos (e.g., Markowitz, Speilman, Sullivan, & Fishman, 2000; Miranda, Azócar, Organista, Dwyer, & Areane, 2003). This growing body of research suggests CBT may be a promising therapeutic modality for integrated care models with Latinos.

Identification and Assessment of Anxiety

The success of behavioral health integration also relies on improving the utilization of mental health screenings. Accurate screening and diagnosis is the first step to ensuring early identification of individuals in need of mental health treatment within primary care. This is particularly true for anxiety disorders, which are often misdiagnosed in these settings (Menninger, 1995) and can lead to significant impairment in both mental and physical health functioning (Revicki, Brandenburg, Matza, Hornbrook, & Feeny, 2008).

Only a handful of screening measures available today have proven feasible in the typically fast-paced primary care setting where limited time and resources are common. The Patient Health Questionnaire (PHQ), 2-item and 9-item version, is commonly used in medical settings and has shown utility in monitoring depression symptom severity and treatment response and remission, even in practices with limited resources (Duffy et al., 2008; Katzelnick et al., 2011). The Overall Anxiety Severity and Impairment Scale (OASIS) is another highly useful screener for primary care settings. It is a 5-item self-report questionnaire that is brief, has demonstrated validity, includes a measure of functional impairment, and is able to capture the severity of any or multiple anxiety disorders (Campbell-Sills et al., 2009). However, it may not discriminate well between depression and anxiety (Campbell-Sills et al., 2009). The Generalized Anxiety Disorder 7-item scale (GAD-7) is also increasingly being used in medical settings, evidencing good sensitivity and specificity as a screener for GAD (Spitzer, Kroenke, Williams, & Lowe, 2006), panic, social anxiety, and post-traumatic stress disorder (PTSD; Kroenke, Spitzer, Williams, Monahan, & Lowe, 2007). Similarly, the Anxiety and Depression Detector (ADD) was developed as a time-efficient screen for GAD, panic disorder, PTSD, social phobia, and depression in primary care settings (Means-Christensen, Sherbourne, Roy-Byrne, Craske, & Stein, 2005). However, the specific items measuring PTSD and social phobia may not be as valid as those for the other anxiety disorders and depression (Chavira, Stein, & Roy-Byrne, 2008). To screen for specific anxiety disorders like PTSD and social phobia, the abbreviated versions of the PTSD Checklist (Lang & Stein, 2006) and the Social Phobia Inventory (SPIN) (Connor, Kobak, Churchill, Katzelnick, & Davidson, 2001) have been useful in primary care. Several of these more commonly used measures have been validated in Latino populations, including the PHQ-9 (Huang, Chung, Kroenke, Delucchi, & Spitzer, 2006) and GAD-7 (Mills et al., 2014). More research is needed in this area to ensure these measures of anxiety are valid in ethnically diverse patient populations.

For a more thorough assessment, The Mini International Neuropsychiatric Interview (MINI) has demonstrated accuracy in diagnosing anxiety disorders such as GAD and panic disorder, is perceived positively by patients, and has been feasibly administered in primary care facilities (Pinninti, Madison, Musser, & Rissmiller, 2003). The MINI also has demonstrated validity as a screener for all the disorders it covers (Lecrubier et al., 1997). The PRIME-MD is also well validated, covers a range of psychiatric disorders, and includes a 26-item self-report screening questionnaire, and a structured interview completed by the provider (Spitzer,

Kroenke, Williams, & Patient Health Questionnaire Primary Care Study Group, 1999). The Brief Symptom Inventory-18 (BSI-18) is a sensitive, well validated measure for psychological distress (Carlson & Bultz, 2003; Degoratis, 2000), though it may be lengthy in comparison to other measures used in primary care settings (Chavira et al., 2008). Such measures are not only important for identifying individuals at risk for mental illness, but also in providing measurement-informed care which is key in tracking progress and outcomes.

Cultural Conceptualizations of Anxiety

The manner in which anxiety manifests may be different for Latinos and should be considered when conducting culturally informed assessments (Benuto, Olmo-Terasa, & Reyes-Rabanillo, 2011). In addition to standard assessments of anxiety, it can be important for a provider to ask questions that allow a patient to explain their understanding of an illness, including causes and expectations of treatment. In doing so, providers will have access to patients conceptualizations of anxiety that may be different from traditional psychiatric and medical explanations. For Latino patients, assessments that include such an approach may improve the strength of the patient-provider relationship and improve detection of problematic anxiety.

Somatic Symptoms

Several studies have found that Latinos are more likely to endorse somatic symptoms as a key feature of anxiety/worry. In particular, findings from clinical samples of patients with anxiety and depressive disorders, suggest that Latinos report more somatic and physiological sensations than their non-Latino white counterparts (Canino, Rubio-Stipec, Canino, & Escobar, 1992; Escobar, Gomez, & Tuason, 1983; Mezzich & Raab, 1980). Some have proposed that Latinos may perceive somatic complaints as less stigmatizing, and therefore more readily report such symptoms. Others have explained that Latinos believe that they are more likely to receive care if they disclose physical problems rather than mental health problems (Canino et al., 1992). Variations in symptom expression across cultures underscore the need for providers to exercise flexibility when assessing Latino patients (Hackethal et al., 2013; Hirai, Stanley, & Novy, 2006; Lewis-Fernandez et al., 2010). Specifically among Latinos (especially Spanish speaking Latinos), physiological/somatic symptoms may be a better indicator of an anxiety disorder, such as GAD, than questions that tap into psychological and cognitive worry.

Ataques de Nervios

Much research surrounds the cultural idiom of distress called ataques de nervios. Translated as "nervous attacks," symptoms of "ataques de nervios" include trembling, crying spells, screaming uncontrollably, and sudden verbal and physical aggression (Lopez & Guarnaccia, 2000). Additional symptoms may include dizziness or fainting, dissociation, and suicidal gestures. These attacks are most prevalent among Puerto Rican and Caribbean populations and episodes often occur after a stressful life event or significant loss (e.g., divorce, death of close family member) (Lopez & Guarnaccia, 2000). Indeed, reports show overlap between ataques de nervios and panic disorder (Lewis-Fernandez et al., 2002; Salman et al., 1998). However, only a third of ataques fulfill DSM-IV criteria for panic attacks and only 17% fulfill panic disorder criteria, suggesting that ataques are not completely accounted for by DSM criteria. While in some cases, ataques may be indicative of an anxiety disorder, in other cases, it may simply be a transient expression of distress among Latinos.

Nervios

"Nervios" is another cultural idiom of distress that is related to anxiety. Nervios differs from ataques as it represents more of a generalized state of distress rather than a discrete episode. Among Latinos, the concept of nervios represents an expression of both physical and emotional distress that often emerges from conflicts in various life domains (family, legal status, parenting, gender roles, etc.) and most often occurs in the context of social disadvantage (Guarnaccia & Farias, 1988). Somatic symptoms associated with nervios include headaches, backaches, trembling, lack of appetite and sleep, fatigue, physical agitation, difficulty breathing, chest pain, gastrointestinal problems, dizziness, blurred vision, fevers, and sweating, among other symptoms (Salgado de Snyder, de Jesus Diaz-Perez, & Maldonado, 1995). Psychological symptoms associated with nervios include irritability, anger, sadness, obsessive ideation, overwhelming concerns, lack of concentration, confusion, crying spells, fears, anxiety, and erratic behavior (Finkler, 1985; Salgado de Snyder et al., 1995).

Questions regarding these expressions of distress should be included in assessments with Latinos. Further, efforts are necessary to educate providers about variations in how Latinos may experience and describe anxiety symptoms. Providers also should be advised that many of these complaints overlap with symptoms of depression and anxiety but are not necessarily synonymous with these disorders.

Cultural Considerations Applied to Evidence-Based Interventions in an Integrated Model of Care

Integrated care efforts in primary care settings may improve the screening and treatment of Latinos with mental health needs simply through accessibility, given they are more likely to seek these services from their primary care providers. Indeed, integrating a consulting psychiatrist and psychological services within primary care has improved access to mental health care among typically underserved minority and low-SES populations (Schreiter et al., 2013). However, access alone does not necessarily improve treatment outcomes (Areán et al., 2008). Culturally appropriate health care practices are necessary to improve diagnosis and quality of care (Young et al., 2001).

Some have proposed that adaptations to interventions are necessary to improve the culturally appropriateness, satisfaction and response rates associated with evidence-based interventions for ethnic/racial minorities. However, debate about the utility of cultural adaptations continues (Benuto & O'Donohue, 2015; Lau, 2006) and few cultural adaptations have been examined in the primary care setting. At present, most findings suggest that Latinos who receive minimally adapted CBT have similarly favorable outcomes as non-Latino whites in both primary care and non-primary care settings (Chavira et al., 2014; Pina, Silverman, Fuentes, Kurtines, & Weems, 2003). Unfortunately, findings are often limited by the fact that most trials have only recruited small proportions of Latinos and many have not been conducted with Spanish speaking or less-acculturated populations. More consistently, data have emerged to suggest potential differences in the social validity (e.g. adherence, engagement) of existing evidence-based interventions such as CBT (Chavira et al., 2014; Lau, 2006) when used with ethnic minorities such as Latinos, underscoring the need for interventions to consider the impact of engagement-related concerns in this group.

Engagement of Latinos in Integrated Models of Care

Studies examining engagement-related outcomes (e.g., treatment uptake, adherence, and attrition) have mostly focused on patients with depression; these studies have found higher attrition rates (drop-out) in both pharmacological and psychosocial interventions for Latinos when compared to whites (Arnow et al., 2007; Chavira et al., 2014; Organista, Muñoz, & Gonzalez, 1994). Problems with medication compliance, CBT attendance, and completion of CBT homework assignments, also have been reported (Aguilera, Garza, & Muñoz, 2010; Miranda & Cooper, 2004). Differences in attendance rates and premature termination have been attributed to logistic (e.g., multiple competing demands, transportation etc.), motivational, and attitudinal factors (e.g., outcome expectancies and stigma) (McCabe, 2002; Miranda, Azócar, et al., 2003). Other factors such as perceived cultural fit of the program, beliefs about causes of mental illness, and therapist-client ethnic match, may also have an impact.

Recommendations for Primary Care

Interventions that are delivered in primary care settings are advised to attend to these differences and utilize strategies to improve engagement in services for Latinos. When working with Latinos in primary care, it is advisable to clarify the need for services and to provide education about the therapy process itself. More specifically, PCPs and behavioral health specialists should be prepared to explain the "therapy" process and to dispel potential myths about therapy (e.g., therapy as long-term, therapy as too difficult, etc.). Further, providers should be active in discussing stigma related concerns, given their frequency in the Latino population. Previous data suggest that stigma associated with mental illness can prevent individuals from seeking care and lead to premature termination and poor adherence (Interian, Martinez, Guarnaccia, Vega, & Escobar, 2007; Nadeem et al., 2007; Sirey et al., 2001). In addition, previous negative experiences with mental health treatment may lead to premature dropout and less future use (McCabe, 2002; McKay, Stoewe, McCadam, & Gonzales, 1998). Important to note, the experience of discrimination has been posited as one explanation for low service use among Latinos with mental health care needs and findings suggest that the perception of discrimination itself, is associated with negative mental health outcomes such as suicidal ideation, state anxiety, trait anxiety, and depression (Hwang & Goto, 2008; Krieger, Smith, Naishadham, Hartman, & Barbeau, 2005).

Barriers such as lack of time, inability to obtain permission to leave work, lack of childcare, and transportation are common logistic barriers that may interfere with initial attendance or ongoing treatment (Alvidrez & Azocar, 1999; Fortuna, Alegria, & Gao, 2010; McKay, McCadam, & Gonzales, 1996; Miranda, Duan, et al., 2003; Miranda & Green, 1999). Such barriers may need to be discussed and problem-solved on a regular basis. In a study of 339 Latino primary care patients with depressive disorders, education sessions, telephone sessions, transportation assistance, and family involvement, were engagement strategies that increased the likelihood of service utilization in this group (Dwight-Johnson et al., 2010). To ensure effective engagement, it is likely that these same issues will need to be addressed in integrated models of care for Latinos with anxiety disorders.

Lastly, bilingual and culturally competent providers as well as well-trained interpreters are necessary in integrated models of mental health care. Unfortunately, recent results from a 10-year perspective examining efforts to diversify the mental health workforce and increase the pool of bilingual providers, suggest that little progress has been made in this area (DeCarlo Santiago & Miranda, 2014). In the absence of a small bilingual mental health workforce, novel models of treatment and service delivery may be required. For example, it is possible that the shortage of bilingual clinicians could be addressed in part through the use of a bilingual and culturally competent paraprofessional workforce (e.g. patient navigators, peer counselors, and/or community health workers/promotoras) to facilitate the delivery of services with Latino communities. Additionally, technological advances including therapies delivered via computer can be translated and used as part of integrated care models for Latinos with anxiety disorders. Future research is necessary to examine such innovations broadly and in primary care models specifically.

Moving toward an integrated health care model that adequately addresses the needs of the Latino population, involves significant administrative, operational, and technical challenges. Leadership and administration are responsible for the development of program protocols that train staff and providers in the fundamentals of integrated care, and also in the fundamentals of culturally competence. Training should focus on how to provide patient-centered health care through the incorporation of the patient's values, needs, and concerns in order to foster a more personalized, culturally appropriate treatment approach. Leadership in primary care must take an active role in reinforcing these messages, with ongoing in-service trainings, and continually encourage the shift away from fragmented, silo-based health care, to one of culturally competent collaboration and information sharing. It is also necessary to ensure that a solid interoperable information technology infrastructure is in place to: (a) promote and monitor collaborative, evidence-based practice, (b) allow for timely sharing of patient health records and treatment plans across providers and care or case managers, and; (c) assist in preventing unnecessary or duplicate procedures and treatments.

Conclusions and Future Directions

Integrated health care has potentially vast implications for improving mental health care amongst the Latino population, especially those who are socially disadvantaged, but more research is required to empirically validate this position. Particularly important is greater examination of cultural factors that may need to be considered in models of integrated care. The current chapter provides a discussion of culturally related assessment and treatment factors that may need to be considered to improve the quality of integrated models of care.

Meeting the aims of current health care reform efforts—to improve quality of care, provide better health for populations, and lower health care expenditures, necessitates the full integration of behavioral health care for underserved populations. The passage of the Affordable Care Act makes it more likely that the number of Latinos with health insurance will increase. In fact, it was recently estimated that the rate of uninsured Latinos has already decreased from 36 to 23 % (Doty, Blumenthal, & Collins, 2014), and increased utilization of mental health by Latinos have been observed (Schreiter et al., 2013). Whether there will be optimal quality mental health services to meet the needs of this population, particularly in primary care settings, remains uncertain. Efforts to improve the availability, accessibility, and quality of behavioral health care for Latinos in primary care, is an important avenue of research that has the potential to deter the chronic course of anxiety that can be so debilitating when left untreated in this population.

References

Aguilera, A., Garza, M. J., & Muñoz, R. F. (2010). Group cognitive-behavioral therapy for depression in Spanish: Culture-sensitive manualized treatment in practice. *Journal of Clinical Psychology, 66*(8), 857–867. doi:10.1002/jclp.20706.

Alegría, M., Canino, G., Ríos, R., Vera, M., Calderón, J., Rusch, D., & Ortega, A. N. (2002). Mental health care for Latinos: Inequalities in use of specialty mental health services among Latinos, African Americans, and non-Latino Whites. *Psychiatric Services*, *53*(*12*), 1547–1555.

Alvidrez, J., & Azocar, F. (1999). Distressed women's clinic patients: Preferences for mental health treatments and perceived obstacles. *General Hospital Psychiatry, 21*(5), 340–347.
Archer, J., Bower, P., Gilbody, S., Lovell, K., Richards, D., Gask, L., & Coventry, P. (2012). Collaborative care for depression and anxiety problems. *Cochrane Database System Review*, *(10)*.
Areán, P. A., Ayalon, L., Jin, C., McCulloch, C. E., Linkins, K., Chen, H., & Estes, C. (2008). Integrated specialty mental health care among older minorities improves access but not outcomes: Results of the PRISMe study. *International Journal of Geriatric Psychiatry, 23(10)*, 1086–1092.
Arnow, B. A., Blasey, C., Manber, R., Constantino, M. J., Markowitz, J. C., Klein, D. N., … Rush, A. J. (2007). Dropouts versus completers among chronically depressed outpatients. *Journal of Affective Disorders, 97(1–3)*, 197–202.
Azocar, F., Areán, P., Miranda, J., & Muñoz, R. F. (2001). Differential item functioning in a Spanish translation of the Beck depression inventory. *Journal of Clinical Psychology, 57*, 355–365.
Benuto, L., & O'Donohue, W. (2015). Is culturally sensitive cognitive behavioral therapy an empirically supported treatment?: The case for Latinos. *International Journal of Psychology and Psychological Therapy, 15*(3), 405.
Benuto, L., Olmo-Terasa, A., & Reyes-Rabanillo, M. (2011). Exploring the factor structure and psychometric properties of a Spanish translation of the clinician-administered PTSD scale. *The International Journal of Educational and Psychological Assessment, 9*(1), 14.
Blanco, C., Patel, S. R., Liu, L., Jiang, H., Lewis-Fernandez, R., Schmidt, A. B., … Olfson, M. (2007). National trends in ethnic Disparities in mental health care. *Medical Care, 45*, 1012–1019.
Breslau, J., Kendler, K. S., Su, M., Gaxiola-Aguilar, S., & Kessler, R. C. (2005). Lifetime risk and persistence of psychiatric disorders across ethnic groups in the United States. *Psychological Medicine, 35*, 317–327.
Campbell-Sills, L., Norman, S. B., Craske, M. G., Sullivan, G., Lang, A. J., Chavira, D. A., & Stein, M. B. (2009). Validation of a brief measure of anxiety-related severity and impairment: The Overall Anxiety Severity and Impairment Scale (OASIS). *Journal of Affective Disorders, 112(1)*, 92–101.
Canino, I. A., Rubio-Stipec, M., Canino, G. J., & Escobar, J. I. (1992). Functional somatic symptoms: A cross-ethnic comparison. *American Journal of Orthopsychiatry, 62*(4), 605–612. doi:10.1037/h0079376.
Carlson, L., & Bultz, B. (2003). Cancer distress screening: Needs, models and methods. *Journal of Psychosomatic Research, 55*, 403–409.
Center for Mental Health Services. (2000). *Cultural competence standards in managed care mental health services; Four underserved/underrepresented racial/ethnic groups*. Retrieved July 28, 2015, from http://www.ce4alliance.com/articles/100124/culturalcompetenceManageCare.pdf.
Chambless, D. L., & Ollendick, T. H. (2001). Empirically supported interventions: Controversies and evidence. *Annual Review of Psychology, 52*, 685–716.
Chavira, D. A., Golinelli, D., Sherbourne, C., Stein, M. B., Sullivan, G., Bystritsky, A., … Craske, M. (2014). Treatment engagement and response to CBT among Latinos with anxiety disorders in primary care. *Journal of Consulting and Clinical Psychology, 82(3)*, 392–403. doi: 10.1037/a0036365.
Chavira, D. A., Stein, M. B., & Roy-Byrne, P. (2008). Managing anxiety in primary care. In *Oxford Handbook of anxiety and related disorders*. New York, NY: Oxford University Press. doi:10.1093/oxfordhb/9780195307030.013.0039.
Collins, C., Hewson, D. L., Munger, R., & Wade, T. (2010). *Evolving models of behavioral health integration in primary care*. New York, NY: Milbank Memorial Fund.
Connor, K., Kobak, K., Churchill, L., Katzelnick, D., & Davidson, J. (2001). Mini-SPIN: A brief screening assessment for generalized social anxiety disorder. *Depression and Anxiety, 14*, 137–140.

Coventry, P. A., Hudson, J. L., Kontopantelis, E., Archer, J., Richards, D. A., Gilbody, S., … Bower, P. (2014). Characteristics of effective collaborative care for treatment of depression: A systematic review and meta-regression of 74 randomised controlled trials. *PLoS One, 9(9)*, e108114.

Craske, M. G. (1999). *Anxiety disorders: Psychological approaches to theory and treatment.* Boulder, CO: Westview Press.

Craske, M. G., Roy-Byrne, P. P., Stein, M. B., Sullivan, G., Sherbourne, C., & Bystritsky, A. (2009). Treatment for anxiety disorders: Efficacy to effectiveness to implementation. *Behaviour Research and Therapy, 47*(11), 931–937.

DeCarlo Santiago, C., & Miranda, J. (2014). Progress in improving mental health services for racial-ethnic minority groups: A ten-year perspective. *Psychiatric Services, 65*(2), 180–185. doi:10.1176/appi.ps.201200517.

Degoratis, L. (2000). *BSI-18: Administration, scoring and procedures manual.* Minneapolis, MN: National Computer Systems.

Derose, K. P., & Baker, D. W. (2000). Limited English proficiency and Latinos' use of physician services. *Medical Care Research Review, 57*, 76–91.

Doty, M. M., Blumenthal, D., & Collins, S. R. (2014). The affordable care act and health insurance for Latinos. *JAMA, 17*, 1735–1736.

Duffy, F. F., Chung, H., Trivedi, M., Rae, D. S., Regier, D. A., & Katzelnick, D. J. (2008). Systematic use of patient-rated depression severity monitoring: Is it helpful and feasible in clinical psychiatry? *Psychiatric Services, 59*, 1148–1154.

Dwight-Johnson, M., Lagomasino, I. T., Hay, J., Zhang, L., Tang, L., Green, J. M., & Duan, N. (2010). Effectiveness of collaborative care in addressing depression treatment preferences among low-income Latinos. *Psychiatric Services, 61(11)*, 1112–1118. doi: 10.1176/appi.ps.61.11.1112.

Ell, K., Katon, W., Xie, B., Lee, P. J., Kapetanovic, S., Guterman, J., & Chou, C. P. (2010). Collaborative Care management of major depression among low-income, Predominantly Hispanic subjects with diabetes. A randomized controlled trial. *Diabetes Care, 33(4)*, 706–713.

Ennis, S. R., Rios-Vargas, M., & Albert, N. G. (2010). *The Hispanic population 2010: 2010 Census briefs.* Retrieved July 28, 2015, from http://www.census.gov/prod/cen2010/briefs/c2010br-04.pdf.

Escobar, J. I., Gomez, J., & Tuason, V. B. (1983). Depressive phenomenology in North and South American patients. *The American Journal of Psychiatry, 140*(1), 47–51.

Finch, B. K., Kolody, B., & Vega, W. A. (2000). Perceived discrimination and depression among Mexican-origin adults in California. *Journal of Health and Social Science Behavior, 4*, 295–313.

Finch, B. K., & Vega, W. A. (2003). Acculturation stress, social support, and self-rated health among Latinos in California. *Journal of Immigrant Health, 5*, 109–117.

Finkler, K. (1985). Symptomatic differences between the sexes in rural Mexico. *Culture, Medicine and Psychiatry, 9*(1), 27–57.

Fortuna, L. R., Alegria, M., & Gao, S. (2010). Retention in depression treatment among ethnic and racial minority groups in the United States. *Depression and Anxiety, 27*(5), 485–494. doi:10.1002/da.20685.

Gilbody, S., Bower, P., Fletcher, J., Richards, D., & Sutton, A. J. (2006). Collaborative care for depression: A cumulative meta-analysis and review of longer-term outcomes. *Archives of Internal Medicine, 166*(21), 2314–2321.

Givens, J. L., Houston, T. K., Van Voorhees, B. W., Ford, D. E., & Cooper, L. A. (2007). Ethnicity and preferences for depression treatment. *General Hospital Psychiatry, 29*, 182–191.

Grant, B. F., Stinson, F. S., Hasin, D. S., Dawson, D. A., Chou, S. P., & Anderson, K. (2004). Immigration and lifetime prevalence of DSM-IV psychiatric disorders among Mexican Americans and Whites in the United States: Results from the National Epidemiologic Survey on alcohol and related conditions. *Archives of General Psychiatry, 61*, 1226–1233.

Guarnaccia, P. J., & Farias, P. (1988). The social meanings of nervios: A case study of a Central American woman. *Social Science & Medicine, 26*(12), 1223–1231.

Hackethal, V., Spiegel, S., Lewis-Fernandez, R., Kealey, E., Salerno, A., & Finnerty, M. (2013). Towards a cultural adaptation of family psychoeducation: Findings from three Latino focus groups. *Community Mental Health Journal, 49*(5), 587–598. doi:10.1007/s10597-012-9559-1.

Hiott, A., Grzywacz, J. G., Arcury, T. A., & Quandt, S. A. (2006). Gender differences in anxiety and depression among immigrant Latinos. *Families, Systems & Health, 24*, 137–146.

Hirai, M., Stanley, M. A., & Novy, D. M. (2006). Generalized anxiety disorder in Latinos: Symptom characteristics and prediction of severity. *Journal of Psychopathology and Behavioral Assessment, 28*(1), 49–56.

Hofmann, S. G., & Smits, J. A. (2008). Cognitive–behavioral therapy for adult anxiety disorders: A meta-analysis of randomized placebo-controlled trials. *Journal of Clinical Psychiatry, 69*, 621–632.

Hovey, J. D. (2000a). Acculturative stress, depression, and suicidal ideation in Mexican immigrants. *Cultural Diversity & Ethnic Minority Psychology, 6*, 134–151.

Hovey, J. D. (2000b). Psychosocial predictors of acculturative stress in Mexican immigrants. *The Journal of Psychology, 134*, 490–502.

Huang, F. Y., Chung, H., Kroenke, K., Delucchi, K. L., & Spitzer, R. L. (2006). Using the Patient Health Questionnaire-9 to measure depression among racially and ethnically diverse primary care patients. *Journal of General Internal Medicine, 6*, 547–552.

Hwang, W.-C., & Goto, S. (2008). The impact of perceived racial discrimination on the mental health of Asian American and Latino college students. *Cultural Diversity and Ethnic Minority Psychology, 14*(4), 326–335. doi:10.1037/1099-9809.14.4.326.

Interian, A., Martinez, I., Guarnaccia, P., Vega, W., & Escobar, J. (2007). A qualitative analysis of the perception of stigma among Latinos receiving antidepressants. *Psychiatric Services, 58*(12), 1591–1594.

Janeway, D. (2009). An integrated approach to the diagnosis and treatment of anxiety within the practice of cardiology. *Cardiology in Review, 17*(1), 36–43.

Kaiser Commission on Medicaid and the Uninsured. (2004). *Covering new Americans: A review of federal and state policies related to immigrants eligibility and access to publicly funded health insurance*. Retrieved July 28, 2015, from http://kff.org/medicaid/report/covering-new-americans-a-review-of-federal/.

Katon, W., Russo, J., Lin, E. H., Schmittdiel, J., Ciechanowski, P., Ludman, E., … Von Korff, M. (2012). Cost-effectiveness of a multicondition collaborative care intervention: A randomized controlled trial. *Archives of general psychiatry, 69*(5), 506–514.

Katon, W., Unützer, J., Wells, K., & Jones, L. (2010). Collaborative depression care: History, evolution and ways to enhance dissemination and sustainability. *General Hospital Psychiatry, 32*(5), 456–464.

Katzelnick, D., Duffy, F. F., Chung, H., Regier, D. A., Rae, D. S., & Trivedi, M. H. (2011). Depression outcomes in a psychiatric clinical practice settings: Using a self-rated measure of depression severity. *Psychiatric Services, 62*, 929–935.

Kessler, R. C., Chiu, W. T., Demler, O., & Walters, E. E. (2005). Prevalence, severity, and comorbidity of 12-month DSM-IV disorders in the National Comorbidity Survey Replication. *Archives of General Psychiatry, 62*, 617–627.

Kessler, R. C., McGongale, K. A., Ahao, S., Nelson, C. B., Hughes, M., Eshelman, S., … Kendler, K. S. (1994). Lifetime and 12-month prevalence of DSM-III-R psychiatric disorders in the United States: Results from the National Comorbidity Study. *Archives of General Psychiatry, 51*, 8–19.

Krieger, N., Smith, K., Naishadham, D., Hartman, C., & Barbeau, E. M. (2005). Experiences of discrimination: Validity and reliability of a self-report measure for population health research on racism and health. *Social Science & Medicine, 61*(7), 1576–1596. doi:10.1016/j.socscimed.2005.03.006.

Kroenke, K., Spitzer, R. L., Williams, J. B., Monahan, P. O., & Lowe, B. (2007). Anxiety disorders in primary care: Prevalence, impairment, comorbidity, and detection. *Annals of Internal Medicine, 146*, 317–325.

Ku, L., & Matani, S. (2001). Left out: Immigrants' access to health care and insurance. *Health Affairs, 20*, 247–256.
Lang, A., & Stein, M. (2006). An abbreviated PTSD checklist for use as a screening instrument in primary care. *Behaviour Research and Therapy, 43*, 585–594.
Lau, A. S. (2006). Making the case for selective and directed cultural adaptations of evidence-based treatments: Examples from parent training. *Clinical Psychology: Science and Practice, 13*(4), 295–310. doi:10.1111/j.1468-2850.2006.00042.x.
Lecrubier, Y., Sheehan, D. V., Weiller, E., Amorim, P., Bonora, I., Harnett Sheehan, K., & Dunbar, G. C. (1997). The mini international neuropsychiatric interview (MINI). A short diagnostic structured interview: Reliability and validity according to the CIDI. *European Psychiatry, 12*(5), 224–231.
Leslie, L. A., & Lietch, M. L. (1989). A demographic profile of recent Central American immigrants: Clinical and service implications. *Hispanic Journal of Behavioral Sciences, 11*, 315–329.
Lewis-Fernandez, R., Guarnaccia, P. J., Martinez, I. E., Salman, E., Schmidt, A., & Liebowitz, M. (2002). Comparative phenomenology of ataques de nervios, panic attacks, and panic disorder. *Culture, Medicine and Psychiatry, 26*(2), 199–223.
Lewis-Fernandez, R., Hinton, D. E., Laria, A. J., Patterson, E. H., Hofmann, S. G., Craske, M. G., ... Liao, B. (2010). Culture and the anxiety disorders: Recommendations for DSM-V. *Depression and Anxiety, 27*(2), 212–229.
Lopez, S. R., & Guarnaccia, P. J. J. (2000). Cultural psychopathology: Uncovering the social world of mental illness. *Annual Review of Psychology, 51*, 571–598. doi:10.1146/annurev.psych.51.1.571.
Markowitz, J. C., Speilman, L. A., Sullivan, M., & Fishman, B. (2000). An exploratory study of ethnicity and psychotherapy outcome among HIV-positive patients with depressive symptoms. *Journal of Psychotherapy Practice and Research, 9*, 226–231.
McCabe, K. M. (2002). Factors that predict premature termination among Mexican-American children in outpatient psychotherapy. *Journal of Child and Family Studies, 11*(3), 347–359. doi:10.1023/a:1016876224388.
McKay, M. M., McCadam, K., & Gonzales, J. J. (1996). Addressing the barriers to mental health services for inner city children and their caretakers. *Community Mental Health Journal, 32*(4), 353–361.
McKay, M. M., Stoewe, J., McCadam, K., & Gonzales, J. (1998). Increasing access to child mental health services for urban children and their caregivers. *Health & Social Work, 23*(1), 9–15.
Means-Christensen, A., Sherbourne, C., Roy-Byrne, P. P., Craske, M. G., & Stein, M. B. (2005). Using five questions to screen for five common mental disorders in primary care. *General Hospital Psychiatry, 28*, 108–118.
Menninger, W. W. (1995). Challenges to providing integrated treatment of anxiety disorders. *Bulletin of the Menninger Clinic, 59*(2, Suppl A), A86–A93.
Mezzich, J. E., & Raab, E. S. (1980). Depressive symptomatology across the Americas. *Archives of General Psychiatry, 37*(7), 818–823.
Mills, S. D., Fox, R. S., Malcarne, V. L., Roesch, S. C., Champagne, B. R., & Sadler, G. R. (2014). The psychometric properties of the generalized anxiety disorder-7 scale in Hispanic Americans with English or Spanish language preference. *Cultural Diversity & Ethnic Minority Psychology, 20*, 463–468.
Minsky, S., Vega, W. A., Miskimen, T., Gara, M., & Escobar, J. (2003). Diagnostic patterns of Latino, African American, and European American psychiatric patients. *Archives of General Psychiatry, 60*, 637–644.
Miranda, J., Azócar, F., Organista, K., Dwyer, E., & Areane, P. (2003). Treatment of depression among impoverished primary care patients from ethnic minority groups. *Psychiatric Services, 54*(2), 219–225.
Miranda, J., & Cooper, L. (2004). Disparities in care for depression among primary care patients. *Journal of General Internal Medicine, 19*, 120–126.

Miranda, J., Duan, N., Sherbourne, C., Schoenbaum, M., Lagomasino, I., Jackson-Triche, M., & Wells, K. B. (2003). Improving care for minorities: Can quality improvement interventions improve care and outcomes for depressed minorities? Results of a randomized, controlled trial. *Health Services Research, 38,* 613–630.

Miranda, J., & Green, B. (1999). The need for mental health services research focusing on poor young women. *Journal of Mental Health Policy and Economics, 2*(2), 73–80.

Muntingh, A., van der Feltz-Cornelis, C., van Marwijk, H., Spinhoven, P., Assendelft, W., de Waal, M., … van Balkom, A. (2013). Effectiveness of collaborative stepped care for anxiety disorders in primary care: A pragmatic cluster randomised controlled trial. *Psychotherapy and psychosomatics, 83(1)*, 37–44.

Nadeem, E., Lange, J., Edge, D., Fongwa, M., Belin, T., & Miranda, J. (2007). Does stigma keep poor young immigrant and U.S.-born Black and Latina women from seeking mental health care? *Psychiatric Services, 58*(12), 1547–1554.

Norton, P. J., & Price, E. C. (2007). A meta-analytic review of adult cognitive-behavioral treatment outcome across the anxiety disorders. *Journal of Nervous and Mental Disorders, 195*, 521–531.

Organista, K. C., & Muñoz, R. F. (1996). Cognitive behavioral therapy with Latinos. *Cognitive and Behavioral Practice, 3*, 255–270.

Organista, K. C., Muñoz, R. F., & Gonzalez, G. (1994). Cognitive-behavioral therapy for depression in low-income and minority medical outpatients: Description of a program and exploratory analyses. *Cognitive Therapy and Research, 18*, 241–259.

Perez, M. C., & Fortuna, L. (2005). Psychosocial stressors, psychiatric diagnosis, and utilization of mental health services among undocumented immigrant Latinos. *Journal of Immigrant and Refugee Services, 3*, 107–123.

Pina, A. A., Silverman, W. K., Fuentes, R. M., Kurtines, W. M., & Weems, C. F. (2003). Exposure-based cognitive-behavioral treatment for phobic and anxiety disorders: Treatment effects and maintenance for Hispanic/Latino relative to European-American youths. *Journal of the American Academy of Child and Adolescent Psychiatry, 42*(10), 1179–1187.

Pinninti, N. R., Madison, H., Musser, E., & Rissmiller, D. (2003). MINI international neuropsychiatric schedule: Clinical utility and patient acceptance. *European Psychiatry, 18*(7), 361–364.

Plante, T. G., Manuel, G. M., Menedez, A. V., & Marcotter, D. (1995). Coping with stress among Salvadoran Immigrants. *Hispanic Journal of Behavioral Sciences, 17*, 471–479.

Portes, A., & Rumbaut, R. G. (2006). *Immigrant America: A portrait*. Berkeley, CA: University of California Press.

Price, D., Beck, A., Nimmer, C., & Bensen, S. (2000). The treatment of anxiety disorders in a primary care HMO setting. *Psychiatric Quarterly, 71*(1), 31–45.

Ramirez, R. R., & de la Cruz, P. G. (2003). *The Hispanic population in the United States: March 2002*. Retrieved July 28, 2015, from http://www.census.gov/prod/2003pubs/p20-545.pdf.

Revicki, D. A., Brandenburg, N., Matza, L., Hornbrook, M. C., & Feeny, D. (2008). Health-related quality of life and utilities in primary-care patients with generalized anxiety disorder. *Quality of Life Research, 17*(10), 1285–1294.

Rollman, B. L., Belnap, B. H., Mazumdar, S., Houck, P. R., Zhu, F., Gardner, W., & Shear, M. K. (2005). A randomized trial to improve the quality of treatment for panic and generalized anxiety disorders in primary care. *Archives of General Psychiatry, 62(12)*, 1332–1341.

Roy-Byrne, P. P., & Cowley, D. S. (2007). Pharmacological treatments for panic disorder, generalized anxiety disorder, specific phobia and social anxiety disorder. In P. E. Nathan & J. M. Gorman (Eds.), *A guide to treatments that work* (3rd ed.). New York, NY: Oxford University Press.

Roy-Byrne, P. P., Craske, M. G., Stein, M. B., Sullivan, G., Bystritsky, A., Katon, W., … Sherbourne, C. D. (2005). A randomized effectiveness trial of cognitive-behavioral therapy and medication for primary care panic disorder. *Archives of General Psychiatry, 62,* 290–298.

Roy-Byrne, P., Craske, M. G., Sullivan, G., Rose, R. D., Edlund, M. J., Lang, A. J., … Stein, M. B. (2010). Delivery of evidence-based treatment for multiple anxiety disorders in primary care: A randomized controlled trial. *JAMA, 303*, 1921–1928. doi: 10.1001/jama.2010.608.

Roy-Byrne, P. P., Katon, W., Cowley, D. S., & Russo, J. (2001). A randomized effectiveness trial of collaborative care for patients with panic disorder in primary care. *Archives of General Psychiatry, 58*(9), 869–876.

Salgado de Snyder, V. N., de Jesus Diaz-Perez, M., & Maldonado, M. (1995). Los nervios de las mujeres Mexicanas de origin rural como motivo para buscar ayuda. *Salud Mental, 18*(1), 50–55.

Salman, E., Liebowitz, M. R., Guarnaccia, P. J., Jusino, C. M., Garfinkel, R., Street, L., ... Klein, D. F. (1998). Subtypes of ataques de nervios: The influence of coexisting psychiatric diagnosis. *Culture, Medicine and Psychiatry, 22(2)*, 231–244.

Schreiter, E. A. Z., Pandhi, N., Fondow, M. D. M., Thomas, C., Vonk, J., Reardon, C. L., & Serrano, N. (2013). Consulting psychiatry within an integrated primary care model. *Journal of Health Care for the Poor and Underserved 24(4)*, 1522–1530.

Sirey, J. A., Bruce, M. L., Alexopoulos, G. S., Perlick, D. A., Friedman, S. J., & Meyers, B. S. (2001). Stigma as a barrier to recovery: Perceived stigma and patient-rated severity of illness as predictors of antidepressant drug adherence. *Psychiatric Services, 52*(12), 1615–1620.

Spitzer, R. L., Kroenke, K., Williams, J. B., & Lowe, B. (2006). A brief measure for assessing generalized anxiety disorder: The GAD-7. *Archives of Internal Medicine, 166*(10), 1092–1097.

Spitzer, R. L., Kroenke, K., Williams, J. B., & Patient Health Questionnaire Primary Care Study Group. (1999). Validation and utility of a self-report version of PRIME-MD: The PHQ primary care study. *JAMA, 282*(18), 1737–1744.

Stein, M. (2005). Anxiety disorders: Somatic treatment. In H. Kaplan & B. Saddock (Eds.), *Comprehensive textbook of psychiatry* (pp. 1780–1788). Baltimore, MD: Williams and Wilkins.

Stockdale, S. E., Lagomasino, I. T., Siddique, J., McGuire, T., & Miranda, J. (2008). Racial and ethnic disparities in detection and treatment of depression and anxiety among psychiatric and primary health care visits, 1995-2005. *Medical Care, 46*, 668–677.

Sullivan, G., Craske, M. G., Sherbourne, C., Edlund, M. J., Rose, R. D., Golinelli, D., & Roy-Byrne, P. P. (2007). Design of the coordinated anxiety learning and management (CALM) study: Innovations in collaborative care for anxiety disorders. *General Hospital Psychiatry, 29(5)*, 379–387.

U.S. Department of Health and Human Services. (2001). *Mental health: Culture, race, and ethnicity. A supplement to mental health: A report of the surgeon general.* Rockville, MD: U.S. Department of Health and Human Services.

Unützer, J., Katon, W. J., Fan, M. Y., Schoenbaum, M. C., Lin, E. H., Della Penna, R. D., & Powers, D. (2008). Long-term cost effects of collaborative care for late-life depression. *The American Journal of Managed Care, 14*(2), 95–100.

Vega, W. A., Alderete, E., Kolody, B., & Aguilar-Gaxiola, S. (1998). Illicit drug use among Mexicans and Mexican Americans in California: The effects of gender and acculturation. *Addiction, 93*, 1839–1850.

Vega, W. A., Kolody, B., Aguilar-Gaxiola, S., & Catalano, R. (1999). Gaps in service utilization by Mexican Americans with mental health problems. *American Journal of Psychiatry, 156*, 928–934.

Vega, W. A., Kolody, B., & Aguilar-Gaxiola, S. A. (2001). Help-seeking for mental health problems among Mexican-Americans. *Journal of Immigrant Health, 3*, 133–140.

Young, A. S., Klap, R., Sherbourne, C. D., & Wells, K. B. (2001). The quality of care for depressive and anxiety disorders in the United States. *Archives of General Psychiatry, 58*, 55–61.

Chapter 12
Integrated Care for Pain Management Among Hispanic Populations

Gwen Sherwood and Jeanette A. McNeill

Introduction

The management of pain continues to challenge health care providers and the health care system with high direct expenditures for medical care and medication related to pain and the indirect costs associated with lost productivity in the work force. This has contributed to a "pain crisis in America" (Meghani, Byun, & Gallagher, 2012, p. 150) and resonates globally. Researchers report community populations may have a pain prevalence as high as 40 % noting minority members are overrepresented and more frequently undertreated (Mossey, 2011). Hispanic populations may present unique considerations that derive from the diversity of multinational backgrounds with strongly held values and beliefs and cultural perspectives. The purpose of this chapter is to explore the pain management experience of Hispanic populations, examine a quality improvement approach, and propose evidence-based integrated care solutions for more effective approaches.

G. Sherwood, Ph.D., R.N., F.A.A.N., A.N.E.F. (✉)
School of Nursing, University of North Carolina at Chapel Hill,
Chapel Hill, NC 27599, USA
e-mail: gwen.sherwood@unc.edu

J.A. McNeill, Dr.P.H., R.N., C.N.E., A.N.E.F.
School of Nursing, University of Northern Colorado, Greeley, CO 80639, USA

© Springer International Publishing Switzerland 2016

L.T. Benuto, W. O'Donohue (eds.), *Enhancing Behavioral Health in Latino Populations*, DOI 10.1007/978-3-319-42533-7_12

Managing Pain in Hispanic Populations

Pain is one of the primary reasons people seek health care; it can be a symptom of a condition in the body requiring treatment. Treating the accompanying pain may be in addition to treating the condition and may invoke other responses and reactions due to both long held beliefs and attitudes on the part of the patient and family but also for health care providers.

Perspectives on Pain

The varied nature of pain is one factor in the conundrum of managing pain effectively, and particularly for vulnerable populations. Pain is a subjective experience with multiple definitions. A common definition comes from the International Association for the Study of Pain which defines pain in terms of an unpleasant and emotional sensory experience associated with actual or potential tissue damage (2012); pain is therefore both a physical experience but also has a psychological and subjective context. McCaffery is credited with an oft quoted classic definition of pain as whatever the person who has pain says it is (Herr, Coyne, McCaffery, Manworren, & Merkel, 2011). As such, pain can best be explained with a biopsychosocial model that begins with the noxious stimulus, awareness that the stimulus is pain, followed by recognition from the brain of these signals as emotional and cognitive factors that determine perceptions of pain; these responses drive how one responds to pain including facial or verbal expressions and ultimately the decision to seek attention to resolve what is happening.

Pain is primarily classified as acute or chronic (International Association for the Study of Pain (IASP), 2012). Accurate assessment is critical as each classification may require unique approaches and behavioral interventions. Acute pain is of short duration, perhaps lasting less than 30 days, and may resolve as the body heals from another condition (Marchand, 2012). Persistent pain lasting more than 6 months may be classified as chronic pain and may be associated with a chronic illness such as arthritis, or may be a condition itself. Pain may also be further delineated between nociceptive (somatic, visceral), neuropathic (results from a disease or lesion affecting the somatosensory nervous system) or cancer related (IASP, 2012).

Managing pain involves several interacting components: pain assessment, strategies and interventions to manage pain, evaluation of effectiveness of pain management, and continuing reassessment of pain. High-quality pain management is collaborative; planning and decision making with the patient and interdisciplinary team lead to best management outcomes. To effectively manage pain, providers are responsible for appropriate comprehensive assessment and delivering treatment that is "efficacious, cost-conscious, culturally and developmentally appropriate, and safe," (Gordon et al., 2010, p. 1173). Providing education and information on pain management is an essential component of an effective management plan. Finally, evaluation and reassessment of response to treatment completes an effective management plan (Fig. 12.1).

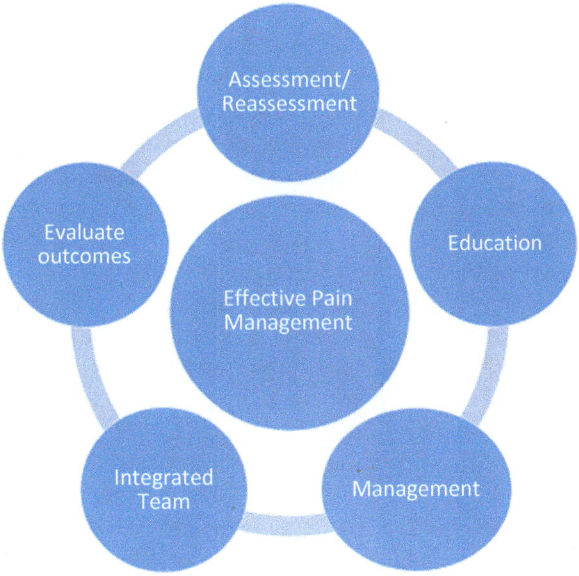

Fig. 12.1 Essentials of effective pain management

Pain and Culture: Biocultural Models of Pain

Few studies have examined the pain experience of Hispanics, yet evidence indicates a multicultural influence on the way people respond and interpret pain. The Biocultural Model of Pain integrates social learning theory into the physiologic explanation of how pain develops and is interpreted (Bates, 1987), therefore, fits with the aims of this book. Bates' biocultural model of pain is an integrated model combining the physiologically based gate-control, social learning, and social comparison theories to more comprehensively describe the pain experience; pain is far more than a strictly physiological experience. The outcome, or pain response, is affected by the physiological processing that occurs as well as the sociocultural influences on the individual. Bates model fits well with McCaffrey's definition of pain based on the subjective experience of the person, meaning pain is influenced by each person's experience, beliefs, and context.

Bates' model questions commonly held assumptions based on research primarily from a Caucasian perspective that the pain experience is the same for all. With worldwide attention on solving the problem of pain and the increasing globalization of health care, issues of disparity in treatment are a significant research topic. Bates' model bridges the narrow medical conception of pain as a symptom of tissue damage with the social and behavioral view of pain as a product of attitude, value, and experience that affects the physiological processes and outcomes involved in pain perception and response (Bates, 1987). Social modeling, group norms, and learned values influence pain perception, the processing of the pain response, and the behavior related to pain. It is assumed that all humans have similar neurophysiological responses to painful stimuli; however, this model exposes factors that influence response, namely social learning processes within ethnocultural groups.

The biocultural model of pain perception proposed by Bates can be applied as a framework for interpreting the influence of cultural context, group characteristics, and language barriers on the pain experience and has been used to better understand pain management among Hispanic populations (McNeill, Sherwood, Starck, & Nieto, 2001). For example, people of Hispanic background may highly value *familismo*, a core value of family attachment such that pain is viewed in terms of family impact. The commitment to family may influence decisions to seek treatment because of not wanting to disrupt family roles and responsibilities. *Personalismo* and *respecto* are other key cultural concepts that focus on mutual respect, empathy, and politeness in interactions, and *simpati*, that values harmonious relationships without interpersonal conflict (Zoucha & Reeves, 1999). Pain is often a symptom of other disease conditions and seeking treatment may focus reluctant attention on the person experiencing pain or lead to a disruption in family life because of care required to address symptoms. Respondents in a qualitative study on the pain experience among Hispanic populations in the southwestern, border area of the US (Sherwood, McNeill, Palos, & Starck, 2003) revealed cultural values and attitudes about pain and its influence within the family unit, and disruption in attending to activities of daily living related to pain, as important influences on decision making regarding obtaining treatment for pain. These findings were consistent with Bates' framework.

Perspectives on Managing Pain in Hispanic Populations

There is wide diversity among Hispanic subgroups and their views regarding health-care treatment often differ from health care providers. Among Hispanics, three basic sets of factors commonly affect world views: (1) core values, as noted above, including the value of family, respect for the individual and authority, and harmonious relationships; (2) the degree of acculturation and assimilation; and (3) the educational, economic, and social status of the individual. Acculturation contrasts with assimilation; acculturation is the ability to function in the new culture whereas assimilation is the adoption of the new host culture's beliefs, values, and practices (Kawaga-Singer, 2012). The most reliable indicators of acculturation that distinguish among Hispanic subgroups include place of origin, ethnic self-identification, and language reported to be preferred or used during an interview (Marin & Marin, 1991).

Several unique characteristics of Hispanic populations must be considered when developing health care interventions and in particular, managing the subjectivity of pain. The heterogeneity of the Hispanic population in the US compounds treatment approaches as the term Hispanic covers wide geographic diversity for country of origin and length of residency in the US. "Hispanic" is an umbrella term for several groups of Spanish speaking peoples, and includes persons of Mexican, Puerto Rican, Central or South American, or other Spanish culture, regardless of race. This broad classification means there are many background factors such as country of origin, time in the United States for acculturation, how well assimilated one is into the local culture and health care delivery system, one's support system such as family near-by, and language. Language is another compounding factor; many speak only Spanish. The limited availability of Spanish language measurement instruments and methods designed specifically for this population limit accurate communication to obtain comprehensive health history and assessment. And, there is general reluctance leading to low rates of participation of Hispanics in research to enhance the evidence base and resolve some of these limitations (Vilaro, 1994).

In spite of the challenge of language, the subjective nature of pain means communication, interpersonal communication, and history taking are important components of pain assessment and intervention. Communication is an important factor in establishing the relationship between health care providers and the patient and family, and language is key. Given that Spanish continues to be the primary language, and perhaps the only language spoken by many in Hispanic populations in the US, providing effective care may be problematic if health care providers are not themselves bilingual or translators are not readily available. Furthermore, Spanish language assessment tools, educational materials, and treatment strategies are limited although hospital regulations now mandate professional translation services to assure accurate communication between providers and patients without relying on family members to translate.

Evidence Base: Pain Outcomes among Hispanic Populations

Reports continue to reveal varying degrees of disparity in treating pain among Hispanic populations (Payne, 2009). Ethical principles in terms of beneficence and justice support the critical value of providing equitable and appropriate distribution of resources in a society. The social determinants of health may in some part help explain the continuing disparity in spite of research that has helped identify evidence and solutions. Disparities in pain treatment may derive from lack of access to health care due to living conditions, location and distance from providers, language, economic status, values and beliefs, and education. As such, the Institute of Medicine (2001) established a quality of care model based on the acronym STEEEP: quality care must be Safe, Timely, Equitable, Effective, Efficient, and Patient-Centered which fits the examination of quality of care for this vulnerable population.

Patient-centered care is the core of effective pain management and fits the emphasis noted previously on communication, relationships, and family that are important tenets in caring for patients from Hispanic populations. A first and critical step in providing patient-centered, effective, and equitable care is language;

communication between patient and provider is the cornerstone of effective treatment. Hispanics with limited English skills may be uncomfortable discussing health concerns if they feel unable to express their feelings about illness appropriately (Gordon et al., 2002). Translation is an important aspect of quality pain management in working with Hispanic patients experiencing pain, both for educational information and for service delivery. Because many Hispanic patients experience limitations of health care coverage, geographic factors or even educational level, providers may fail to establish collaborative partnerships with the patient and family. Effective pain treatment is grounded in a collaborative, integrated, interdisciplinary approach in which the patient and provider share decision making (Novy, Ritter, & McNeill, 2009). Language appropriate communication and tools help promote a collaborative partnership between members of the interdisciplinary team and the patient and family.

Evidence on the nature and prevalence of disparity in pain management among Hispanics is unclear. Historically, studies have reported that ethnic minority populations experience poorer pain management than white, non-Hispanics (Bonhan, 2001; Cleland et al., 1994; Ng, Dimsdale, Schragg, & Deutsch, 1996; Payne, 2009; Todd, Samaroo, & Hoffman, 1993). A more recent study by Meghani et al. (2012) reports that while Hispanics were prescribed some type of analgesic for acute pain, they were significantly less likely to be prescribed an opioid than non-Hispanic whites. This may be interpreted as a lack of collaboration with the Hispanic individual experiencing moderate to severe pain in working with providers due to misunderstanding, education, or language. In contrast, Bijur, Berard, Esses, Calderon, and Gallagher (2008) reported no evidence of a relationship between receiving analgesics, specifically opioid analgesics, and race or ethnicity of emergency department patients. A comprehensive analysis is reported in a meta-analysis of analgesic treatment disparities covering a 20 year period based on 34 qualifying studies (Meghani et al., 2012). While there were no overall disparities in use of analgesics for Hispanics, the use of opioid analgesia was significantly lower among Hispanics; they were 22 % less likely than white counterparts to receive treatment with opioids (OR 0.78, $p=0.006$).

This evidence points to lingering questions about the role providers have in managing pain and the role of the partnership between patient and provider in accurate assessment and consideration of treatment choices. A study of analgesia in childbirth by Atherton, Feeg, and El-Adham (2004) found that Hispanic women were twice as likely *not* to receive an epidural procedure during childbirth, although the authors note that decision making in childbirth is influenced not only by provider choice but also by mothers' decision making in accordance with cultural expectations.

Communication has a pivotal role in establishing a partnership role between patients and their healthcare providers for most effective pain management, and so does education and information about pain management. Katz et al. (2011) interviewed focus groups of Hispanic and Non-Hispanic white patients with knee and back pain regarding management of their pain problem and preferences for decision making in relation to treatment. Hispanic participants reported a general preference for allowing their physicians to take the primary role in decision making, as well as the importance of faith and religion in coping with their pain and disability. This may indicate a need for more current education about pain management to improve care outcomes.

Provider bias may also contribute to ineffective or inadequate management of pain (Payne, 2009). Stepanikova (2012) found that two potential factors affecting the occurrence of disparities involve implicit biases and pressures related to time to treat. Eighty-one family physicians and general internists were provided a case vignette of a patient with chest pain; the clinicians were advised regarding the time they had for decision-making as well as treatment possibilities such as diagnosis and referral. Among the findings, perceived bias regarding race and ethnicity led to increased likelihood that Hispanic and African American patients were not diagnosed with serious pain, and were not referred to specialists. These reports confirm the need to continue to study the complex issues surrounding pain management in ethnic populations and to provide education and information to both providers and patients.

Measuring Pain Management Quality: Key to Improvement

Language may pose a significant barrier for Hispanics seeking health care. Spanish assessment tools and educational materials are limited. Hispanics with limited English skills may be uncomfortable discussing health concerns if they feel unable to express their feelings about illness appropriately (Gordon et al., 2002). Bonhan (2001) noted that because the majority of studies have found a disparity in pain treatment by ethnic group, further study of language in the communication about pain will help to unravel the causes of these disparities. The Joint Commission on the Accreditation of Healthcare Organizations, (2003) recognized the need for linguistically appropriate pain assessment tools to have available Spanish versions of the numeric scale (continuum with 0 no pain graduating up to 10 as worst pain), FACES in both English and Spanish (Wong-Baker FACES Foundation (2015). Wong-Baker FACES® Pain Rating Scale. Retrieved September 19, 2015 with permission from http://www.WongBakerFACES.org) (Fig. 12.2), and pain location diagrams. Another is the Spanish version of the Brief Pain Inventory (Cleland, 2009). However, until recently, there were no tools developed for Hispanics that were both culturally and linguistically appropriate for assessment of the experience of pain for Hispanic individuals of a range of cultural traditions (Mexican American, Puerto Rican, etc.) (Table 12.1).

National regulations (The Joint Commission, 2003, 2012) emphasize the need to assess the effectiveness of pain management and specify components of an acute pain management program for health care (The Joint Commission, 2012). Culturally appropriate approaches are essential to achieve effective pain management for any cultural group. Language is crucial; communication is the cornerstone of accurate pain assessment (Juarez, Ferrell, & Borneman, 1998). Although Bonham

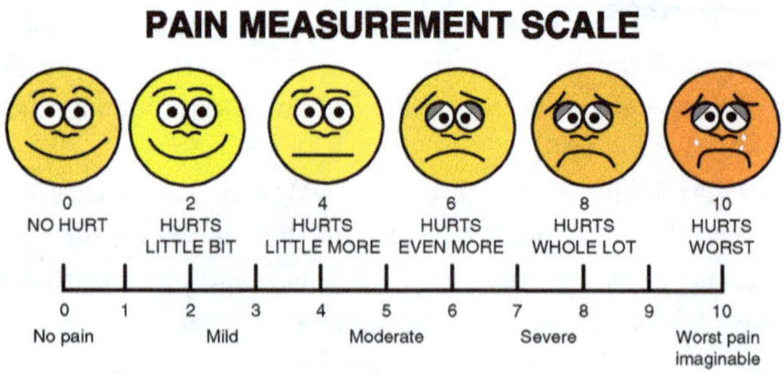

Fig. 12.2 FACES pain measurement scale for adults or children (Wong-Baker FACES Foundation (2015). Wong-Baker FACES® Pain Rating Scale. Retrieved September 19, 2015 with permission from http://www.WongBakerFACES.org) in English and Spanish

Table 12.1 Measuring outcomes of pain management: spanish language tools

Instrument focus	Instrument title	Available in Spanish
Unidimensional measures of pain intensity	Numeric pain intensity scale, verbal intensity scale, FACES scale (Wong-Baker and others)	Yes
Multidimensional measures of pain	Brief Pain Inventory	Yes
	American Pain Society-Patient Outcome Questionnaire-Revised	Yes
Acute pain	Houston Pain Outcome Instrument (HPOI)	Yes
Multidimensional measures of pain	Chronic Pain Acceptance Questionnaire (CPAQ) (Rodero et al., 2010)	Yes
Chronic (Fibromyalgia)	Pain Self Perception Scale for Fibromyalgia (Garcia-Campayo et al., 2010)	Yes

recommended as early as 2001 that further study of language to communicate about pain will help to unravel the causes of continuing reports of disparities, still there are reports of disparity and inadequate treatment. Hispanics experiencing pain are not consistently managed in accordance with the components of quality proposed by Gordon et al. (2005) nor by the IOM STEEEP model for quality care (2001). For example, assessment may lack language interpretation and thus overlook critical information. Pain management disparities, then, can derive from the linguistic challenges in the assessment process as well as the underreporting of pain intensity among minority individuals (Mossey, 2011).

Components of Quality Pain Management

Questions about pain management can be evaluated in terms of quality (Zoega, Gunnarsdottir, Wilson, & Gordon, 2016). The acronym STEEEP proposed by the Institute of Medicine in 2001, cited above, provides a framework for examining quality of care relevant to pain management among Hispanic populations that fits the goals of this chapter. STEEEP examines health care in terms of care that is safe, timely, effective, equitable, efficient, and patient-centered. Increasingly, patient-centered care is recognized as the foundation for delivering quality care because it addresses cultural perspectives. Additionally, safety is a closely linked concept to quality; quality measures safety and safe care is concerned with quality. There are inherent safety issues in managing pain, and in fact, pain mismanagement is described as a medical error (Starck, Sherwood, Adams-McNeill, & Thomas, 2001) when not delivered according to standards of care to meet the unique needs of the patient (McNeill, Sherwood, & Starck, 2004) or address the quality aims described previously in the STEEEP model.

Measurement of Effective Pain Management in Hispanic Populations

Differing results in reporting the effectiveness of pain management among Hispanic populations may be attributed to the lack of effective measures, the variability among Hispanic populations, reluctance to participate in research studies, and assumptions and attitudes of researchers and clinicians about pain management (McNeill et al., 2003). Evidence supports the importance of using language appropriate tools and strategies to achieve best outcomes; see Table 12.2 below. Two comprehensive quality management tools are presented that have been field tested in Spanish language with Hispanic populations to meet the need for linguistically appropriate measurement tools, the American Pain Society—Patient Outcome Questionnaire and the Houston Pain Outcome Instrument.

American Pain Society-Patient Outcome Questionnaire

The most reported measure of pain management is the American Pain Society-Patient Outcome Questionnaire (APS-POQ) (2001). Comprehensive studies using the APS-POQ have consistently revealed patient reports of moderate to severe pain

Table 12.2 A quality pain management approach (Adapted from Porche, 2010)

• Appropriate assessment and management
• Initial assessment upon admission/provider contact and on-going assessment
• Documentation of assessment and reassessment
• Relevant treatment plan consistent with patient pain severity, duration, and level
• Education and information about pain management and resources
• Discharge information, resources, and options
• Knowledgeable, informed providers
• Monitoring health care delivery organization effectiveness of pain management outcomes

intensity and interference ratings, and high satisfaction ratings among general populations (Gordon et al., 2002). The APS-POQ was revised in 2010 as the American Pain Society-Patient Outcome Questionnaire-Revised (APS-POQ-R) (Gordon et al., 2010). However, data was not reported on Hispanic populations in these studies. The APS-POQ-R is available in 11 languages, including Spanish, on the American Pain Society web-site (http://americanpainsociety.org/education/2010-revised-outcomes-questionnaire).

McNeill et al. (2001) reported using the original APS-POQ with a sample from Hispanic populations. They found that 98 % of patients ($n = 104$) in a rural sample of Mexican American postoperative medical/surgical patients in a regional hospital on the U.S.-Mexico border reported pain in the preceding 24 h. Mean current pain and usual pain ratings were in the moderate range, while worst pain ratings and pain-related interference for activities associated with recovery from surgery were in the severe range. Satisfaction ratings were moderately high (4.67) (on a 1–6 scale with 6 being very satisfied) in spite of pain. From these findings and realizing the importance of language, this research team pursued development of a Spanish language instrument to better understand issues in pain management for Hispanic populations, described below.

Houston Pain Outcome Instrument (HPOI)

Modeled on the prototype APS-POQ, the Houston Pain Outcome Instrument (HPOI) derived from a qualitative study on the experience of pain among Hispanics in a sample of 35 Hispanics from urban and rural sites in Texas who were between 18 and 70 years of age (Sherwood et al., 2003). The qualitative interviews were conducted in Spanish and translated as the first phase of the project to develop a linguistically appropriate pain assessment instrument for Spanish speakers. Data from the interviews describe Hispanic individuals' past experiences with pain, attitudes toward pain and attention to pain stimuli. These descriptions are consistent with Bates' biocultural model in which social learning processes regarding pain integrate with cognitive awareness and physiological variables.

Participants' responses were categorized into five themes, which then formed the basis for organization of the new, Spanish language instrument: Characteristics of pain experiences, Managing pain, Information about pain, Interactions with providers, and Cultural considerations.

- Characteristics about pain were described by sharing attitudes, beliefs, and expectations; responses to pain; effects of pain on their lives; and descriptions of the pain itself.
- Managing pain included multiple approaches to pain and descriptions of the effectiveness of formal prescribed interventions and those not prescribes, such as nonpharmacological. While most participants described use of analgesics, many also described nonpharmacological approaches such as meditation and prayer, special teas, and support of family.

- Information about pain included sources and types of information, whether from providers, family, or multimedia; language preferences; and, effectiveness of information received.
- Interactions with providers included both how providers approached and responded to the participants' pain, but also how patients responded to the providers, hence the relationship mattered.
- Cultural considerations included gender-specific considerations, religious beliefs and approaches, specific ethnicity, and other factors such as acculturation and assimilation.

Using these findings, researchers developed the Houston Pain Outcome Instrument (HPOI) as a culturally sensitive assessment tool to measure satisfaction with pain management, or also known as the *Cuestionario de Houston Sobre el Dolor*. The HPOI was systematically developed in Spanish, translated from Spanish into English, and then back translated by a professional translation service. The resulting instrument was pre-tested to assess Spanish and English forms for clarity, content, and linguistic equivalence, and to estimate the time and ease of administration, and adapted to a final version with 27 items that assess pain intensity, pain interference, satisfaction, and barriers to effective management. It differs from the APS-POQ by including items that reflect culturally specific opinions that may pose barriers to pain management due to language or cultural perspectives. Items were expanded to assess pain interference with emotional well-being, expectations about pain, sources of information about pain and ways of managing pain. The HPOI is available from the chapter authors.

The HPOI was administered to a sample of postoperative, self-identified adult Hispanics drawn from three hospitals in the Rio Grande Valley and Houston ($N=95$) (Sherwood, McNeill, Hernandez, Penarrieta, & Peterson, 2005). Mean age was 41 years, 74 % were female, over 50 % had less than a high school education, and 33 % were first generation Hispanics in the US. With 0 meaning no pain and 10 worst pain, results indicated that post-surgical patients expected pain (mean rating 7.8), and expected relief from pain (mean rating of 7.5). The pain intensity level for worst pain matched this expectation, 7.9, although reported current and usual pain intensity ratings were somewhat lower. Generally, pain was reported as moderately interfering with mood and physical function. Opinions about pain and pain management ranged from a low of 1.7 for "Showing pain makes me lose the respect of family/friends," to greatest agreement for "Pain medicine is the only way to relieve pain," 7.0. Satisfaction with pain management was high, ranging from 9.2 for comfort in talking to doctor or nurse about pain and pain management to 8.2 for the inclusion of family and friends in the care given for pain and also for education about pain management with means >8. The results of this study are unique in assessing pain with an instrument developed specifically for use in Spanish language and tested with this population.

Content validity was assessed by 14 cultural and pain experts, who served as advisors to the project. The reliability of the HPOI was assessed using Chronbach's alpha to determine its internal consistency. Internal consistency for the entire instrument was estimated at 0.87 using Chronbach's Alpha. Specific items, particularly those related to Opinions about pain and pain management, tended to negatively influence overall reliability. Using this procedure, all subscales achieved an internal consistency reliability of >0.75 (Unpublished data available from authors).

Integrated Approaches to Effective Pain Management in Hispanic Populations

A multilevel approach is necessary to achieve an integrated quality approach to pain management (Fig. 12.3). First, there must be a system commitment to effectively manage pain for all patients, in-patient and out-patient. This includes an educational approach for providers and for patients and families. To initiate effective management, culturally appropriate approaches must be available and used. Communication is the cornerstone of pain assessment, and assessing and documenting language preference is crucial. Management strategies are many and varied so much fit the patient and family expectations and goals.

Systems Approach to Quality Pain Management

To address the complexities of pain management requires a multimodel systems approach to include the institution, providers, and the patient and family. Tables 12.3 (Institution), 4 (Providers), and 5 (Patient and Family) present strategies for implementing a systems approach. A basic tenet of a systems approach to pain management is based on quality (Beck et al., 2010; Gordon et al., 2010; Starck et al., 2001). Gordon et al. (2002) defined quality pain management as the appropriate assessment of pain parameters coordinated by an interprofessional team that encourages shared decision making with the patient. Assessment is both broad and detailed

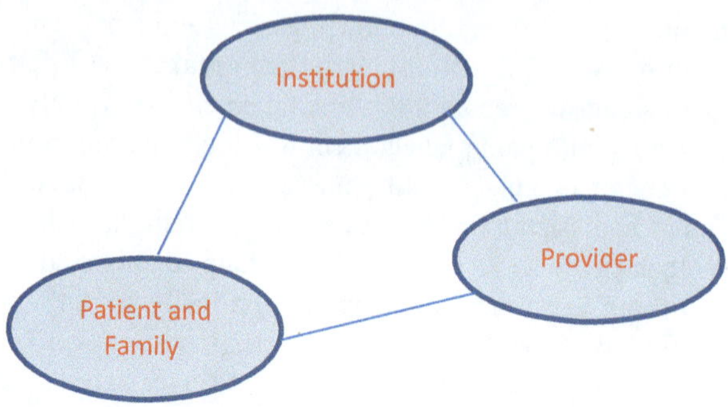

Fig. 12.3 Comprehensive systems approach to pain management involves the institution, providers, and patient/family

Table 12.3 Stage 1: Institutional approach to quality culturally appropriate pain management

First stage: Institutional approach to quality culturally appropriate pain management
1. Determine benchmarks for pain management
2. Approve best practice standards and protocols based on professional and regulatory standards
3. Determine management strategies
4. Measure status of pain management based on STEEEP (IOM, 2001)
(a) Safe: Are pain management strategies delivered without harm to the patient? Are errors disclosed, analyzed, and the system corrected?
(b) Timely: Are pain management interventions, including assessment/reassessment, completed according to the treatment plan?
(c) Effective: What measures are in place to determine effectiveness of pain management interventions both at the individual patient level and at the system level?
(d) Efficient: What is the cost benefit ratio of care delivery to achieve pain management goals?
(e) Equitable: Are there population disparities in pain management strategies and outcomes?
(f) Patient-centered: What is the assurance that pain management assessment, management, education, and outcome measures respect culturally appropriate patient goals, expectations, beliefs, and values about pain?

such as presence of pain; the presence of pain requires comprehensive assessment to examine history, type, level and type of pain followed by periodic reassessment to monitor patient responses. To achieve quality outcomes, treatment should follow the STEEEP guidelines for safe, timely, effective, efficient, equitable, and patient-centered care as an effective model to assure quality pain management. The Joint Commission which accredits hospitals and other clinical settings outlined a systems approach for pain management strategies (Porche, 2010) (Table 12.2) to assure quality care.

One hospital system used a report card or dashboard for baseline expectations (Starck, Adams-McNeill, Sherwood, & Thompson, 2000). The report card helped system administrators consider the prevalence, intensity, and duration of pain experienced by patients in their hospital and discuss with front-line providers the issues confronted in alleviating patient pain. Using a dashboard to report standard outcomes across units can be help raise awareness, improve commitment to education about pain, and foster patient and family engagement in pain management and indicate gaps that may be at the institutional level, in the provider approach, or implementation with patients and family.

Institution

The institution or system sets expectations for its commitment to quality and outcome goals (Blizzard, 2013). Table 12.3 illustrates the important of organizational commitment to resolving pain by providing the resources for providers to have the latest knowledge and best practices for assessing and treating pain from a multicultural perspective. Organizations must also demonstrate commitment to continuous

Table 12.4 Stage 2 of a comprehensive organizational approach to effective pain management: Provider education and implementation

Second stage: Provider education and engagement
1. Update education about pain models and theories, their own beliefs and values about pain, and cultural perspectives about pain reporting and management
2. Set expectations about pain management goals
3. Determine pain management protocols and standards
(a) Discipline-specific roles and responsibilities
(b) Pharmacologic measures
(c) Nonpharmacologic strategies
4. Plan patient education approach
5. Agree on measurements for benchmarks
6. Re-assessment and continuous evaluation
7. Determine out-patient plans
(a) Interdisciplinary team planning
(b) Discharge education
Out-patient pain management

quality improvement by measuring the outcomes of pain management and examine gaps that emerge to resolve care issues. Table 12.4 presents a comprehensive educational approach to assure that all providers have the training and education needed to accurately assess pain as a subjective person based experience while recognizing the impact of culture and the social determinants of health. Table 12.5 completes this three prong approach for addressing pain management with an evidence-based, patient-centered approach and specifically addressing language-specific needs.

Providers

Providers often lack education about comprehensive, patient-centered, quality approaches to pain management. Education to reduce myths about pain helps to reduce the stigma often attached to patients who report continuing issues with pain to better assess, intervene medically and nonmedically, and recognize cultural beliefs and values that impact pain reporting and management. Pain management requires an interdisciplinary team approach that includes primary and behavioral health collaboration such as counselors and behavioral health specialists (Main, Keefe, Jensen, Vlaeyen, & Vowles, 2014).

Patients and Families

The third stage of a comprehensive approach to effective patient-centered pain management is a patient- and family-centered approach that considers patient perspectives and engagement. To achieve quality goals outlined in a systems approach, a

Table 12.5 Stage 3 of a comprehensive organizational approach to effective pain management: A stepped approach for culturally appropriate care for patient and family

Third Stage: Patient and family approaches
Level 1: Assessment and Education
1. Determine language and health literacy for individualized approach
2. Cultural background related to health beliefs and values
3. Translation service as appropriate
4. Language appropriate tools
5. Overall goals for health
(a) Complete accurate medical history for intervening factors
• Family history for genetic/familial traits
• Social support system
• Potential sources of stress
• Health history
(b) Assess pain history and current status
• Characteristics of pain: onset, duration, quality, triggers/stimuli, intensity
• Interference with daily activities
• Management strategies
(c) Operationalize pain management
• Assess expectations for pain management and relief
• Goals for pain intensity, duration, and interference with quality of life
• Preferences for pharmacologic and nonpharmacologic management
Level 3

stepped approach enables providers to work with each patient based on their individual needs and preferences. Table 12.5 offers a culturally sensitive quality approach to pain management that defines each step of the care process. A stepped approach is not necessarily linear, but provides a checklist in working with each patient and family and may include multiple sessions, repeated education to assure understanding, and repeated assessments. Education, assessment, and care management are discussed in greater detail to guide implementation of a stepped approach.

Pain is a broad area of symptom management, and patients present from multiple experiences, pain severity, longevity of symptoms, and accompanying diagnoses that range from the need for surgical intervention to chronic pain, or long term cancer pain, any of which can escalate to the need for integrated behavioral interventions. A four level plan to pain management can accommodate the variety of patient experiences and needs (Table 12.6). Level 1 is primarily bibliotherapy, an approach of providing education and information according to the patient's background, language, and health literacy. The majority of patients who present with acute pain will be effectively managed with Level 1 and Level 2 which is primarily assessment and intervention managed by a primary health care team. Level 3 provides access to

Table 12.6 Integrated Behavioral Health care applied to pain management intervention

Assessment	Assessment
1. Determine language, health literacy, beliefs and values	Level 1 patient education
	Level 2 (group counseling)
2. Gather medical and family history, pain history, previous pain management approaches, and effectiveness	Level 1
	Level 2
	Level 3 (individual counseling, psychiatric services)
3. Management	Level 1 and Level 2 approaches for patient/family members
Operationalize plan	Level 3 and Level 4 (team approach) for patient/family
Set pain relief goals	
Pharmacologic	
Nonpharmacologic/behavioral	
4. Evaluation and Re-assessment	Evaluation
Note outcomes—patient satisfaction, achievement of pain and pain relief goals, physiologic and Activities of Daily Living (ADL)	Continue stepped approach to maintain desired pain relief, support patient/family
	Level 1—continued patient/family education
	Level 2—group counseling as needed
	Level 3—individual counseling
	Level 4—Team approach with consultation as needed

group intervention with a behavioral health care specialist. Level 4 includes a team-based approach with a psychiatrist and behavioral healthcare specialist. A case study illustrates the overlay of a comprehensive approach to pain management as described in Table 12.5, with an overlay of a four level approach to integrate behavioral health care to the complexity of pain management.

Education. Patients and families often lack education about current standards and treatment options to replace myths or misunderstandings. Research among Hispanic populations reveals many individual members have beliefs and values about pain that affect pain management and family participation and engagement (McNeill et al., 2003). Patients who lack education about pain management may not realize most acute pain can be managed with careful attention to symptoms, a combination of pharmacologic and nonpharmacologic approaches, and partnerships with providers. Patients who have language or communication issues or are not provided effective translation services are at higher risk for ineffective pain management. There may be limited Spanish language education materials and assessment tools available for patients from Hispanic populations with limited communication skills in English.

Assessment. Pain is subjective, therefore patients are the only reliable source about their pain. All patients should be assessed for pain. Observable behavioral and physiological indicators are not reliable measures of pain, although they may be useful when assessing patients unable to communicate. Assessing language preference is the first step in working with Hispanic populations to assure selection of appropriate assessment tools for the patient, whether for language, cognitive impairment, or age. Many health care systems have found that holding scheduled clinic hours for Spanish speakers contributes to integrated care by staffing with bilingual providers.

Establishing rapport with the patient is important for accurate assessment, so that patients are willing to share their histories, signs, and symptoms. With Hispanic populations that includes family constellation and involvement in care, country of origin, assimilation and/or time in the US, and treatment goals. Pain is most often associated with other conditions or illnesses; accurately diagnosing and managing underlying condition is dependent on a true and revealing history and assessment. Information should include past medical and psychosocial history, pain history and characteristics, and patient expectations and goals for seeking treatment.

Because pain is an unpleasant sensory experience that may also have an emotional response, assessment must be more than the widely practiced pain as a fifth vital sign in which patients may only be asked to rate pain on a numeric scale. Questions must probe deeper to learn the true nature and experience of pain, thus integrating care from behavioral health specialists can help assure effective approaches, and in particular for those with chronic pain (Main et al., 2014). Questions include the onset of pain, the duration, location, type of pain such as sharp or dull, pain triggers, and intensity. Appropriate language is critical; for Hispanic patients, using words other than pain may reveal more information, such as hurt or ache. Providers should ask the patient and family members about management strategies, any relevant medical or family history that helps understand the patient's pain, the impact of pain on the patient's activities of daily living, and expectations for managing the pain.

Re-assessment of pain and evaluation of pain management includes both the assessment of the patient's response to the treatment approach and patient satisfaction with care related to pain, as well as the overall evaluation of a pain management program in an institution or population setting. While there has been purposeful inclusion of both types of evaluation approaches in pain management guidelines (APS, 2001) there has been little research on this aspect of pain management, or its differential application for Hispanic populations, except in the area of development of Spanish language instruments used for evaluation.

Management. Patients may require varied approaches for pain that is acute (AHRQ, 2015) such as post-operative (ASA, 2012), or chronic pain associated with long term illness or behavioral issues (Main et al., 2014), or for pain that is cancer related (WHO, 2012) (materials also in Spanish). Numerous standards of care are available from the American Pain American Pain Society (2001), The Joint Commission (2003, 2012), the Institute of Medicine (2011), the International Association for the Study of Pain (2012), and others. A comprehensive list of available guidelines for various types of pain is available from the Agency for Healthcare Research and Quality (AHRQ, 2015).

Analgesic treatment is complex and is prescribed according to the reason the patient has pain, whether in-patient or out-patient, pain severity, expectations for pain relief, tolerance/side effects. Interference with activities and mood, preference for pharmacologic and/or nonpharmacologic interventions, and other contextual factors (AHRQ, 2015). Prescription is based on holistic assessment that includes patient attitudes and beliefs about pain and desires to include nonpharmacologic adjuvant therapy. Patients and providers must work together to determine pharmacologic and nonpharmacologic treatment regimens that enable patients to attain their pain relief goals and expectations, manage side effects, and anticipate future management for chronic or unrelieved disease manifestations.

To determine an effective management plan requires providers to take into account the patient's sociocultural framework, prior pain experiences, cognitive understanding, and physiological components are important components of an effective approach with the Hispanic patient, and family to effectively manage the pain experience. High-quality pain management is collaborative and based on careful planning and decision making with the patient and interdisciplinary team. To effectively manage pain, culturally sensitive care includes appropriate comprehensive assessment and treatment that is "efficacious, cost-conscious, culturally and developmentally appropriate, and safe," (Gordon et al., 2010, p. 1173). Evaluation. Evaluation and reassessment of response to treatment completes an effective management plan. Reliable and valid measures which are culturally and linguistically appropriate will assure that the strategies are effective and acceptable to the patient and family. The evaluation step is critical in an effective plan leading to improved approaches for individuals and quality improvement in pain management for Hispanic populations. Providing education and tailored information on pain management is an essential component of an effective management plan.

The Case of Ms. Santos Illustrates the Stepped Care Approach for Pain Management

Ms. Santos is a 68 year old woman with a 15 year history of osteoarthritis, and a recent back injury resulting from a fall. She is otherwise healthy with no other chronic illnesses. She is a recent widow, and has three grown children and seven grandchildren. She lives with one of her daughters and family and helps take care of three small grandchildren. Her pain has been managed in the past with over the counter (OTC) medications for her osteoarthritis and some natural remedies, according to her daughter who visits daily while her mother has been in the hospital. She is being treated in the hospital for the fall injury, but is refusing additional pain medicine for her back despite the doctors and nurses urging her to take something. The possible need for back surgery has been explained to her and her daughter. When asked about her pain she rates it as a 3 on a 10 point numeric scale (1 being no pain and 10 the worst pain imagineable), but is moaning softly, restless, and has not been able to sleep. While she speaks English, the nurses overhear her speaking Spanish to her daughter. She is anxious to go home and is concerned about the care of her grandchildren. In order to provide comprehensive, and culturally appropriate care for Ms. Santos, her primary provider would employ a systematic, stepped care, pain management approach. A stepped care approach would begin with Level 1, patient education, and progress if needed to Level 2, group counseling approaches. Depending on the patient response and pain management outcomes, Level 3, provision of behavioral health services on an individual basis, would be employed; finally Level 4 might be used, consisting of a team-based approach with a psychiatrist and behavioral healthcare specialist working with the patient and family.

Stepped care, **Level 1 and 2**. Assessment—this would be a first step toward pain management and also for meeting patient and family educational needs. AT this step the priority is conducting a comprehensive pain assessment in order to plan care, and beginning patient and family education.

1. Gathering a medical and social history including Ms. Santos's language preferences, and her understanding of her past pain problems and the impact of the new injury.
2. Obtain translation services if needed. Note: her daughter may be present at the interview but should not be the main translator for her mother.
3. Have an appropriate pain assessment tool on hand such as the numeric scale with Spanish anchors, the faces or verbal rating scale, in Spanish.
4. Inquiring as to her expressed cultural background and health beliefs/values—specifically ask about natural remedies for pain that Ms. Santos feels may be helpful—for example, heat application, prayer, or relaxation.
5. Asking about goals for health—ask what Ms. Santos's goals are for recovery from the back injury, ask how she feels she can manage the new pain related to the injury
6. Complete the history for intervening factors—such as any genetic/familial traits (may influence response to analgesics), Social support system, Potential sources of stress, and verifying health history
7. Specifically assess pain history and current status
    (a) Characteristics of pain: onset, duration, quality, triggers/stimuli, intensity
    (b) Interference with daily activities

    Management strategies she has already tried; again give the opportunity and permission to talk about traditional remedies, indicating acceptance of these as important and valuable to her. Based on the assessment, provide patient education materials (**Level 1**) on nonpharmacologic and pharmacologic therapy and possible side effects. Refer Ms. Santos and her daughter to web based materials, such as the American Pain Society website, the Agency for Healthcare Research and Quality site related to pain management; assure that all information is available in both English and Spanish.

8. Inquire of Ms. Santos and/or her daughter's interest in participating in a group therapy (**Level 2**) situation for chronic pain patients. Working with social services and the psychologist for the pain service, assure that a group is available in Spanish for Ms. Santos.

Stepped care, **Level 2, 3, and 4**. Plan and Operationalize pain management interventions

1. Reinforce the fact that a group approach to chronic pain care will be a valuable addition to any pain management plan. Follow-up with Ms. Santos regarding participation in a Spanish speaking group.

2. Gather information about expectations and goals for pain relief

   (a) Inquire as to Ms. Santos's expectations for pain management and relief—her goals for pain relief; for instance, does she feel she can go about her daily activities with a low level of pain (up to a 3 on a 0–10 scale)?
   (b) Ask about her tolerance for pain—what pain intensity, duration, she feels would interfere with her quality of life

3. Working in partnership with Ms. Santos and her daughter, discuss their preferences regarding pharmacologic and nonpharmacologic management
4. Reinforce the **Level 1** stepped approach regarding education about pain management—provide information, printed and web-based according to their preference and in English and/or Spanish for Ms. Santos and her daughter about both pharmacologic and nonpharmacologic approaches that could be tried, and the advantages/disadvantages of each approach being suggested for her—(for example. a certain type of medication, scheduled vs. as needed dosing, possibility of using the medication at home, expected side effects and how these would be managed.) If nonpharmacological approaches are her preference, discuss various ones and try to agree on a trial of these to see if effective for her.
5. Reinforce the use of a **Level 2** intervention by referral to an appropriate group.
6. Put the plan into effect in the hospital setting and have providers monitor closely, using language appropriate pain assessment scales.
7. Consider social and spiritual needs and refer to these providers as needed.
8. Refer to a behavioral health specialist (**Level 3**) for assistance with monitoring pain management, effective use of nonpharmacologic approaches, and enhanced understanding of her beliefs about pain.

Reassess and evaluate effectiveness of approaches

1. After each dose of pain medication, reassess for level and quality of pain from her perspective.
2. Note presence of side effects; specifically note gastrointestinal disturbance such as nausea or vomiting, check on occurrence of constipation and be sure to institute a bowel management program for any prolonged use of opiates (longer than 3 days or so)
3. If nonpharmacological approaches are being used, note frequency of use, combination or instead of pharmacological approaches, effectiveness and Ms. Santos's satisfaction with the approach.
4. Plan together with Ms. Santos and her daughter regarding continuation of the pain management program throughout the acute injury period, and when at home.
5. If evaluation of the overall management approach indicates ineffective management of her recurring pain from the osteoarthritis, and the acute pain related to the fall and imminent surgical intervention, Ms. Santos and her daughter may be referred to the interdisciplinary team for **Level 4** care to further explore the use of nonpharmacological approaches, assure that the pain management plan is acceptable to Ms. Santos and culturally appropriate, and prepare her for the

possibility of surgical treatment. It may be that she could benefit from more intensive attention to her beliefs about pain, use of analgesic therapy, and exploration of her concerns about surgery and further pain treatment.

Conclusions and Summary

Education for both providers and patients can help to eliminate perceived and actual disparities, and lead to more effective assessment and management (IOM, 2011). Understanding the role of culture in managing pain is the foundation for patient-centered, quality safe care. Cultural values related to family as well as family support in managing pain are important considerations for Hispanics experiencing pain. Hispanics' disagreement with the statement, "Pain makes me want to be left alone," has not been explored but is congruent with the emphasis on family support in this cultural group, and impacts intervention protocols and planning for the overall hospital experience.

Nonpharmacologic methods require continued investigation. For example, prayer was a pain management strategy reported in two samples including Hispanics (Anderson et al., 2000; McNeill et al., 2001). To improve care, providers must tailor pain management approaches to each person's experience to promote self-management. Collaboration among all team members, then, can coordinate this complex aspect of patient care.

An integrated team approach to improving the pain management of Hispanics in the health care system is imperative. A system approach that establishes pain management as an ethical principle will follow with educational resources to assure the integrated team as well as patients and their families have the information and tools needed to achieve quality outcomes. While reports do not agree whether outcomes of pain management across ethnic groups is equitable and effective, continued research on specific assessment and treatment among Hispanics populations is essential. Establishing consistent goals and assessment strategies can standardize treatment and measurement so that the goals of the STEEEP model are applied throughout the health care delivery system.

References

Agency for Healthcare Research and Quality (AHRQ). (2015). *Pain guidelines*. Retrieved July 20, 2015, from http://www.guideline.gov/search/search.aspx?term=pain+guidelines.

American Pain Society. (2001). *Pain: Current understanding of assessment, management and treatments*. American Pain Society and National Pharmaceutical Council. Retrieved from http://www.npcnow.org/system/files/research/download/Pain-Current-Understanding-of-Assessment-Management-and-Treatments.pdf.

American Society of Anesthesiologists (ASA) Task Force on Acute Pain Management. (2012). Practice guidelines for acute pain management in the perioperative setting: An updated report by the American Society of Anesthesiologists (ASA) Task Force on Acute Pain Management. *Anesthesiology, 116*(2), 248–273.

Anderson, K. O., Mendoza, T. R., Valero, V., Richman, S. P., Russell, C., Hurley, J., et al. (2000) Minority cancer patients and their providers: Pain management attitudes and practice. Cancer, 88, 1929–1938.

Atherton, M. J., Feeg, V. D., & El-Adham, A. F. (2004). Race, ethnicity and insurance as determinants of epidural use: Analysis of a national sample survey. *Nursing Economics, 22*(1), 6.

Bates, M. (1987). Ethnicity and pain: A biocultural model. *Social Science in Medicine, 24*(1), 47–50.

Beck, S., Towsley, G., Pett, M., Berry, P., Smith, E., Brant, J., & Guo, J. (2010). Initial psychometric properties of the Pain Care Quality Survery (PainCQ). *The Journal of Pain, 11(12)*, 1311–1319.

Bijur, P., Berard, A., Esses, D., Calderon, Y., & Gallagher, J. (2008). Face, ethnicity and management of pain from long-bone fractures: A prospective study of two academic urban emergency departments. *Academic Emergency Medicine, 15*, 589–597.

Blizzard, R. (2013). *How hospitals can effectively manage patients' pain.*

Bonhan, V. L. (2001). Race, ethnicity, and pain treatment: Striving to understand the causes and solutions to the disparities in pain treatment. *Journal of Law, Medicine & Ethics, 29*, 52–68.

Cleland, C. (2009). *Brief pain inventory*. Retrieved from http://prc.coh.org/pdf/BPI%20Short%20Version.pdf.

Cleland, C., Gonnin, R., Hatfield, A. K., Edmonson, J. H., Blum, R. H., Stewart, J. A., & Pandya, K. J. (1994). Pain and its treatment in outpatients with metastatic cancer. *New England Journal of Medicine, 330*(9), 592–596.

Garcia-Campayo, J., Rodero, B., Lopez del Hoyo, Y., Luciano, J. V., Alda, M., & Gili, M. (2010). Validation of a Spanish language version of the pain self-perception scale in patients with fibromyalgia. *BMC Musculoskeletal Disorders, 11*, 255. doi:10.1186/1471-2474-11-255.

Gordon, D., Dahl, J., Miaskowski, C., McCarbeerg, B., Todd, K. H., Paice, J. A., … Carr, D. B. (2005) American Pain Society recommendations for improving the quality of acute and cancer pain management. *Archives of Internal Medicine, 165*, 1574–1580.

Gordon, D., Pellino, T., Miaskowski, C., Mcneill, J., Paice, J., Laferriere, D., & Bookbinder, M. (2002). A 10 year review of quality improvement monitoring pain management: Recommendations for standardized outcome measure. *Pain Management Nursing, 3(4)*, 116–130.

Gordon, D. B., Polomano, R. C., Pellino, T. A., Turk, D. C., McCracken, L. M., Sherwood, G., … Farrar, J. T. (2010) Revised American Pain Society Patient Outcome Questionnaire (APS-POQ-R) for quality improvement of pain management in hospitalized adults: Preliminary psychometric evaluation. *Journal of Pain, 11*, 1172–1186.

Herr, K., Coyne, P., McCaffery, M., Manworren, R., & Merkel, S. (2011). Pain assessment in the patient unable to self-report. Position statement with clinical practice recommendations. *Pain Management Nursing, 12*(4), 230–250. doi:10.1016/j.pmn.2011.10.002.

Institute of Medicine. (2001). *Crossing the quality chasm: A new health system for the 21st century*. Committee on Quality of Health Care in America. Washington, DC: National Academy Press.

Institute of Medicine. (2011). *Relieving pain in America: A blueprint for transforming patient care, education and research*. Washington, DC: National Academy Press.

International Association for the Study of Pain. (2012). *IASP taxonomy*. Retrieved from http://www.iasp-pain.org/Taxonomy?navItemNumber=576.

Juarez, G., Ferrell, B., & Borneman, T. (1998). Influence of culture on cancer pain management in Hispanic patients. *Cancer Practice, 6*(5), 262.

Katz, J. N., Lyons, N., Wolff, L. S., Silverman, J., Emrani, P., Holt, H. L., … Losina, E. (2011). Medical decision-making among Hispanics and non-Hispanic Whites with chronic back and knee pain: A qualitative study. *BMC Musculosketetal Disorders, 12*, 78.

Kawaga-Singer, M. (2012). Applying the concept of culture to reduce health disparities through health behavior research. *Preventive Medicine, 55*(5), 356–361.
Main, C., Keefe, F., Jensen, M., Vlaeyen, J., & Vowles, K. (Eds.). (2014). *Fordyce's behavioral methods for chronic pain and illness: Republished with invited commentaries*. Alphen aan den Rijn, Netherlands: Wolters Kluwer Health.
Marchand, S. (2012). *The phenomenon of pain*. Seattle, WA: IASP Press.
Marin, B. V. O., & Marin, G. (1991). *Research with Hispanic populations*. Newbury Park, CA: Sage Publications.
McNeill, J. A., Sherwood, G., Starck, P., Palos, G., Disnard, G., & Rodriguez, T. (2003). Design strategies in pain management research with Hispanics. *Hispanic Health Care International, 2*(2), 73.
McNeill, J. A., Sherwood, G., Starck, P., & Nieto, B. (2001). Pain management outcomes in hospitalized Hispanic patients. *Pain Management Nursing, 2*, 26–35.
McNeill, J., Sherwood, G., & Starck, P. (2004). The hidden error of mismanaged pain: A systems approach. *Journal of Pain and Symptom Management, 25*(1), 47–58.
Meghani, S. H., Byun, E., & Gallagher, R. (2012). Time to take stock: A meta-analysis and systematic review of analgesic treatment disparities for pain in the United States. *Pain Medicine, 13*, 150–174.
Mossey, J. M. (2011). Defining racial and ethnic disparities in pain management. *Clinical Orthopedic Related Research, 469*, 1859–1870.
Ng, B., Dimsdale, J., Schragg, G. P., & Deutsch, R. (1996). Ethnic differences in analgesic consumption for postoperative pain. *Psychosomatic Medicine, 58*, 125–129.
Novy, D., Ritter, L. M., & McNeill, J. (2009). A primer of ethical issues involving opioid therapy for chronic nonmalignant pain in a multidisciplinary setting. *American Academy of Pain Management, 10*(2), 356–363.
Payne, R. (2009). Racially based disparities in pain management: Something old, something new, but what to do? *Pain Medicine, 10*(3), 432–434.
Porché, R. A. (Ed.). (2010). Approaches to pain managment. An essential guide for clinical leaders (2 ed.). Oakbrook (Il): The Joint Commission.
Rodero, B., García-Campayo, J., Casanueva, B., del Hoyo, Y. L., Serrano-Blanco, A., & Luciano, J. V. (2010). Validation of the Spanish version of the Chronic Pain Acceptance Questionnaire (CPAQ) for the assessment of acceptance in fibromyalgia. *Health and Quality of Life Outcomes, 12*, 37. doi:10.1186/1477-7525-8-37.
Sherwood, G., McNeill, J., Hernandez, L., Penarrieta, I., & Peterson, J. (2005). A multinational study of pain management among Hispanics. An evidence-based approach. *Journal of Research in Nursing, 10*, 403–423.
Sherwood, G., McNeill, J., Palos, G., & Starck, P. (2003). Perspectives on pain: A qualitative analysis of the Hispanic pain experience. *Nursing Times Research, 8*(5), 364–377.
Starck, P., Adams-McNeill, J., Sherwood, G., & Thompson, C. (2000). What nursing administrators need to know: Pain management report cards. *Nursing Administration Quarterly, 24*(3), 78–81.
Starck, P., Sherwood, G., Adams-McNeill, J., & Thomas, E. (2001). Identifying and addressing medical errors in pain mismanagement. *Joint Commission Journal on Quality Improvement, 27*(4), 191–199.
Stepanikova, I. (2012). Racial-ethnic biases, time pressure and medical decisions. *Journal of Health and Social Behavior, 53*(3), 329–343.
The Joint Commission. (2003). *Improving the quality of pain management through measurement and action*. Oakbrook, IL: Joint Commission Resources.
The Joint Commission. (2012). *Pain management: A systems approach to improving quality and safety*. Oakbrook, IL: Joint commission Resources.
Todd, K. H., Samaroo, N., & Hoffman, J. R. (1993). Ethnicity as a risk factor for inadequate emergency department analgesia. *Journal of the American Medical Association, 269*, 1537–1539.

Vilaro, F. M. (1994). *Methodological issues in the implementation of research in a Latino population. Nursing Research and Under-served Populations. Third National Conference on Cancer Nursing Research.* Newport Beach, CA: American Cancer Society.
Wong-Baker FACES Foundation. (2015). *Wong-Baker FACES® Pain Rating Scale.* Retrieved September 19, 2015, with permission from http://www.WongBakerFACES.org.
World Health Organization (WHO). (2012). *Treatment guidelines on pain.* Retrieved July 20, 2015, from http://www.who.int/medicines/areas/quality_safety/guide_on_pain/en/.
Zoega, S., Gunnarsdottir, S., Wilson, M., & Gordon, D. (2016). Quality pain management in adult hospitalized patients: A concept evaluation. *Nursing Forum, 51*, 3. doi:10.1111/nuf.12085.
Zoucha, R., & Reeves, J. (1999). A view of professional caring as personal for Mexican Americans. *International Journal for Human Caring, 3*, 14–20.

Chapter 13
Using Integrated Care for Addressing Tobacco Use Among Latino Populations

Virmarie Correa Fernández and Yessenia Castro

Prevalence and Patterns of Tobacco Use

Tobacco use, mainly in the form of cigarette smoking, is the principal health hazard in the United States (US; CDC, 2004), and epidemiological data indicate that 12.1 % of Latino adults smoke cigarettes (CDC, 2014). Although overall smoking prevalence among Latinos is lower compared with some other racial/ethnic groups [19.4 % for non-Latino whites, 18.3 % African Americans, 26.1 % American Indian/ Alaska Natives; (CDC, 2014)], smoking is linked to the two leading causes of death among this population [i.e., heart disease and cancer; (American Cancer Society, 2012; CDC, 2015)]. As such, there is a pressing need to effectively intervene on smoking among U.S. Latinos in order to decrease the burden of tobacco-related health consequences in the U.S.

Latino smokers share many of the same characteristics as the general population of smokers. For example, like the general population of smokers, Latino smokers are more likely to be single, younger, male, and have other smokers in the home (Cooper, Rodríguez de Ybarra, Charter, & Blow, 2011; Cox, Feng, Cañar, Ford, & Tercyak, 2005; Kaplan et al., 2014; Rodríguez-Esquivel, Cooper, Blow, & Resor, 2009; Wilkinson et al., 2005). In contrast, common socioeconomic correlates of smoking among the general population (e.g., education, income, employment status) have not been consistently related to smoking among Latinos (Abraído-Lanza, Chao, & Flórez, 2005; Kaplan et al., 2014; Lorenzo-Blanco & Cortina, 2013a; Reitzel et al., 2009).

V. Correa Fernández, Ph.D. (✉)
Department of Psychological, Health and Learning Sciences College of Education, University of Houston, 411 Farish Hall, Houston, TX 77204, USA
e-mail: vcorreaf@central.uh.edu

Y. Castro, Ph.D.
1925 San Jacinto Blvd, R5100, Austin, TX, 78748 USA

© Springer International Publishing Switzerland 2016

L.T. Benuto, W. O'Donohue (eds.), *Enhancing Behavioral Health in Latino Populations*, DOI 10.1007/978-3-319-42533-7_13

Smoking rates among Latinos differ by nativity (whether the person was born in the US or another country), country of origin, and gender. The smoking prevalence rate is 17.7 % for US-born Latinos and 10.3 % for Foreign-born (CDC, 2015). The prevalence of smoking is higher among U.S. Latinos of Puerto Rican and Cuban descent (21.6 % and 18.2 % respectively), followed by those of Mexican (13.0 %) and Central/South American descent (9.2 %). Also, within Latinos, substantially more men than women smoke (17.7 % vs. 8.9 %, respectively), and that pattern is similar in all sub-ethnic groups (American Cancer Society, 2012; CDC, 2015; Kaplan et al., 2014).

The smoking patterns of Latinos smokers also differ from other racial/ethnic groups of smokers and across Latinos subgroups. A considerable number of Latino adult smokers report that they are social/occasional (known in the literature as intermittent or non-daily) and/or light smokers; that is, they smoke cigarettes only some days rather than on a daily basis, and tend to smoke fewer cigarettes on the days they smoke (i.e. about 10 cigarettes per day) compared to the general population of smokers (Cupertino et al., 2011; Fagan, Shavers, Lawrence, Gibson, & Ponder, 2007; Moolchan et al., 2007; Perez-Stable et al., 2001; Trinidad et al., 2009; Trinidad, Perez-Stable, White, Emery, & Messer, 2011; Zhu, Pulvers, Zhuang, & Baezconde-Garbanati, 2007). This pattern of non-daily and light smoking has been reported by nearly all age groups, gender, and backgrounds, although it is more common among younger adults and persons of Mexican and Central American origin. An exception to this is Cuban daily smokers, whose smoking intensity is the highest among sub-ethnic groups (e.g. about half men and 1/3 of females consume >20 cigarettes per day; Kaplan et al., 2014). Latinos also wait longer after waking to smoke their first cigarette of the day (Benowitz, Bernert, Caraballo, Holiday, & Wang, 2009; Daza et al., 2006; Trinidad et al., 2011). However, it is important to note that there is no safe amount of smoking. Both intermittent and light smoking are still associated with negative health outcomes (e.g. chronic diseases) when compared with former or never-smokers (Bjartveit & Tverdal, 2005).

Although cigarettes are still the most prevalent tobacco product, experimentation with a variety of non-cigarette tobacco products (e.g. cigars, little cigars, hookah, smokeless tobacco, e-cigarettes) is widespread, partially due to misperceptions of safety. Latinos generally acknowledge the adverse health effects of tobacco use; however, some gaps in knowledge have been identified including uncertainty about how different tobacco products vary with respect to health risks (Foraker, Patten, Lopez, Croghan, & Thomas, 2005; Richter, Pederson, & O'Hegarty, 2006). In recent surveys, Latino youth report high rates of smokeless tobacco and hookah use compared to teens of other race/ethnicities (Lauterstein et al., 2014; Wilkinson et al., 2015). Except for cigars, ever use of most non-cigarette tobacco products is lowest among foreign-born Latino young adults aged 18–34, and similarly high among US-born Latino, Non-Latino Blacks, and Non-Latino Whites (Lariscy et al., 2013). These patterns are similar for both men and women. Current use of other tobacco products is very low among foreign-born Latino women and there is no difference between US-born Latino and Whites (Lariscy et al., 2013). Among men, current use of other tobacco products do not significantly differ by race/ethnicity or nativity. In addition, some perceived benefits of smoking identified by Latinos include: stress and anxiety relief, pleasure, help to make friends, improved ability to focus, and weight loss. These perceived benefits have been found to differ by gender, age, and education level (Constantine et al., 2009). Even though there is a general warning that no tobacco product is safe, more research is needed regarding the health effects of all tobacco products in order to better inform the population and provide guidance to health care professionals (Kozlowski & Edwards, 2005; Noonan & Kulbok, 2009).

Culturally relevant factors that correlate with smoking include acculturation and experience of discrimination. Acculturation refers to a process of multiple behavioral and ideological changes experienced by individuals as a result of contact between one or more cultures (Schwartz, Unger, Zamboanga, & Szapocznik, 2010). Acculturation toward mainstream U.S. culture (as indicated by more years lived in the U.S., greater proportion of life lived in the U.S., English language preference or proficiency, etc.) is related to higher smoking prevalence among Latina women, but unrelated to prevalence among Latino men (Abraído-Lanza et al., 2005; Bethel & Schenker, 2005). Also, the experience of discrimination is a risk factor for smoking among Latinos (Lorenzo-Blanco & Cortina, 2013a, 2013b; Nguyen, Subramanian, Sorensen, Tsang, & Wright, 2012). Currently, scarce published research exists that examines how or why acculturation and discrimination might lead to increased smoking among Latinos, and the limited available research focuses on Latino youth. Generally, experience of discrimination is suspected to increase stress or negative emotions, which in turn increases the odds of smoking (Unger, Schwartz, Huh, Soto, & Baezconde-Garbanati, 2014) and greater acculturation is suspected to lead to higher odds of smoking both by increasing the experience of certain stressors (e.g. acculturative stress, discrimination, family conflict; Lorenzo-Blanco & Cortina, 2013b), but also by influencing the adoption of beliefs and attitudes that are more accepting of smoking (Bethel & Schenker, 2005).

Tobacco Cessation and Treatment-Related Characteristics

Compared to smoking prevalence and patterns, much less is known about what predicts success in quitting smoking among Latino smokers, but many factors relevant to White smokers and the general population of smokers are also relevant to Latino smokers. For example, older age, having a spouse/partner, partner support for quitting, the presence of children in the home (Brothers & Borrelli, 2011; Kaplan et al., 2014; Nevid & Javier, 1997), all increase odds of quitting, while stress (Businelle et al., 2010) and withdrawal from cigarettes (Castro, Kendzor et al., 2011) decrease odds of quitting among Latino smokers as they do among the general population of smokers.

Unlike the general population of smokers, success with quitting smoking does not seem to differ by gender (Bock, Niaura, Neighbors, Carmona-Barros, & Azam, 2005; Castro et al., 2009; Kaplan et al., 2014) and experiencing depressive symptoms does not appear to be associated with quitting among Latino (Castro, Costello, et al., 2011; Kiviniemi, Orom, & Giovino, 2011; Munoz, Marin, Posner, & Perez-Stable, 1997). Also, traditional indications of socioeconomic status (education, income, employment) have not been consistently associated with quitting among Latinos in the U.S. (Businelle et al., 2010; Chiang & Borrelli, 2014; Kaplan et al., 2014).

As noted earlier, Latinos differ notably from the general population in behavioral smoking patterns, namely, daily versus non-daily smoking, cigarettes smoked per day, and the amount of time elapsed between waking and one's first cigarette of the day. These smoking patterns are widely used as behavioral markers of tobacco dependence (Heatherton, Kozlowski, Frecker, Rickert, & Robinson, 1989), but this practice may have limited utility for Latino smokers. Specifically, Latino's observed smoking patterns may suggest that they are less likely to be dependent on cigarettes, which would in turn lead to the assumption that they would be more successful at quitting. In fact, the quit rates of Latino smokers are lower or no different from non-Latino White smokers (CDC, 2002, 2011). There is a strong relationship between physical dependence and success at quitting smoking among non-Latino White smokers (Ferguson et al., 2003; Foulds et al., 2006; Rohsenow, Martin, Tidey, Monti, & Colby, 2013), but not among Latinos (Bock et al., 2005; Reitzel et al., 2009; Woodruff, Talavera, & Elder, 2002). This phenomenon among Latino smokers is not well-understood, but one possibility is that physiological aspects of dependence, may not be strong motivators for tobacco use among Latino smokers. This is consistent with the common occurrence of light and social/occasional smoking among Latino smokers. Nonphysiological aspects of dependence (e.g., social/environmental cues, cognitive factors such as outcome expectancies) may be more important motivators for smoking among Latinos (Castro et al., 2012, 2014; Foraker et al., 2005), but more research in this area is needed. Generally, indicators of physical dependence may not be useful prognostic indicators for Latino smokers trying to quit.

Acculturation toward mainstream U.S. culture may be related to greater likelihood of quitting (Bock et al., 2005) especially among men (Castro et al., 2009; Wetter et al., 2007). Lifetime experience of discrimination, particularly major discriminatory events, may reduce the probability of quitting among Mexican Americans (Kendzor et al., 2014). Research on how cultural variables influence cessation is limited and relatively new, but such knowledge can be used to identify and target at-risk groups.

Latinos experience notable disparities related to healthcare support for smoking cessation. In particular, Latinos consistently report extremely limited use of cessation aides compared to non-Latino Whites (Cupertino et al., 2011; Fu et al., 2005; Levinson, Perez-Stable, Espinoza, Flores, & Byers, 2004; Rodríguez-Esquivel et al., 2009; Trinidad et al., 2011). Socioeconomic condition likely plays some role in this disparity. For example, among Latino former smokers, use of prescriptions and over-the-counter medications for smoking cessation is more common among those with health insurance compared with those without insurance (Kaplan et al., 2014). Other studies have also demonstrated that socioeconomic factors may partly explain Latinos lesser use of cessation aids but these factors do not fully account for the disparity (Levinson et al., 2004; Thorndike, Biener, & Rigotti, 2002). Avoidance of medications and misconceptions about their use and effectiveness have also been reported (Foraker et al., 2005; Webb, Rodriguez-Esquivel, & Baker, 2010).

Latinos are also less likely compared to Whites to be asked whether or not they smoke and, if they do smoke, are less likely to receive advice to quit or be counseled about quitting during a healthcare encounter (CDC, 2011; Cokkinides, Halpern, Barbeau, Ward, & Thun, 2008; Houston, Scarinci, Person, & Greene, 2005; Levinson et al., 2004; Lopez-Quintero, Crum, & Neumark, 2006). This is particularly troubling because receiving physician advice (Kreuter, Chheda, & Bull, 2000; Whitlock, Orleans, Pender, & Allan, 2002) increases the probability of making a quit attempt and using cessation aids (Levinson et al., 2004). As these disparities in cessation support apply to actual encounters with healthcare professionals, they are clearly not an issue of lack of access to healthcare providers. Furthermore, the disparity in receiving advice to quit does not appear to be explained by the patients' English language proficiency (Lopez-Quintero et al., 2006).

Finally, there is a dearth of information regarding the efficacy of behavioral and pharmacological smoking cessation interventions among Latinos. Recent report found that, in contrast to the hundreds of smoking cessation intervention trials in existence (Fiore et al., 2008), fewer than 20 published studies directly target Latino smokers (Cox, Okuyemi, Choi, & Ahluwalia, 2011; Webb et al., 2010). The limited available evidence suggests that pharmacological and behavioral interventions for smoking cessation among Latinos are effective at the end of treatment, but their effects tend to wane beyond end of treatment (Webb et al., 2010). Additional research devoted to enhancing tobacco cessation interventions among Latinos is needed.

Assessment of Tobacco Use and Dependence

Screening for Tobacco Use

Health care practitioners are well-positioned to assess and intervene with patients that use tobacco. Depending on their particular work setting (e.g., primary care versus substance abuse treatments), one-third to three-fourths of practitioners' caseloads may be smokers (Fiore et al., 2008). Irrespective of a provider' specialty or treatment context, identifying tobacco users is the first step in treating tobacco use and dependence among patients in any health care setting. Given the high work demands experienced by some clinics coupled with lack of training for providers and staff, tobacco use assessments (TUAs) have historically seldom been included as a standard clinical practice and have often depended on the discretion of the practitioner. As a result, the documentation and delivery of tobacco cessation interventions has often been inconsistent and suboptimal. Fortunately, with the adoption of the Patient Protection and Affordable Care Act, there has been a dramatic increase in both the emphasis on and coverage for preventive care, including tobacco cessation (American Lung Association). Such changes are expected to positively impact the frequency and quality of TUAs and treatment in healthcare settings. Moreover, there are research-based recommendations for screening protocols that can facilitate a clinic's adoption and implementation of structured TUAs and subsequent tobacco cessation support (Fiore et al., 2008; Warren et al., 2014). Healthcare settings are encouraged to treat "smoking as a vital sign" (McCullough, Fisher, Goldstein, Kramer, & Ripley-Moffitt, 2009) to be assessed systematically and in every patient encounter. As few as two questions integrated into a healthcare setting's electronic health records (EHR) system ("current smoker?" and "plans to quit?") dramatically increases both the number of smokers who are identified and those who receive cessation counseling (McCullough et al., 2009). In fact, even screenings comprised of just a few more questions can enable the identification of a large number of patients that use tobacco and promote referrals to specialized cessation programs without sacrificing significant additional time (Warren et al., 2014). An example of a short TUA is below.

For new patients, a *positive screen* results if a patient answers "every day" or "some days" to question 1, answers YES to either question 2 or 3, or responds that s/he has used tobacco during the last 30 days (question 4).

1. Do you currently smoke cigarettes every day, some days, or not at all?
2. Do you currently use any other tobacco products such as cigars, pipes, chewing tobacco, e-cigarettes, snuff, snus, bidis, etc?
3. Are you currently using any medication or nicotine replacement therapy (like gum, patches) to try to quit tobacco?
4. About how long ago did you last smoke a cigarette, even a puff or used other tobacco products?
5. Are you interested in stopping tobacco use or speaking with a team member (e.g. nurse, counselor, tobacco cessation specialist) about it?

When considering TUAs with Latino patients, it will be important to be mindful of the common practice of intermittent and light smoking among this population. This pattern of smoking may not be perceived as sufficiently frequent for the patient to identify him/herself as a tobacco user. Indeed, as many as 25 % of light and intermittent smokers under-report the amount they smoke (Perez-Stable, Marin, Marin, & Katz, 1990). Deliberate deception should not be assumed; patient reports are likely well-intended even when inaccurate. Questions like those above, which focus on the frequency of smoking behavior and that do not impose a label such as "smoker" or "nonsmoker" may be more helpful.

Tobacco Dependence and Withdrawal

Substance *dependence* refers to when a person cannot control the impulse to use a drug, such as tobacco, even in the face of negative consequences, and there are changes in the brain's natural inhibition and reward centers (National Institute of Drug Abuse). People with tobacco dependence may or may not also exhibit *physical dependence*. Physical dependence is characterized by either *tolerance* (need for increased amounts of a drug to achieve the desired effect or a diminished effect with continued use of the same amount of the drug) or *withdrawal* (the characteristic set of symptoms that occur when use of a drug is stopped or continued use of the drug to avoid withdrawal symptoms). It is important to note that not all smokers are tobacco dependent, and that the degree to which tobacco dependence develops varies significantly across individuals. Although the diagnosis of tobacco dependence requires only two of 10 possible symptoms, only about half of regular smokers meet criteria for a *tobacco use disorder* according to the Diagnostic and Statistical Manual of Mental Disorders, fifth Edition (DSM-5; American Psychiatric Association, 2013; Breslau, Johnson, Hiripi, & Kessler, 2001), a widely used tool for assessing dependence and withdrawal.

Although documenting a *tobacco use disorder* (previosuly labeled as *nicotine use disorder*; DSM-IV-TR; American Psychiatric Association, 2000) or *tobacco withdrawal* may be required and useful for insurance-related purposes, examining all of the DSM-5 diagnostic criteria is not always feasible in a health care setting. In fact, its appropriateness for use in clinical settings as well as its validity to predict important outcomes (e.g. likelihood of quitting, response to treatment) has been questioned by experts in the field (Baker, Breslau, Covey, & Shiffman, 2012). Consequently, researchers have developed alternative instruments that better identify persons with tobacco dependence and that can be administered in shorter periods of time. The Fagestrom Test for Nicotine Dependence (FTND; Heatherton, Kozlowski, Frecker, & Fagerstrom, 1991) and the Heaviness of Smoking Index (HSI; Heatherton et al., 1989) are examples of such instruments. The FTND is a widely used instrument to measure tobacco dependence in both research and practice. Comprised of six items, it is a brief instrument that can be easily used in any health care setting. Ranges from 0 to 10, with higher scores indicative of higher dependence. Table 13.1 presents the items and scoring interpretation of the FTND.

Alternatively, the HSI consists of two items from the FTND: time to the first cigarette after waking up (TTFC; item 1) and number of cigarettes smoked per day (CPD; tem 4; Heatherton et al., 1989; Heatherton et al., 1991). When combined, these items comprise the HSI scale which ranges from 0 to 6 (Borland, Yong, O'Connor, Hyland, & Thompson, 2010). Higher scores indicate higher dependence. It is important to reiterate here that measures such as these, which assess physical dependence, have shown limited utility for predicting smoking treatment outcomes among Latino smokers (Bock et al., 2005; Brothers & Borrelli, 2011; Reitzel et al., 2009; Woodruff et al., 2002), and so we caution against using such measures for prognostic judgements among this population. However, such measures are still useful for documenting smoking behavior and physical dependence among Latinos, which is useful for treatment planning. Essentially, patients with low dependence (FTND = 0–4) may benefit from brief interventions [see Brief Interventions section], while patients with moderate to high dependence (FTND = 5–10) may require more intensive counseling and pharmacotherapy in order to increase their chances of quitting [see Intensive Interventions section].

Table 13.1 Fagerstrom test for nicotine dependence (FTND)/HSI

Item	Response options	Score
1. How soon after you wake up do you smoke your first cigarette?	(a) after 60 minutes	0
	(b) 31–60 minutes	1
	(c) 6–30 minutes	2
	(d) within 5 minutes consists of two items	3
2. Do you find it difficult to refrain from smoking where it is forbidden?	No	0
	Yes	1
3. Which cigarette would you hate most to give up?	(a) The first one in the morning	1
	(b) Any others	0
4. How many cigarettes per day do you smoke?	(a) 10 or less	0
	(b) 11–20	1
	(c) 21–30	2
	(d) 31 or more	3
5. Do you smoke more frequently during the first hours after waking than during the rest of the day?	No	0
	Yes	1
6. Do you smoke even if you are so ill that you are in bed most of the day? (no/yes)	No	0
	Yes	1
Total Score (0–10)		

Source. Heatheron TF, Kozlowski LT, Frecker RC, Fagerstrom K (1991). The Fagerstrom Test for Nicotine Dependence: a Revision of the Fagerstrom Tolerance Questionnaire. British Journal of Addiction; 86: 1119–1127

Note. Scoring: Sum up the scores of all items and interpret the total score as follows: 0–2 very low dependence; 3–4 low dependence; 5 moderate dependence; 6–7 high dependence; and 8–10 very high dependence

Comprehensive Assessment of Tobacco Use

Screening for tobacco use is a very important first step in intervening with tobacco users. However, once in treatment, helping smokers quit usually requires more extensive assessments, particularly among those highly dependent and/or with comorbid psychiatric conditions. Comprehensive TUAs involve getting to know the patient's tobacco use, smoking patterns, as well as reasons to smoke and reasons to quit. They guide the clinician to determine the most effective intervention that meets the patient's particular needs and to help formulate a treatment plan. TUAs can take the form of questionnaires that the patients complete by themselves or can be done by the practitioner in an interview format. They can take place in any treatment context, even if the focus of treatment is not smoking cessation. The time and resources available to administer the assessments and the complexity of the smoker's profile will help determine the length and breadth of the comprehensive TUA. Importantly, as with screening, a comprehensive TUA is an ongoing and dynamic process rather than a one-time clinical activity. As such, a comprehensive TUA should be completed throughout multiple visits and updated as the patient progresses in his/her quitting process.

In the comprehensive TUAs is important to ask questions about the patient's views regarding their history with tobacco, as well as their beliefs about, struggles with, and aspirations for behavior change. The purpose of the comprehensive TUA is to go beyond simply eliciting answers to the set of questions, but to facilitate a discussion that motivates behavior change. Furthermore, because physical dependence might be less important as a motivator for smoking among Latinos, broader conversations about a Latino patient's lived experience with smoking may uncover other, more relevant motivators for smoking that can be targeted in treatment. Indeed, limited evidence suggests that a "multiple motives" approach to tobacco dependence that takes into account contextual and psychological motivators for smoking (Piper et al., 2004) may be more useful for predicting smoking outcomes among Latinos (Castro et al., 2012).

Biological Assessment. Carbon monoxide (CO) in the breath, and nicotine and its metabolite cotinine in saliva, urine, or blood, can be used to measure the extent of tobacco or nicotine use (APA, 2013). CO is one of the most deadly chemicals found in cigarette smoke. Burning cigars, cigarettes, and pipes all produce CO. CO takes the place of oxygen in the red blood cells, decreasing the actual amount of oxygen available causing strain on the heart and body, putting smokers at increased risk for having cardiovascular disease, especially heart attacks. Although CO is very deadly, it lasts in the body only a short time. Thus, its effect is reversible if the person stops smoking. The body can eliminate CO within 24 h but more likely within 2–3 days after a person quits smoking. The CO will go back down to the same level as that of someone who hast never smoked. CO meters measure expired CO from smoke exposure as either CO in parts per million (ppm) or percent carboxyhemoglobin (%COHb). Such devices provide immediate feedback on smoking level or confirmation of abstinence, and such feedback could serve as a motivator for the patient. A chart can help the patient to visualize CO effects (Table 13.2):

In sum, typical domains to be included in comprehensive TUAs are: (a) current tobacco use and intentions to quit, (b) past quit attempts (with particular attention to withdrawal symptoms), (c) social and contextual factors (that facilitate or hinder quitting), (d) medical history and biological assessment, (e) psychological assessment (e.g. psychiatric comorbidity, motivations to quit, self-efficacy, outcome expectancies). Examples of recommended measures and instruments to incorporate in a comprehensive TUA can be found in the *Smoking Initiative* of the Patient-Reported Outcome Measurement Information System (PROMIS; http://www.nihpromis.org/default.aspx). This initiative aims to develop, evaluate, and standardize item banks to assess smoking behavior and associated psychosocial constructs for both daily and nondaily smokers (Edelen et al., 2014; Shadel, Edelen, & Tucker, 2011). Some, although not all, of the recommended measures have been translated into Spanish and validated among Latinos.

Table 13.2 Meaning of CO levels

CO level	Meaning
0–8	Normal or very low (normal is 0–3 ppm)
8–12	Worry. Person is affecting their health
12–25	Cause for alarm. The person is harming themselves
25–40	Danger and hazard to health
Over 40	Severe danger—take immediate action (person can get lethargic)

Brief Interventions for Tobacco Cessation

The Public Health Service Clinical Practice Guideline *Treating Tobacco Use and Dependence: 2008 Update* (PHS Guidelines; Fiore et al., 2008) provides clear recommendations regarding interventions for patients that are willing to make a quit attempt as well as for those that are not ready to make a quit attempt. The Guidelines are available in both English and Spanish and can be retrieved from http://www.ahrq.gov/professionals/clinicians-providers/guidelines-recommendations/tobacco/clinicians/update/index.html. Brief interventions for tobacco cessation are characterized by a practical counseling encounter that lasts no more than 10 min. They are intended to be used by any health care provider in either outpatient or inpatient settings. Brief interventions for patients willing to make a quit attempt are best known as the 5A's (Ask-Advise-Assess-Assist-Arrange).

Interventions for Patients Willing to Make a Quit Attempt

ASK about tobacco use. Implement a clinic-wide system that ensures that every patient at every clinical encounter is queried about their tobacco use and that their smoking status is documented in their medical record. The main recommended identification system is simply to expand the Vital Signs to include tobacco use. Other alternatives include adding reminders to indicate tobacco use status through the EHR or "stickers" in the patient's charts.

Example: *Tobacco use (circle one): Current–Former–Never*

ADVISE the patient to quit. In a professional manner, offer the patient a strong advice to quit, emphasizing reasons to quit that are personally relevant to the patient and clearly emphasize the benefits of quitting. Beginning the conversation with assurance that providing this advice is standard practice for all tobacco users and that it is the professional responsibility of the provider may minimize the patient's perception of being judged or criticized. For example, "As your provider, it is my responsibility to let you know that stopping smoking (or using tobacco) is the best thing you can do for your own and your family's health and well-being. It will reduce your blood pressure, and reduce the asthma episodes in your child, and it will even allow you to save money. Cutting down is not enough. We are here to help you."

ASSESS willingness to make a quit attempt. Assess patient's willingness to make a quit attempt at the present time or the near future. For example, "How do you feel about trying to quit smoking within the next 2 weeks? Would you be willing to give it a try?"

If the patient is willing to make a quit attempt within the next 2 weeks, congratulate him/her for the decision and proceed to the next step, ASSIST.

If the patient is not willing to make a quit attempt within the next 2 weeks, evaluate their willingness to make the attempt within the next 30 days and assist accordingly.

If the patient is not willing to make a quit attempt in the near future, use a motivational approach and the 5R's model (discussed later) to increase the probability of a future quit attempt.

ASSIST in making a quit attempt. *For patients willing to make a quit attempt*, provide evidence-based intervention options to help them quit. Assistance includes provision or referral to counseling services as well as a prescription or recommendation to use medication. This step requires the provider to be knowledgeable in evidence-based interventions for smoking cessation as well as local smoking cessation resources. For example, if someone other than a physician is providing the 5 A's intervention, open communication must exist between the physician and the 5 A's provider regarding the feasibility of and physician's willingness to provide cessation aids that require a prescription. Providers should be familiar with the telephone Quitline services and be prepared to refer or connect patients with it [see Quitlines section]. In addition, there are numerous freely available self-help materials in English and Spanish that can be provided to the patient. Finally, local community organizations, clinics, and hospitals often have free or low cost smoking cessation counseling services available to community members. Beyond providing resources and referrals, there is much the provider can do immediately during the encounter to assist the patient with a quit attempt:

1. *Help the patient to prepare a quit plan.* Common steps to prepare for quitting include: (a) Setting a quit date, ideally, within 2 weeks; (b) Telling friends, family, and coworkers about intentions to quit and request their support. It may be particularly important to help the patient prepare for this if they have many other smokers in their social network; (c) Removing all tobacco-related products from the environment, including ashtrays, lighters, matches, and any other materials that promote smoking. If has not already been done, this is the time to make the home and car smoke-free. Prior to the quit day, the patient can practice changing their routine to disrupt their smoking pattern, and practice not smoking in places or situations where they frequently smoke. Patients should urge other smokers in the household to also quit or to not smoke in their presence; (d) Anticipating the challenges that will likely occur in the few weeks following the quit date, particularly nicotine withdrawal symptoms. The patient can make a list of these potential challenges and identify alternatives to deal with them; (e) Writing down the reasons why they are motivated to quit. Some people find useful to put that list in a visible place as a constant reminder; and (f) Determining if they want to start reducing the amount of cigarettes smoked per day in preparation for the quit day or if they will maintain their current smoking level and stop completely on the quit day. This preference varies by person, their previous experience quitting and their level of dependence. In general, lower socioeconomic status has been associated with gradual quitting.
2. *Provide practical counseling based on problem-solving/skills training*. Striving for complete abstinence is essential. Even one puff after quitting is discouraged. Capitalize on the patient's previous experience with quitting to identify what helped him/her to succeed and what factors provoked a relapse (e.g. increased

Table 13.3 Summary of the 5 A's model for treating tobacco use and dependence

Component	Description
ASK about tobacco use	For *every* patient at *every* visit, identify and document current and past tobacco use at the time that other vital signs are assessed
ADVISE to quit	In a clear, strong, and personalized manner, urge every tobacco user to quit (and encourage former smokers to stay quit)
ASSESS willingness to make a quit attempt	Inquire patient's interest in trying to quit
ASSIST in making a quit attempt	Aid the patient in quitting
ARRANGE follow-up	Ensure follow up contact

Main source: Fiore MC, Jaen CR, Baker TB, et al. Treating Tobacco Use and Dependence: 2008 Update. (May 2008). Clinical Practice Guideline. Rockville, MD: U.S. Department of Health and Human Services. Public Health Service

physical activity and reducing coffee intake may have helped during previous quit attempts). The patient should plan to reduce stressful situations as much as possible and increase mood management and self-control skills [see Intensive Interventions].

3. *Recommend approved medications for cessation*, except when is contraindicated or with specific populations for which there is insufficient evidence of its effectiveness (Fiore et al., 2008). Approved medications are listed in a section below.
4. *Provide intra-treatment social support*; that is, providing general encouragement of the patient's quit attempt and be receptive to their questions.

ARRANGE a follow-up. Tobacco use is a chronic condition and should be treated as such. *For patients interested in making a quit attempt*, arrange for follow-up contacts, either in person or via telephone. Ideally, the follow-up contact should occur on the quit day or the day before. Other follow-ups should occur within a week after the quit day. During these follow-up contacts, discuss problems and challenges that have been encountered, and ways to address them. Assess medication use and any related issues. If patient is abstinent, congratulate them for their success! If they have smoked, congratulate them for the effort, revisit the challenges and strategies used and encourage a new attempt. *For patients unwilling to make a quit attempt* at a particular visit, continue addressing tobacco use/dependence and interest in quitting at the next clinic visit (Table 13.3).

Ask-Advice-Refer and Ask-Advice-Connect Models

In an effort to integrate brief interventions for tobacco cessation at the clinic level and after considering that often even the 5As approach is challenging to fully implement in a busy health care setting, briefer models started to emerge. The *Ask-Advise-Refer* (AAR) model is a health care-based smoking cessation initiative promoted nationally and recommended by several professional organizations (i.e. surgeons, dental hygienists; www.askadviserefer.org). Providers using this model ask their patients about their tobacco use, advise them to quit and then make a standard recommendation providing the patient with a business/referral card to a state quitline or another local cessation service. Certainly, implementation of the AAR has been a major step in the right direction and represents an improvement compared to outdated practices where assessment of tobacco use was not part of the clinical encounter. Unfortunately, the implementation of AAR has not been found to yield the expected results and only a small proportion of referred persons actually enroll in the recommended cessation program.

In an attempt to address clinic and patient-level barriers to effectively linking smokers to treatment, telephone care coordination programs and fax/email referral programs have been developed wherein quitlines receive patients' contact information from providers with the patient's permission, and the quitline proactively contacts the patient (Lichtenstein, Zhu, & Tedeschi, 2010). This eliminates the onus of initiating contact from the patient. One such program is the *Ask-Advise-Connect* (AAC) approach, which is designed to link smokers with quitline services through an automated system within the clinic's EHR (Vidrine, Shete, Cao, et al., 2013). In the AAC model, connections to the quitline are made by medical assistants and licensed vocational nurses, distributing the workload among various providers. Personnel are trained to *ask* every patient about their smoking status at the time that vital signs are assessed, *advise* all smokers to quit, offer cessation *assistance* via the quitline, and *connect* to the quitline those willing to receive help. With the patient's permission, the quitline proactively calls the patient.

Research has been conducted in both private and safety-net health care systems comparing AAR and AAC approaches (Vidrine, Shete, Li, et al., 2013; Vidrine, Shete, Cao, et al., 2013). In both sectors, AAC has proven to significantly increase treatment enrollment when compared with AAR (a 13-fold and 30-fold increase for private and safety-net sectors, respectively). Of note, even when a high proportion of smokers declined to be connected to the quitline or were unreachable, the streamlined and automated nature of the AAC approach dramatically enhanced the potential for cessation treatment enrollment. In sum, research suggests that active connecting-to-quitline programs should be favored over passive referral approaches (Vidrine, Shete, Li, et al., 2013; Warren et al., 2014).

Quitlines. Quitlines are telephone-based tobacco cessation services that help tobacco users quit and that are available for free throughout the U.S. The main services include counseling and coaching by trained staff, mailing of self-help materials, and referral to local resources. The counseling offered can be reactive or active. Quitlines with a reactive counseling approach only respond to incoming calls; whereas proactive quitlines respond to incoming calls and also generate outbound and follow-up calls to interested individuals. In addition, quitlines differ in their level of sophistication and resources; as such, they vary in the intensity of the counseling schedule (e.g. from 1 to 10 sessions), and time of operations (e.g. some are available 24 h a day, 7 days a week, and most holidays, while others operate only during typical business hours). Currently, the majority of quitlines offer web-based services, and some may also include provision of free nicotine replacement therapy (NRT) and training to healthcare providers. In addition, evidence-based internet smoking cessation interventions have been shown to produce good abstinence rates among Spanish speakers (Muñoz et al. 2009).

The North American Quitline Consortium (NAQC; http://www.naquitline.org/) is a nonprofit membership organization that seeks to promote evidence-based quitline services across diverse communities in North America. NAQC had set a goal for all quitline service providers in the U.S. to have the capacity for receiving referrals from EHRs by 2016. NAQC collects monthly data on call attempts to all quitlines in the U.S. and its territories and provinces. At present, NAQC does not collect quit rate data, but is planning to do it going forward. Notably, one of its goals is to "Increase the quality and cultural appropriateness of quitlines in North America". To achieve this goal, NAQC aims to deliver services to 6 % of each priority populations, including Latinos. At present, some states (e.g., Texas, Washington) provide services in Spanish and services are available in at least 15 additional languages through a third party. For services in English, callers may contact 1-800-QUIT-NOW (1-800-784-8669), which is the national portal number that routes callers to their respective state quitline. For services in Spanish, persons should call 1-855-DEJELO-YA (1-855-335-3569) or access http://espanol.smokefree.gov

Research has shown that quitlines are highly effective in helping tobacco users quit (Fiore et al., 2008; Lichtenstein et al., 2010). They can double or even triple an individual's chances of successfully quitting smoking. Importantly, given that the vast majority of people and households have phone services (U.S. Bureau of the Census), quitlines are an intervention modality with extremely broad reach. Nevertheless, they can reach only 1–2 % of smokers annually (Borland & Segan, 2006). In addition, few data is available regarding the reach, caller satisfaction, and effectiveness of the quitlines by diverse race/ethnic groups, including Latinos. While one study reported low reach among a Latino subgroup (Ortiz et al., 2008), another study reported that their state quitline services were as well received and effective for Latinos as they were for other race/ethnic groups (Maher et al., 2007). Moreover, the efficacy of clinical trials utilizing telephone-based smoking cessation counseling among Latinos (Correa-Fernández et al., submitted; Wetter et al., 2007) speaks about the potential of quitlines with this population.

Pharmacotherapy for Treating Tobacco Dependence

Current national guidelines for smoking cessation interventions recommend that all smokers be offered tobacco dependence treatment (TDT) that includes both behavioral counseling and pharmacotherapy (Fiore et al., 2008). The rationale for using pharmacotherapy in TDT is that nicotine, the main constituent in tobacco products, rapidly reaches and accumulates in the reward centers of the brain, promoting and maintaining the physical component of tobacco dependence. Thus, the main purpose of pharmacotherapy is to ease the withdrawal symptoms from nicotine. Currently, there are 7 medications approved by the Food and Drug Administration and that are considered first-line medications to treat tobacco use and dependence. Two of the approved medications are oral medicines and need a physician's prescription, and the others are NRT. Two of the NRT are available with prescription and three can be obtained over the counter (OTC). The OTC medications are the most commonly used pharmacotherapy for tobacco cessation (Table 13.4).

Table 13.4 Pharmacotherapy guidelines for tobacco use and dependence among adults

Medication	Dosage	Duration of treatment
Nicotine patch[a]	21 mg/24 hour[b]	8 week treatment (step-down)
	14 mg/24 hour	21 mg × 4 weeks
	7 mg/24 hour	14 mg × 2 weeks
		7 mg × 2 weeks
Nicotine gum[a]	2 mg piece (less than 20 cpd)	1 piece every 1–2 h for 6 weeks (and up to 12 weeks)
	4 mg piece (more than 20 cpd)	
Nicotine lozenge[a]	2 mg piece (TTF[c] more than 30 min)	Approx. 9 lozenges daily in the first 6 weeks (and up to 12 weeks)
	4 mg piece (TTF less than 30 min)	
Nicotine inhaler	Dose = 1 puff or inhalation	Up to 6 month; taper dosage during last 3 months
	1 cartridge = 4 mg or 80 inhalations	
	6–16 cartridges a day	
Nicotine nasal spray	Dose = 1 mg (0.5 mg per nostril)	3–6 months
	1–2 doses per hour, increasing as needed	
	Minimum = 8 doses/day; Maximum = 40 doses per day	
Bupropion SR	150 mg every morning × 3 days; then	Begin 1–2 weeks before the quit date. For long term treatment, 150 mg daily for up to 6 months.
	150 mg twice daily × 7–12 weeks	
Varenicline	0.5 mg/daily × 3 days	Begin 1 week before the quit date. For long term treatment, up to 6 months.
	0.5 mg/twice daily × 4 days	
	1 mg twice daily × 3 months	

[a]OTC = over the counter
[b]Patients consuming less than 20 CPD can start with a lower dose patch
Main source: Fiore MC, Jaen CR, Baker TB, et al. Treating Tobacco Use and Dependence: 2008 Update. (May 2008). Clinical Practice Guideline. Rockville, MD: U.S. Department of Health and Human Services. Public Health Service
[c]TTF = time to first cigarette/tobacco consumption

The type of pharmacotherapy will depend on whether the patient is ready to make a quit attempt or not, and considering potential contraindications. For example, nicotine patches works well for cessation treatment whereas nicotine gum and lozenges may be used for cessation and also to encourage tobacco reduction among those not ready to fully quit (Piper et al., 2014). Although the research documenting the efficacy of pharmacotherapy for TDT among Latinos is in its infancy, there is evidence for the use of the nicotine patch, and the acceptability of bupropion and varenicline (Cox et al., 2011; de Dios, Anderson, Stanton, Audet, & Stein, 2012).

Interventions for Patients Not Willing to Make a Quit Attempt

For patients not willing to make a quit attempt at the moment, a combination of brief motivational interventions and the 5R's model are recommended (Fiore et al., 2008).

Motivational Interviewing

Research has shown that when a patient is not ready to make a behavioral change, clinician's lectures and exhortations to modify their behavior are very unlikely to promote behavior change compared to when the patient voices his/her own concerns and reasons for a change (Amrhein, Miller, Yahne, Palmer, & Fulcher, 2003). Motivational Interviewing (MI) is a goal-oriented, patient-centered counseling intervention that aims to strengthen personal motivation for and commitment to achieve a specific goal (Miller & Rollnick, 2013). With tobacco users, the overall objective of the MI approach is to explore tobacco user's beliefs, feelings, and values regarding tobacco use, identify any ambivalence about the use and elicit an intrinsic motivation for behavior change. By using MI, the clinician would pay particular attention to the *language of change*, which would be expressions of any desire, ability, reasons, and need to stop tobacco use, as well as verbalizations of commitment to quit and any actions or steps toward change. Although MI comprises several specialized techniques that may be more suitable to use within Intensive Interventions (see section below), its fundamental principles (e.g., collaboration, evocation, and autonomy) should be applied in any encounter with tobacco users not ready to quit. Of note, specific applications of MI in health care has been published (see Rollnick, Miller, & Butler, 2008). In their book, Rollnick and colleagues compare MI with a *guiding* communication style and suggest that health care providers use this approach (instead of the other extreme approaches of *directing* or *following*) when having conversations with the patient about behavior change. A guiding style makes a good balance of three communication skills: *asking*, *listening, and informing*. Thus, practitioners can engage in the MI spirit by asking the patient about their tobacco use and intentions to quit, listening nonjudgmentally to their reasons and barriers to quit, and informing them about the benefits of quitting and the resources available.

Research has generally supported the use of MI for smoking cessation, including single sessions, short sessions and those delivered by general practitioners and trained counselors (Lindson-Hawley, Thompson, & Begh, 2015). Although some of the research included in meta-analyses (studies that combine information from multiple intervention studies in order to estimate overall effect) have included Latinos in their sample, we are unaware of specific published research evaluating the efficacy of brief motivational interventions for Latino smokers not willing to quit.

The 5R's Model

The 5R's model provide the content areas that should be addressed within an MI framework. This model appears to increase future quit attempts (Carpenter, Hughes, Solomon, & Callas, 2004; Fiore et al., 2008). However, its particular usefulness among Latino populations have not been reported.

RELEVANCE. Providing information about tobacco use has the greatest impact when it is related to the patient's particular characteristics and situation. These include age, gender, his/her family (e.g., effects of smoking on children), health issues (e.g., high blood pressure, dental problems), social issues (e.g., tobacco-free workplace policies), among others. Help the patient reflect on why quitting is personally relevant.

RISKS. Help the patient to identify potential negative consequences of tobacco use (U.S. Department of Health and Human Services, 2014), and suggest additional ones that seem relevant to the patient. For example, short term health risks include: shortness of breath, risk of respiratory infections, and exacerbation of asthma, impotence, fertility problems, bad smell, skin aging, and harm to pregnancy. Long term health risks include: several cancers (e.g., lung, oral cavity, larynx, pancreas, etc.), heart attacks and strokes, chronic obstructive pulmonary disease. Importantly, practitioners should also emphasize that smoking may negatively affect others in the household through second hand smoke (e.g. ear and respiratory infections in children, risk of lung cancer and heart disease in partners), and that smoking low tar/low nicotine cigarettes or other tobacco products still represent a risk.

REWARDS. Inquire about the patient's perceived benefits of stopping tobacco use, and suggest additional ones that seem relevant to the patient's situation. Rewards range from health improvements to other personal/social benefits including: improved sense of smell and taste, improved overall health and reduction of risk of chronic diseases, improved breath, improved smell of one's home/car, clothing will smell better, improved health of children and people in one's household, saving money, greater performance in physical activities, better appearance, feeling better about oneself (sense of success and control), and being a role model for one's children.

ROADBLOCKS. Explore perceived barriers and challenges for quitting tobacco, and provide strategies to cope with them. Typical barriers include: withdrawal symptoms; stress, anxiety, or depressed mood; tobacco is embedded in their routine/habit; gratification of tobacco use; other smokers in the environment; lack of support to quit; concurrent alcohol or other substance use; other psychological comorbidities; fear of failure; and lack of knowledge about effective treatment options.

REPETITION. Repeat the motivational messages to every patient that is not motivated or ready to quit, every time he/she attends the clinical setting (Table 13.5).

Table 13.5 The 5R's model for enhancing motivation to quit tobacco use

Component	Description
RELEVANCE	Providing information about tobacco use that is relevant for the patient.
RISKS	Help the patient to identify potential negative consequences of tobacco use, and provide additional information when needed.
REWARDS	Inquire the patient about perceived benefits of stopping tobacco use, and suggest additional ones that seem relevant to the patient's situation.
ROADBLOCKS	Explore perceived barriers and challenges for quitting tobacco, and provide strategies to cope with them.
REPETITION	Repeat the motivational messages to every patient that is not motivated or ready to quit, every time he/she attends the clinical setting.

Main source: Fiore MC, Jaen CR, Baker TB, et al. Treating Tobacco Use and Dependence: 2008 Update. (May 2008). Clinical Practice Guideline. Rockville, MD: U.S. Department of Health and Human Services. Public Health Service

Intensive Interventions

Intensive interventions for TDT last more than 10 min in duration per clinical encounter and are characterized by greater depth and breadth in the assessment and counseling of tobacco use when compared with brief interventions. These are suitable for tobacco cessation clinics, substance abuse programs, psychology practices, and any other health care setting with trained personnel and time allocated for more intensive behavioral interventions. Intensive interventions are ideal for more complex patients, including individuals with higher tobacco dependence, and with comorbid physical or mental health conditions. These interventions include an extension of the 5A's model, with a particular focus on motivational interviewing techniques as well as cognitive behavioral treatment and problem solving/skills training approaches (Abrams et al., 2003; Rollnick et al., 2008). Importantly, a tobacco use treatment approach that combines pharmachotherapy/nicotine replacement with behavioral coping skills training outperforms the use of either treatment alone and this combined approach is recommended in the guidelines (Fiore et al., 2008). Further, although studies that specifically target Latino tobacco users are very few, the limited evidence suggests these treatment approaches are efficacious among Latinos (Webb et al., 2010).

Cultural Considerations

It has been consistently demonstrated that behavioral health interventions, including substance-use interventions, that are adapted for racial/ethnic minority populations tend to be more effective than non-adapted interventions. In fact, meta-analytic studies of culturally adapted interventions indicate that culturally adapted behavioral health interventions are approximately 20 % more effective than non-adapted interventions (Benish, Quintana, & Wampold, 2011; Smith, Rodríguez, & Bernal, 2011). Furthermore, it is widely regarded as an ethical responsibility for healthcare professionals to understand and consider factors associated with culture in order to effectively provide services (American Medical Association; American Psychological Association, 2002; National Association of Social Workers). As such, to incorporate cultural considerations into intensive interventions for TDT for Latinos is ethical and will increase the probabilities of positive outcomes.

Although still in its infancy, available evidence on cultural adaptations of TDT for Latinos seems promising (Wetter et al., 2007; Woodruff et al., 2002). Examples of elements that have been incorporated in the content and delivery of culturally adapted smoking cessation interventions for Latinos include: language appropriate content (e.g. for individuals with Limited English Proficiency (LEP) or attending to nuances in Spanish-terminology across subgroups), culturally specific images and stories (in written or audiovisual materials), and integration of common cultural values (e.g. *familismo* [family involvement], *personalismo* [positive personal relationship], *respeto* [respect]) (Cox et al., 2011; Webb et al., 2010). Nevertheless, the usefulness of specific elements have not been directly tested. Hence, there is still a need to further examine the extent to which culturally relevant components are potential moderators of treatment effects on smoking abstinence and/or intermediate outcomes (e.g. motivation to quit, reduction of smoking rates, and quitting attempts). Additionally, given the different patterns of smoking behaviors among Latino ethnic subgroups and acculturation levels, researchers and practitioners should consider that effectiveness of cultural adaptations may differ by groups. For example, emphasis on traditional Latino values may be important for less acculturated persons but less relevant for more acculturated individuals.

Program Structure

The design of an intensive TDT program may vary depending on the resources available at a particular health care setting as well as the population being served. Specific aspects to consider include format (e.g., individual or group; in-person or telephone-based), total number of sessions, time allocated per session, length of the program and structure. For instance, programs can use individual (e.g., phone or face-to-face) or group format (or a combination of both), include 5–20 sessions, last from 10 min to 2 h (depending on format), and be conducted within 5 weeks to 6 months of duration. Many tobacco users may not be interested in committing to long programs, so shorter programs in between 6 and 10 sessions may be more appealing to a broader group of individuals. In terms of structure, it is typical for programs to go from weekly sessions to sessions every other week, and a final one that takes place a month after the penultimate one. Some programs are structured to have more sessions devoted to the preparation before the quit date, while others allocate more sessions after the quit day to help address withdrawal and prevent relapse. Whenever possible, the timing of the service should be relapse-sensitive, including one or more sessions before the quit date ("preparation phase"), one session on the quit day and one or more sessions after the quit date ("quitting phase"), another session a week after the first post-quit session, and additional sessions generally occurring at 2–3 weeks intervals thereafter ("maintenance").

Below we describe the core components of an intensive cessation program. These components can be incorporated in either group and individual formats, as well as both face-to-face and phone modalities. In-depth details on the procedures and treatment content are available in treatment handbooks such as those by Abrams et al., 2003 and Peterson, Vander Weg, & Jaen, 2010.

Therapeutic Approach

Motivational Interviewing. As previously discussed, MI is an approach especially suited for patients who are not willing or ready to change their tobacco use. The MI principles can be incorporated in any type of counseling encounter (e.g., brief intervention), but their specific techniques may be more feasible to use within intensive interventions. Also, given that motivation for change can fluctuate during the quitting process, an MI approach can be incorporated at any time and can be easily integrated with other therapeutic approaches (Vidrine, Reitzel, Figueroa, et al., 2013). Among the several counseling strategies utilized in MI, the *rulers* is the most common. The "rulers" (Figure) inquire about how important is a behavior change for the person. For example, the clinician would ask the patient "*In a scale from 1 to 10, how important it is for you to quit smoking*?" After the patient select a number, and let's assume they chose a "6", the clinician would follow with "*Why did you select a "6" and not a "4"*?" By inquiring about why a patient didn't select a lower number, a clinician is encouraging the patient to talk about why stopping is important. After discussing the reasons to quit smoking, the clinician could follow with "*What would you need to go from "6" to an "8"*?" Asking about how the patient would get to a higher number will encourage the discussion about potential challenges and patient's needs. Similar procedures should follow to explore both confidence and readiness to quit (Figure). Additional details on MI-based strategies can be found elsewhere (Miller & Rollnick, 2013).

MI has been found to be effective in treating a variety of substance-use disorders. Among Latinos, it has shown to be efficacious for the reduction of problematic drinking (Clair et al., 2013). Also, when integrated with other approaches, MI has significantly increased continuous smoking abstinence in various underserved Latino populations (Borrelli, McQuaid, Novak, Hammond, & Becker, 2010; Clarke et al., 2013). Further implementation and testing of MI-based smoking cessation interventions among this population is warranted.

Rulers exercise utilized in Motivational Interviewing

Importance

1	2	3	4	5	6	7	8	9	10
Not at all Important			Average Importance				Extremely Important		

Readiness

1	2	3	4	5	6	7	8	9	10
Not at all Ready			Average Readiness				Extremely Ready		

Confidence

1	2	3	4	5	6	7	8	9	10
Not at all Confident			Average Confidence				Extremely Confident		

Cognitive Behavioral/Social Learning model. The cognitive-behavioral/social learning model has proven to be an evidence-based approach to treat tobacco dependence (Fiore et al., 2008) and has shown promise for Latino populations (Clarke et al., 2013; Webb Hooper & Kolar, 2015) This model conceptualizes smoking as a learned behavior that is acquired through classical and operant conditioning principles and cognitive processes (e.g. modeling other's behaviors, beliefs, self-control mechanisms, self-efficacy and outcome expectations). For instance, several cognitive, affective, and contextual cues can trigger the desire to smoke. Once the person smokes, they experience rewarding effects that reinforce smoking. Thus, the general rationale for treatment is that with behavioral skills training and practice, the smoker can unlearn the automatic sequence of events that leads to smoking and replace it with more adaptive patterns (Abrams et al., 2003). The learning of new skills involves actual practice both inside and outside of the counseling session. As such, homework in between sessions is encouraged as a way of helping the patient gaining insight regarding their tobacco use patterns and practice with quitting.

Below is a description of core components of cognitive behavioral interventions that have been recommended for TDT programs and have been positively related to smoking cessation (West, Walia, Hyder, Shahab, & Michie, 2010). Additional empirical support for the generalizability of current evidence-based practices for TDT among Latinos is warranted.

1. *Concept of dependence*. Social-cognitive model conceptualizes dependence on tobacco as motivated by mood management and learned automatic habits and patterns, as well as physical dependence. As such, the intervention should incorporate: (a) Discussion of the extent to which tobacco use is a way to cope with unpleasant feelings such as anger, frustration, depression, and anxiety; or when it is used to enhance an already positive experience (e.g., celebrations); (b) Identification of situations and behaviors that prompt the patient to smoke (i.e., triggers, urges), and; (c) The rationale and options for nicotine fading (e.g., changing brands, reducing number of cigarettes per day), and/or the use of pharmacotherapy. Information on approved medications should be offered. Nicotine fading addresses both pharmacological and psychological factors. The rationale is that, given that nicotine is physically addictive, gradually reducing its intake will reduce the intensity of withdrawal symptoms, making it less difficult to quit. Nicotine fading can serve as an alternative to pharmacological approaches for those interested in a nonpharmacological approach to quitting, or for whom medications are contraindicated. Importantly, patients need to be reminded that withdrawal symptoms may last for 2–3 weeks but that they are more intense during the first week, that urges/cravings only last minutes, and that cravings usually increase when exposed to triggers. Smokers often erroneously believe that urges to smoke will not cease until they succumb to smoke; thus they should be instructed of other ways to cope (see skills training).
2. *Conceptualization of quitting as a process*. Quitting is a long-term process that can be learned. For the majority of smokers it requires multiple quit attempts to finally achieve long-term abstinence. Ambivalence and mixed feelings about quitting are normal and the motivation to quit can wax and wane as smokers go through the quitting process and diverse life circumstances.

3. *Self-monitoring of smoking behavior.* A written record of cigarettes per day allows the patient to increase their awareness of their current smoking pattern. They are encouraged to keep a log of each cigarette smoked, time of the day, what they were doing, and their mood. This information will reveal factors that trigger smoking (e.g., situations, behaviors, thoughts, and feelings) which can be future high-risk situations for relapse. Considerations should be taken with smokers with low literacy as they may need assistance from a family/friend in completing a written log. Alternatively, the provider will work with the patient during the session to identify the patient's smoking pattern.
4. *Selection of a quit date.* Choosing a quit day gives the patient a specific day to work toward, and allows the patient to physically and mentally prepare to quit, as well as have time to acquire the skills needed to succeed. Typically, the target quit day is between 2 and 4 weeks from the treatment start date, but can be set before or after that timeframe depending on patient's readiness. Usually, quit days coincide with special occasions (e.g., holidays, birthdays, anniversaries) or particular days of the week when the patient is less stressed (e.g., after major work/school deadlines).
5. *Identification of steps to take in preparation for quitting.* Small behavioral changes that represent practice or preparation for quitting should be introduced prior to the quit day. Ideally, specific behavioral changes should come from the patient. However, typical examples that can be shared with them are: stop smoking in the car and/or inside the home, buy fewer quantities of cigarettes at a time, reduce the quantity of cigarettes smoked per day by eliminating the "least important cigarette of the day", change the smoking routine, eliminating cues from the environment, tell other people about the plans to quit, or write the reasons to quit and put in a visible place at home. The day before the quit day, it is important that the patient remove all cigarettes from their environments before going to bed, identify sources of support, and quit smoking upon awakening. Ideally, the patient should have an hour-by-hour plan for not smoking on the first day.
6. *Planning to manage triggers.* Setting short-term goals and planning in advance to manage triggers is key to success. Prior to goal setting and planning, it is important to differentiate *self-control* from *willpower*. Provider should discourage the common notion of willpower and introduce the concept of self-control. Willpower is "trying to exert absolute will over quitting without any particular plan or strategy", whereas self-control entails the "development of a systematic and strategic plan to manage trigger situations without smoking" (Abrams et al., 2003, p. 137). Self-control strategies fall under three main types. They are: (a) *avoid trigger situations*: for example, avoid being around other smokers near the time of usual smoking breaks, avoid common "smoke break" locations or hangouts, avoid social situations that include alcohol and/or the presence of other smokers; (b) *alter trigger situations*: for example, if the patient normally smokes while drinking their morning coffee, they might try drinking hot chocolate or juice instead, go for a walk during break time instead of smoking a cigarette, or practice positive self-talk such as "I don't need a cigarette in this

situation" when confronted with a stressful situation; (c) *use an alternative or substitute behavior instead of a cigarette*: for example, eating sugarless candy or chewing gum, cinnamon sticks, or a straw; also, eating a fruit, practicing breathing techniques, engaging in physical activity, drinking water, calling a friend, or painting can all help to keep one both physically and mentally distracted when an urge to smoke strikes. The practice of self-control strategies is key to treatment. Elicit from the patients their ideas on how to refrain from smoking in trigger situations. After quitting, discuss which strategies patients have found useful and which not, and remind them that they can fine-tune or change a strategy that has not worked. Remind the patient that managing triggers is a trial-and-error process for each person, but that *avoiding* triggers is the most effective coping strategy and should be used whenever possible. However, providers should be aware that sometimes the patient may discount the notion of avoiding cues/situations altogether because they believe they should expose themselves to the trigger and be able to not smoke ("willpower"); or they simply do not want to give up multiple pleasurable experiences at the same time (e.g. drinking coffee, consuming alcohol, socializing). Of note, although triggers related to negative emotions (e.g., stress boredom) and social situations (e.g., at parties, at a bar) appear to be equally important triggers for Latino and non-Latino white smokers, triggers that represent habitual or unpremeditated behaviors (e.g., smoking while driving, while on the phone, when drinking coffee) seem to be less salient to Latino smokers (Marin, Marin, Perez-Stable, Sabogal, & Otero-Sabogal, 1990). Importantly, stress related to acculturation processes and instances of discrimination may be particularly relevant for some Latinos.

7. *Self-efficacy*. High levels of self-efficacy is one of the best predictors of successful quitting in various populations (Businelle et al., 2010; Correa-Fernández et al., 2012). Self-efficacy can be increased by encouraging the patient to think about moments in their lives when they have been successful in making changes or accomplishing goals and how they did it. Reassure the patient that they can apply those abilities to quitting as well. It is expected that with the practice of new coping skills, patients will increase their self-efficacy for quitting. However, is important to note that, as with motivation, self-efficacy to quit may fluctuate at different stages of the quitting process and in different situations.
8. *Social support and social influences*. Initiate discussion about the role of social support for not smoking, and maximize support for quitting. Help the patient differentiate positive and negative social influences and support. For example, a positive social influence is someone who volunteers to talk over the phone or go for a walk when the patient is experiencing a craving to smoke. In contrast, a negative social influence could be someone who undermines the smoker's ability or determination to quit. Patients should identify what kinds of behaviors from others they find not supportive regarding quitting, and which ones they do find supportive. Then, help the patient to identify people who can be supportive and to practice asking for positive social support from others. Discourage the contact with other smokers and ask the patient how they will reduce or eliminate contact

to negative and non-supportive behaviors from others that interfere with their quitting efforts. For patients that live with other smokers or whose partner uses tobacco, quitting can be particularly challenging. Ideally, these individuals would quit together. Otherwise, the patient needs to practice assertiveness skills to be able to request instrumental support from these persons (e.g., not smoking in their presence or leaving tobacco-related paraphernalia visible or accessible).

The role of social support may be of particular importance with Latino smokers as the Latino cultural value of *familismo* may influence their quitting process in either direction. In particular, family conflict and low family cohesion have been associated with elevated smoking risk among Latinos (Lorenzo-Blanco & Cortina, 2013a, 2013b). On the one hand, high family support and cohesion can be a great motivator and support for quitting, but on the other hand, low levels of these can produce stress that triggers relapse. Anecdotally, it has been the experience of the first author that high family support and cohesion may also inhibit success, especially if family members are quitting together and one of them relapses. For example, in one instance family members quit together and when one person slipped to smoking, soon the other person lapsed even though they were doing well. The second person's reasons for returning to smoke included not wanting to succeed while the other person failed. In the patient own words: "We are together in this, and I feel bad being quit when he lapsed. We will try together again. (Correa-Fernández, Agosto, Sánchez, & Diaz-Toro, Unpublished manuscript).

9. *Skills training*. Techniques to manage negative mood, stress, and craving will be useful in the quitting process, particularly during the first weeks after the quit day. For example, advise patients to identify safe places and activities when they do not smoke. Also, engage daily in a relaxing and enjoyable activity for at least 45–60 min. It can be a hobby or an activity that can be done easily, that does not require a lot of mental energy, and has some value for the smoker (e.g. reading, exercising, dancing, playing with their children). Also, relaxation techniques, such as deep breathing, is a practice the can be used on a daily basis as well as in specific stressful situations. Coping imagery may be particularly useful to cope with urges or craving to smoke. For example, patients can imagine urges as a rollercoaster ride that rises and falls. Encourage patients to create their own metaphors and images and to practice letting the urge pass. Reductions in distress levels pre-to-postcognitive behavioral therapy have been linked with increased smoking abstinence among treatment-seeking Latinos (Webb Hooper & Kolar, 2015).
10. *Relapse prevention*. The ability to cope with high risk situations determines an individual's probability of maintaining abstinence. As such, discussion of how to cope with a lapse and avoid a relapse is highly warranted. First, help the patient understand that a lapse or slip (an instance of smoking after the quit date) is different from relapse (returning to smoking at levels similar to those before the quit date). Second, help the patient recognize that the typical response to an instance of smoking following the quit day is one of negative emotional reactions (e.g., sadness, guilt) and self-defeating attributions (e.g., considering oneself a failure or weak for slipping), which may result in

resumption of regular smoking. This normalization of slipping is not permission to slip, but an opportunity to view it as a mistake, rather than a failure. Now the objective is to prevent a lapse from becoming a relapse, by not smoking the next cigarette and by strengthening coping strategies. Introduce the relapse-prevention concept of identifying and coping with high-risk situations (i.e., a situation that can lead to resumption of smoking). Highlight that the major high risk situations for relapse are: (a) cravings; (b) negative mood; (c) social interactions with other smokers, and (d) positive mood, especially social situations involving alcohol use. However, patients should identify their own risk situation and for each situation, they should develop a full set of coping strategies (see *Plans to Manage Triggers*) to deal with the situation without smoking.

11. *Weight control*. A modest and usually temporary weight gain is common among people that quit smoking, and many smokers, especially women, relapse to smoking due to concerns about perceived or actual weight gain. Increasing physical activity, making healthy food choices, drinking a lot of water, snacking on fruits, vegetables, and low calorie foods will help control weight gain, and can be addressed as a lifestyle change.
12. *Rewards*. As a positive reinforcement, patients should be encouraged to plan rewards for a day of not smoking, as well as after a week, a month, or a year. An option is to calculate the amount of money saved for not smoking and choose a reward with similar value.
13. *Benefits of quitting*. For patients that become abstinent, exploring the benefits of quitting could serve as a motivator to continue without smoking. Examples include feeling proud of themselves, saving money, breathing more easily, increased taste and smell, etc. Benefits and reasons for quitting should be generated by the patient, but some examples that have been shown to be significantly more relevant to Latino smokers compared to non-Latino white smokers include: being criticized by family, burning clothes, damaging children's health, bad breath, family pressure, and being a good example to children (Pérez-Stable, Marín, & Posner, 1998).
14. *Lifestyle changes that support quitting*. For many smokers, quitting is a lifestyle change that can be enhanced and maintained by the simultaneous change in other areas. Common lifestyle changes recommended include: stress management, maintain a positive social support network, healthy diet, weight control, and physical activity. Most of these changes have been described above. Also, there has been some evidence that physical activity enhance smoking cessation and maintenance (Ussher, Taylor & Faulkner, 2014). Since exercise is usually incompatible with simultaneous smoking, it can serve as a substitute behavior. It may also be a good alternative to control weight gain, attenuate withdrawal symptoms, and decrease mood changes (such as anxiety and depression). For a vigorous exercise regimen the patient should consult a physician. Additionally, be aware of a panic reaction when patients think they are quitting for the rest of their lives. Encourage thinking of it as one day at a time, or an hour at a time. Offer information on resources for later support.

Innovative approaches that fully integrate MI and Cognitive-Behavioral models for smoking cessation has been documented (Vidrine, Reitzel, Figueroa, et al., 2013) and utilized among Latinos with positive results (Clarke et al., 2013; Correa-Fernández et al., submitted). Additionally, contemporary forms of cognitive-behavioral therapies, such as Acceptance and Commitment Therapy, has also shown promise for the treatment of tobacco dependence (Bricker, Mann, Marek, Liu, & Peterson, 2010; Gifford et al., 2011).

Provider and Clinic Changes in Integrated Health Care Settings

The occurrence of both medical and behavioral health problems is disproportionately higher among tobacco users compared to the general population, which puts them at further increased risk of mortality (Colton & Manderscheid, 2006). In particular, it is estimated that 44 % of the cigarettes smoked in the U.S. are consumed by people with a behavioral health disorders. As such, there is a call to designate smokers with behavioral health comorbidities as a specific tobacco use disparity group (Williams, Steinberg, Griffiths, & Cooperman, 2013). Fortunately, the benefits of quitting smoking encompass improvements in both physical and mental health status of the patient.

Programs that include quality interventions at both the provider- and clinic-level are more likely to increase the reach and effectiveness of TDT. As discussed, regular screening for tobacco use and the provision of cessation counseling and pharmacotherapy are evidence-based practices known to reduce tobacco use among Latino patients, including those with behavioral health disorders. Moreover, the adoption of clinic-level policies and interventions, such as tobacco-free workplace regulations and the provision of TDT to employees, are also effective in assisting patients quit (Anderson & Hughes, 2000). Importantly, these provider- and clinic-level approaches are likely to reduce patient-level barriers to care.

Below, we offer a number of recommendations for clinic-level and integrated approaches to successfully incorporate and support TDT. These recommendations are grounded in evidence-based practices as well as in our clinical experience with integrated care programs (Cahill & Lancaster, 2014; Correa-Fernández, et al., submitted; Fiore et al., 2008).

Environment

- *Develop and implement a tobacco-free workplace policy*. The objective of this policy is to support health initiatives by completely prohibiting the use of any form of tobacco on the worksite property. This regulation not only protects all individuals (including nonsmokers) from environmental tobacco smoke, but also helps former smokers maintain abstinence by eliminating smoking cues and temptations in the environment. If possible, add to the policy cessation services for employees. Although this is not a standard component in all tobacco-free workplace policies, those policies that do include these services have positive impact on the reduction of tobacco use behaviors.

Support the implementation of a tobacco user identification system. The practitioner's intentions to systematically provide brief interventions for cessation must be supported by a clinic-wide system where the identification of every tobacco user can be documented. This can be accomplished my modifying the EHR or paper progress notes. Also, allowing time for tobacco-related education and training is another way of supporting this efforts.

Personnel

- *Provide training in TDT to all personnel.* All the personnel, including the administrative assistants or people making the appointments, should be trained in the basics TDT. This will promote shared values and a culture of change for tobacco use. Moreover, more specialized training for physicians and other health care providers is warranted. Research has shown that some of the barriers for assisting smokers to quit include providers' lack of knowledge and confidence in providing TDT. Conversely, there is evidence that having had cessation training is positively associated with performing some components of the 5A's and that intensive training programs for behavioral health professionals can increase the delivery of TDT as well as patient attempts to quit. Booster training sessions are often useful and can be done both in-person or through webinars. Also, peer-led audit and feedback increases the frequency of documenting cessation counseling and the appropriateness of NRT prescriptions (Kisuule, Necocheax, Howe, & Wright, 2010).
- *Designate a TDT coordinator ("tobacco champion").* A tobacco champion would be a person trained in tobacco dependence and treatment that would take the lead in initiating and/or maintaining all initiatives related to tobacco-free workplace regulations as well as TDT. The person's responsibilities would vary depending on the treatment setting but could include following up with clinic's signage related to tobacco use, surveying providers and patients about their needs, ensuring the systematic identification of smokers, distributing NRT when available, and peer-leading trainings and booster sessions.

Use of an interdisciplinary team. The involvement of multiple health care professionals in TDT is effective and should be utilized. An approach could be to have a physician providing advice to quit in relation to the patient's health issues and offering pharmacotherapy, and having a behavioral specialist providing the counseling component (using recommended brief or intensive interventions). When available, other health professionals can be incorporated to provide additional education or support (e.g. nutritionist to address weight gain, health educator, and pharmacist).

Services

- Use a *patient-centered model of care* including logistics and practical aspects of the services. For instance:
  - Whenever possible, have an administrative assistant dedicated to the scheduling and logistic aspects of the TDT program. When that is not feasible, distribute the tasks among various professionals so no one is particularly burdened.
  - Show respect for the patient's time. Do not schedule more patients that clinicians are available to see at a given time point. Ideally, avoid the "first come, first serve" approach and instead schedule appointment for a specific time. Individuals that are not abstinent would likely be anxious if have to wait too long, especially if that alters their smoking routine, and this event may risk them leaving and missing the appointment.
  - Have the availability of making appointments by phone or internet, and allow for walk-in services when possible. If a patient stops by to inquire about cessation services, it is crucial to capitalize on that moment's motivation and at least offer a brief intervention.
  - Have flexible/extended hours of service, such as in the evening or weekends. For recent immigrants or Latinos of low SES, factors such as having multiple jobs, family obligations, and lack of transportation may be obstacles to attend sessions at normal business hours.
  - Maintain complete transparency about the program from the initial phone call or contact. Explain the services to the patient including how long it will take, which practitioners will see him/her and an overall structure of the program.
  - If smoking is allowed in the clinic premises, explain to patients exactly where they can or cannot smoke during the visit. If the clinic is tobacco-free, remind the patient.
  - Maximize privacy as much as possible. Tobacco use could be a source of a shame for some individuals, including less acculturated Latino women and persons from higher SES status or in the health fields.
  - Provide follow-up calls and reminders. Calls to confirm the appointment, and calls after a patient misses an appointment to check in on how they are doing and to reschedule are examples of intra-treatment support, which is recommended in the PHS guidelines (Fiore et al., 2008).
- Use a *patient-centered model of care in the content and structure* of the service. For instance:
  - Emphasize to patients from the beginning that they can and should keep coming to the visits, irrespective of their smoking status. Is not uncommon for Latino patients to withdraw from the program if they resume smoking due to shame and guilt of letting the provider down.
  - Implement a streamlined intake system, where information can be collected through questionnaires in the waiting room. Whenever possible, have help available for those who had difficulty reading/writing, have low literacy or LEP.

- Establish an EHR system and incorporate tobacco use modules and questions into it. This will facilitate communication among all health care providers.
- Be aware that Latino patients, particularly recent immigrants, less acculturated persons, or those with LEP can come to the visit accompanied with one or more relatives. Be prepared to incorporate them to any particular session at the request of the patient. However, use your clinical judgment to identify when is preferred to have individual sessions only with the patient and kindly communicate that to him/her.
- Provide an effective service at each visit. Enhance motivation and provide a service that is useful even if the patient does not return to the next visit.

Every health care setting has particular needs and resources, and the level and timing in which they can incorporate evidence-based practices varies. Nevertheless, these practices can be implemented in a gradual manner and evaluated for its effectiveness until a satisfactory integrated system is reached. Providing evidence-based practices through integrated care is a tremendous avenue for achieving tobacco use cessation in Latinos so its careful implementation should not be underestimated but pursued.

References

Abraído-Lanza, A. F., Chao, M. T., & Flórez, K. R. (2005). Do healthy behaviors decline with greater acculturation?: Implications for the Latino mortality paradox. *Social Science and Medicine, 61*(6), 1243–1255.

Abrams, D., Niaura, R., Brown, R., Emmons, K., Goldstein, M., & Monti, P. (2003). *The tobacco dependence treatment handbook. A guide to best practices*. New York, NY: The Guilford Press.

American Cancer Society. (2012). *Cancer facts & figures for Latinos/Latinos 2012–2014*. Atlanta, GA: American Cancer Society.

American Lung Association. *Tobacco cessation and the affordable care act*. Retrieved August 28, 2015.

American Medical Association. *American Medical Association's code of ethics*. Retrieved August, 2015, from http://www.ama-assn.org/ama/pub/physician-resources/medical-ethics/code-medical-ethics.page.

American Psychiatric Association. (2000). *Diagnostic and statistical manual of mental disorders text revised* (4th ed.). Washington, DC: Author.

American Psychiatric Association. (2013). *Diagnostic and statistical manual of mental disorders 5* (5th ed.). Washington, DC: Author.

American Psychological Association. (2002). *Ethical principles of psychologists and code of conduct*. Washington, DC: American Psychological Association.

Amrhein, P. C., Miller, W. R., Yahne, C. E., Palmer, M., & Fulcher, L. (2003). Client commitment language during motivational interviewing predicts drug use outcomes. *Journal of Consulting and Clinical Psychology, 71*(5), 862–878.

Anderson, P., & Hughes, J. R. (2000). Policy interventions to reduce the harm from smoking. *Addiction, 95*(Suppl 1), S9–S11.

Baker, T. B., Breslau, N., Covey, L., & Shiffman, S. (2012). DSM criteria for tobacco use disorder and tobacco withdrawal: A critique and proposed revisions for DSM-5. *Addiction, 107*(2), 263–275.

Benish, S. G., Quintana, S., & Wampold, B. E. (2011). Culturally adapted psychotherapy and the legitimacy of myth: A direct-comparison meta-analysis. *Journal of Counseling Psychology, 58*(3), 279–289.

Benowitz, N. L., Bernert, J. T., Caraballo, R. S., Holiday, D. B., & Wang, J. (2009). Optimal serum cotinine levels for distinguishing cigarette smokers and nonsmokers within different racial/ethnic groups in the United States between 1999 and 2004. *American Journal of Epidemiology, 169*(2), 236–248.

Bethel, J. W., & Schenker, M. B. (2005). Acculturation and smoking patterns among Latinos: A review. *American Journal of Preventive Medicine, 29*(2), 143–148.

Bjartveit, K., & Tverdal, A. (2005). Health consequences of smoking 1-4 cigarettes per day. *Tobacco Control, 14*(5), 315–320.

Bock, B. C., Niaura, R. S., Neighbors, C. J., Carmona-Barros, R., & Azam, M. (2005). Differences between Latino and non-Latino White smokers in cognitive and behavioral characteristics relevant to smoking cessation. *Addictive Behaviors, 30*(4), 711–724.

Borland, R., & Segan, C. J. (2006). The potential of quitlines to increase smoking cessation. *Drug and Alcohol Review, 25*(1), 73–78.

Borland, R., Yong, H. H., O'Connor, R. J., Hyland, A., & Thompson, M. E. (2010). The reliability and predictive validity of the Heaviness of Smoking Index and its two components: Findings from the International Tobacco Control Four Country study. *Nicotine & Tobacco Research, 12*(Suppl), S45–S50.

Borrelli, B., McQuaid, E. L., Novak, S. P., Hammond, S. K., & Becker, B. (2010). Motivating Latino caregivers of children with asthma to quit smoking: A randomized trial. *Journal of Consulting and Clinical Psychology, 78*(1), 34–43.

Breslau, N., Johnson, E. O., Hiripi, E., & Kessler, R. (2001). Nicotine dependence in the United States: Prevalence, trends, and smoking persistence. *Archives of General Psychiatry, 58*(9), 810–816.

Bricker, J. B., Mann, S. L., Marek, P. M., Liu, J., & Peterson, A. V. (2010). Telephone-delivered Acceptance and Commitment Therapy for adult smoking cessation: A feasibility study. *Nicotine & Tobacco Research, 12*(4), 454–458.

Brothers, B. M., & Borrelli, B. (2011). Motivating Latino smokers to quit: Does type of social support matter? *American Journal of Health Promotion, 25*(5 Suppl), S96–S102.

Businelle, M. S., Kendzor, D. E., Reitzel, L. R., Costello, T. J., Cofta-Woerpel, L., Li, Y., … Wetter, D. W. (2010). Mechanisms linking socioeconomic status to smoking cessation: A structural equation modeling approach. *Health Psychology, 29(3)*, 262–273.

Cahill K, Lancaster T. (2014). Workplace interventions for smoking cessation. *Cochrane Database Syst Rev, 26*(2), CD003440. doi:10.1002/14651858.CD003440.pub4. Review.

Carpenter, M. J., Hughes, J. R., Solomon, L. J., & Callas, P. W. (2004). Both smoking reduction with nicotine replacement therapy and motivational advice increase future cessation among smokers unmotivated to quit. *Journal of Consulting and Clinical Psychology, 72*(3), 371–381.

Castro, Y., Businelle, M. S., Correa-Fernández, V., Kendzor, D. E., Mazas, C. A., Cofta-Woerpel, L., & Wetter, D. W. (2012). Associations between indicators of acculturation and tobacco dependence among Spanish-speaking Latino smokers. *Addictive Behaviors, 37(10)*, 1101–1108.

Castro, Y., Correa-Fernández, V., Cano, M. A., Mazas, C., Gonzalez, K., Vidrine, D. J., … Wetter, D. W. (2014). Failure to replicate the structure of a Spanish-language brief Wisconsin Inventory of Smoking Dependence Motives across three samples of Latino smokers. *Nicotine & Tobacco Research, 16*(9), 1277–1281.

Castro, Y., Costello, T., Correa-Fernández, V., Heppner, W. L., Reitzel, L. R., Cofta-Woerpel, L., … Wetter, D. W. (2011). Differential effects of depression on smoking cessation in a diverse sample of smokers in treatment. *American Journal of Preventive Medicine, 41(1)*, 84–87.

Castro, Y., Kendzor, D. E., Businelle, M. S., Mazas, C. A., Cofta-Woerpel, L., Cinciripini, P. M., & Wetter, D. W. (2011). Structural and predictive equivalency of the Wisconsin Smoking Withdrawal Scale across three racial/ethnic groups. *Nicotine & Tobacco Research, 13(7)*, 548–555.

Castro, Y., Reitzel, L. R., Businelle, M. S., Kendzor, D. E., Mazas, C. A., Li, Y., … Wetter, D. W. (2009). Acculturation differentially predicts smoking cessation among Latino men and women. *Cancer Epidemiology Biomarkers Prevention, 18(12)*, 3468–3475.

CDC. (2002). Cigarette smoking among adults --- United States, 2000. *Morbidity and Mortality Weekly Report, 51*(29), 642–645.

CDC. (2004). *The health consequences of smoking: A report of the Surgeon General*. Washington, DC: Atlanta, GA: Department of Health and Human Services, Centers for Disease Control and Prevention, National Center for Chronic Disease Prevention and Health Promotion, Office on Smoking and Health.

CDC. (2011). Quitting smoking among adults--United States, 2001–2010. *MMWR. Morbidity and Mortality Weekly Report, 60*(44), 1513–1519.

CDC. (2014). Current cigarette smoking among adults--United States, 2005-2013. *MMWR. Morbidity and Mortality Weekly Report, 63*(47), 1108–1112.

CDC. (2015). Vital signs: Leading causes of death, prevalence of diseases and risk factors, and use of health services among Latinos in the United States—2009–2013. *Morbidity and Mortality Weekly Report, 64*(17), 469–478.

Chiang, K., & Borrelli, B. (2014). Income predictors of smoking cessation among Latinos. *Journal of Health Psychology, 19*(7), 869–876.

Clair, M., Stein, L. A., Soenksen, S., Martin, R. A., Lebeau, R., & Golembeske, C. (2013). Ethnicity as a moderator of motivational interviewing for incarcerated adolescents after release. *Journal of Substance Abuse Treatment, 45*(4), 370–375.

Clarke, J. G., Stein, L. A., Martin, R. A., Martin, S. A., Parker, D., Lopes, C. E., … Bock, B. (2013). Forced smoking abstinence: Not enough for smoking cessation. *JAMA Internal Medicine, 173(9)*, 789–794.

Cokkinides, V. E., Halpern, M. T., Barbeau, E. M., Ward, E., & Thun, M. J. (2008). Racial and ethnic disparities in smoking-cessation interventions: Analysis of the 2005 National Health Interview Survey. *American Journal of Preventive Medicine, 34*(5), 404–412.

Colton, C. W., & Manderscheid, R. W. (2006). Congruencies in increased mortality rates, years of potential life lost, and causes of death among public mental health clients in eight states. *Preventing Chronic Disease, 3*(2), A42.

Constantine, M. L., Rockwood, T. H., Schillo, B. A., Castellanos, J. W., Foldes, S. S., & Saul, J. E. (2009). The relationship between acculturation and knowledge of health harms and benefits associated with smoking in the Latino population of Minnesota. *Addictive Behaviors, 34*(11), 980–983.

Cooper, T. V., Rodríguez de Ybarra, D., Charter, J. E., & Blow, J. (2011). Characteristics associated with smoking in a Latino college student sample. *Addictive Behaviors, 36*(12), 1329–1332.

Correa-Fernández, V., Agosto, J., Sánchez, A., & Diaz-Toro, E. C. Integrating an interdisciplinary tobacco cessation clinic in a School of Dental Medicine. Unpublished manuscript.

Correa-FernÃ¡ndez, V., DÃaz-Toro, E. C., Reitzel, L. R., Guo, L., Chen, M., Li, Y.,.. Wetter, D. W. (2016). *Combined treatment for smoking cessation and at-risk drinking in Latinos*. Paper presented at the Society for Research on Nicotine and Tobacco, Chicago, IL.

Correa-Fernández, V., Ji, L., Castro, Y., Heppner, W. L., Vidrine, J. I., Costello, T. J., … Wetter, D. W. (2012). Mediators of the association of major depressive syndrome and anxiety syndrome with postpartum smoking relapse. *Journal of Consulting and Clinical Psychology, 80(4)*, 636–648.

Cox, L. S., Feng, S., Cañar, J., Ford, M. M., & Tercyak, K. P. (2005). Social and behavioral correlates of cigarette smoking among mid-Atlantic Latino primary care patients. *Cancer Epidemiology, Biomarkers & Prevention, 14*(8), 1976–1980.

Cox, L. S., Okuyemi, K., Choi, W. S., & Ahluwalia, J. S. (2011). A review of tobacco use treatments in US ethnic minority populations. *American Journal of Health Promotion, 25*(5), S11–S30.

Cupertino, P. A., Cox, L. S. C., Garrett, S., Suarez, N., Sandt, H., Mendoza, I., & Ellerbeck, E. F. (2011). Tobacco use and interest in smoking cessation among Latinos attending community health fairs. *Journal of Immigrant and Minority Health, 13(4)*, 719–724.

Daza, P., Cofta-Woerpel, L., Mazas, C., Fouladi, R. T., Cinciripini, P. M., Gritz, E. R., & Wetter, D. W. (2006). Racial and ethnic differences in predictors of smoking cessation. *Substance Use and Misuse, 41(3)*, 317–339.

de Dios, M. A., Anderson, B. J., Stanton, C., Audet, D. A., & Stein, M. (2012). Project Impact: A pharmacotherapy pilot trial investigating the abstinence and treatment adherence of Latino light smokers. *Journal of Substance Abuse Treatment, 43*(3), 322–330.

Edelen, M. O., Stucky, B. D., Hansen, M., Tucker, J. S., Shadel, W. G., & Cai, L. (2014). The PROMIS smoking initiative: Initial validity evidence for six new smoking item banks. *Nicotine & Tobacco Research, 16*(Suppl 3), S250–S260.

Fagan, P., Shavers, V., Lawrence, D., Gibson, J. T., & Ponder, P. (2007). Cigarette smoking and quitting behaviors among unemployed adults in the United States. *Nicotine & Tobacco Research, 9*(2), 241–248.

Ferguson, J. A., Patten, C. A., Schroeder, D. R., Offord, K. P., Eberman, K. M., & Hurt, R. D. (2003). Predictors of 6-month tobacco abstinence among 1224 cigarette smokers treated for nicotine dependence. *Addictive Behaviors, 28*(7), 1203–1218.

Fiore, M. C., Jaen, C. R., Baker, T. B., Bailey, W. C., Benowitz, N. L., Curry, S. J., … Goldstein, M. G. (2008). *Treating tobacco use and dependence: 2008 Update. Clinical practice guideline.* Rockville, MD: U.S. Department of Health and Human Services, Public Health Service.

Foraker, R. E., Patten, C. A., Lopez, K. N., Croghan, I. T., & Thomas, J. L. (2005). Beliefs and attitudes regarding smoking among young adult Latinos: A pilot study. *Preventive Medicine, 41*(1), 126–133.

Foulds, J., Gandhi, K. K., Steinberg, M. B., Richardson, D. L., Williams, J. M., Burke, M. V., & Rhoads, G. G. (2006). Factors associated with quitting smoking at a tobacco dependence treatment clinic. *American Journal of Health Behavior, 30(4)*, 400–412.

Fu, S. S., Sherman, S. E., Yano, E. M., van Ryn, M., Lanto, A. B., & Joseph, A. M. (2005). Ethnic disparities in the use of nicotine replacement therapy for smoking cessation in an equal access health care system. *American Journal of Health Promotion, 20*(2), 108–116.

Gifford, E. V., Kohlenberg, B. S., Hayes, S. C., Pierson, H. M., Piasecki, M. P., Antonuccio, D. O., Palm, K. M. (2011). Does acceptance and relationship focused behavior therapy contribute to bupropion outcomes? A randomized controlled trial of functional analytic psychotherapy and acceptance and commitment therapy for smoking cessation. *Behaviour Therapy, 42(4)*, 700–715.

Heatherton, T. F., Kozlowski, L. T., Frecker, R. C., Rickert, W., & Robinson, J. (1989). Measuring the heaviness of smoking: Using self-reported time to the first cigarette of the day and number of cigarettes smoked per day. *British Journal of Addiction, 84*(7), 791–799.

Heatherton, T. F., Kozlowski, L. T., Frecker, R. C., & Fagerstrom, K. O. (1991). The Fagerstrom test for nicotine dependence: A revision of the Fagerstrom tolerance questionnaire. *British Journal of Addiction, 86*(9), 1119–1127.

Houston, T. K., Scarinci, I. C., Person, S. D., & Greene, P. G. (2005). Patient smoking cessation advice by health care providers: The role of ethnicity, socioeconomic status, and health. *American Journal of Public Health, 95*(6), 1056–1061.

Kaplan, R. C., Bangdiwala, S. I., Barnhart, J. M., Castaneda, S. F., Gellman, M. D., Lee, D. J., … Giachello, A. L. (2014). Smoking among US Latino/Latino adults. The Latino Community Health Study/Study of Latinos. *American Journal of Preventive Medicine, 46(5)*, 496–506.

Kendzor, D. E., Businelle, M. S., Reitzel, L. R., Castro, Y., Vidrine, J. I., Mazas, C. A., … Wetter, D. W. (2014). The influence of discrimination on smoking cessation among Latinos. *Drug and Alcohol Dependence, 136*, 143–148.

Kisuule, F., Necocheax, A., Howe, E. E., & Wright, S. (2010). Utilizing audit and feedback to improve hospitalists' performance in tobacco dependence counseling. *Nicotine & Tobacco Research, 12*(8), 797–800.

Kiviniemi, M. T., Orom, H., & Giovino, G. A. (2011). Psychological distress and smoking behavior: The nature of the relation differs by race/ethnicity. *Nicotine & Tobacco Research, 13*(2), 113–119.

Kozlowski, L. T., & Edwards, B. Q. (2005). "Not safe" is not enough: Smokers have a right to know more than there is no safe tobacco product. *Tobacco Control, 14*(Suppl 2), ii3–ii7.
Kreuter, M. W., Chheda, S. G., & Bull, F. C. (2000). How does physician advice influence patient behavior? Evidence for a priming effect. *Archives of Family Medicine, 9*(5), 426–433.
Lariscy, J. T., Hummer, R. A., Rath, J. M., Villanti, A. C., Hayward, M. D., & Vallone, D. M. (2013). Race/ethnicity, nativity, and tobacco use among US young adults: Results from a nationally representative survey. *Nicotine & Tobacco Research, 15*(8), 1417–1426.
Lauterstein, D., Hoshino, R., Gordon, T., Watkins, B. X., Weitzman, M., & Zelikoff, J. (2014). The changing face of tobacco use among United States youth. *Current Drug Abuse Reviews, 7*(1), 29–43.
Levinson, A. H., Perez-Stable, E. J., Espinoza, P., Flores, E. T., & Byers, T. E. (2004). Latinos report less use of pharmaceutical aids when trying to quit smoking. *American Journal of Preventive Medicine, 26*(2), 105–111.
Lichtenstein, E., Zhu, S. H., & Tedeschi, G. J. (2010). Smoking cessation quitlines: An underrecognized intervention success story. *American Psychologist, 65*(4), 252–261.
Lindson-Hawley, N., Thompson, T. P., & Begh, R. (2015). Motivational interviewing for smoking cessation. *Cochrane Database System Review, (3)*, CD006936.
Lopez-Quintero, C., Crum, R. M., & Neumark, Y. D. (2006). Racial/ethnic disparities in report of physician-provided smoking cessation advice: Analysis of the 2000 National Health Interview Survey. *American Journal of Public Health, 96*(12), 2235–2239.
Lorenzo-Blanco, E. I., & Cortina, L. M. (2013a). Latino/a depression and smoking: An analysis through the lenses of culture, gender, and ethnicity. *American Journal of Community Psychology, 51*(3-4), 332–346.
Lorenzo-Blanco, E. I., & Cortina, L. M. (2013b). Towards an integrated understanding of Latino/a acculturation, depression, and smoking: A gendered analysis. *Journal of Latina/o Psychology, 1*(1), 3–20.
Maher, J. E., Rohde, K., Dent, C. W., Stark, M. J., Pizacani, B., Boysun, M. J., … Yepassis-Zembrou, P. L. (2007). Is a statewide tobacco quitline an appropriate service for specific populations? *Tobacco Control, 16*, I65–I70.
Marin, G., Marin, B. V., Perez-Stable, E. J., Sabogal, F., & Otero-Sabogal, R. (1990). Changes in information as a function of a culturally appropriate smoking cessation community intervention for Latinos. *American Journal of Community Psychology, 18*(6), 847–864.
McCullough, A., Fisher, M., Goldstein, A. O., Kramer, K. D., & Ripley-Moffitt, C. (2009). Smoking as a vital sign: Prompts to ask and assess increase cessation counseling. *Journal of the American Board of Family Medicine, 22*(6), 625–632.
Miller, W. R., & Rollnick, S. (2013). *Motivational interviewing: Helping people change* (3rd ed.). New York, NY: The Guilford Press.
Moolchan, E. T., Fagan, P., Fernander, A. F., Velicer, W. F., Hayward, M. D., King, G., & Clayton, R. R. (2007). Addressing tobacco-related health disparities. *Addiction, 102(Suppl 2)*, 30–42.
Muñoz, R. F., Barrera, A. Z., Delucchi, K., Penilla, C., Torres, L. D., Pérez-Stable, E. J. (2009). International Spanish/English Internet smoking cessation trial yields 20% abstinence rates at 1 year. *Nicotine & Tobacco Research, 11*(9), 1025–1034.
Munoz, R. F., Marin, B. V., Posner, S. F., & Perez-Stable, E. J. (1997). Mood management mail intervention increases abstinence rates for Spanish-speaking Latino smokers. *American Journal of Community Psychology, 25*(3), 325–343.
National Association of Social Workers. *Code of ethics of the National Association of Social Workers*. Retrieved August, 2015, from http://www.socialworkers.org/pubs/code/code.asp.
Nevid, J. S., & Javier, R. A. (1997). Preliminary investigation of a culturally specific smoking cessation intervention for Latino smokers. *American Journal of Health Promotion, 11*(3), 198–207.
Nguyen, K. H., Subramanian, S. V., Sorensen, G., Tsang, K., & Wright, R. J. (2012). Influence of experiences of racial discrimination and ethnic identity on prenatal smoking among urban black and Latino women. *Journal of Epidemiology and Community Health, 66*(4), 315–321.
Noonan, D., & Kulbok, P. A. (2009). New tobacco trends: Waterpipe (hookah) smoking and implications for healthcare providers. *Journal of the American Academy of Nurse Practitioners, 21*(5), 258–260.

Ortiz, A. P., Diaz-Toro, E. C., Calo, W. A., Correa-Fernandez, V., Cases, A., Santos-Ortiz, M. C., … Wetter, D. W. (2008). Characteristics of smokers accessing the Puerto Rico Quitline. *Puerto Rico Health Sciences Journal, 27(3)*, 213–219.

Perez-Stable, E. J., Marin, G., Marin, B. V., & Katz, M. H. (1990). Depressive symptoms and cigarette smoking among Latinos in San Francisco. *American Journal of Public Health, 80*(12), 1500–1502.

Pérez-Stable, E. J., Marín, G., & Posner, S. F. (1998). Ethnic comparison of attitudes and beliefs about cigarette smoking. *Journal of General Internal Medicine, 13*(3), 167–174.

Perez-Stable, E. J., Ramirez, A., Villareal, R., Talavera, G. A., Trapido, E., Suarez, L., … McAlister, A. (2001). Cigarette smoking behavior among US Latino men and women from different countries of origin. *American Journal of Public Health, 91*(*9*), 1424–1430.

Peterson, A., Vander Weg, M., & Jaen, C. (2010). *Nicotine and tobacco dependence*. Ashland, OH: Hogefre Publishing.

Piper, M. E., Piasecki, T. M., Federman, E. B., Bolt, D. M., Smith, S. S., Fiore, M. C., & Baker, T. B. (2004). A multiple motives approach to tobacco dependence: The Wisconsin Inventory of Smoking Dependence Motives (WISDM-68). *Journal of Consulting and Clinical Psychology, 72*(*2*), 139–154.

Piper, M. E., Schlam, T. R., Cook, J., Smith, S. S., Jorenby, D. E., Mermelstein, R. J., … Baker, T. B. (2014). *Identifying optimal smoking cessation intervention components for smoking cessation*. Paper presented at the 22nd Annual Meeting of the Society for Prevention Research (SPR), Washington, DC.

Reitzel, L. R., Costello, T. J., Mazas, C. A., Vidrine, J. I., Businelle, M. S., Kendzor, D. E., … Wetter, D. W. (2009). Low-level smoking among Spanish-speaking Latino smokers: Relationships with demographics, tobacco dependence, withdrawal, and cessation. *Nicotine & Tobacco Research, 11*(*2*), 178–184.

Richter, P. A., Pederson, L. L., & O'Hegarty, M. M. (2006). Young adult smoker risk perceptions of traditional cigarettes and nontraditional tobacco products. *American Journal of Health Behavior, 30*(3), 302–312.

Rodríguez-Esquivel, D., Cooper, T. V., Blow, J., & Resor, M. R. (2009). Characteristics associated with smoking in a Latino sample. *Addictive Behaviors, 34*(*6–7*), 593–598.

Rohsenow, D. J., Martin, R. A., Tidey, J. W., Monti, P. M., & Colby, S. M. (2013). Comparison of the Cigarette Dependence Scale with four other measures of nicotine involvement: Correlations with smoking history and smoking treatment outcome in smokers with substance use disorders. *Addictive Behaviors, 38*(8), 2409–2413.

Rollnick, S., Miller, W. R., & Butler, C. C. (2008). *Motivational interviewing in health care: Helping patients change behavior*. New York, NY: The Guilford Press.

Schwartz, S. J., Unger, J. B., Zamboanga, B. L., & Szapocznik, J. (2010). Rethinking the concept of acculturation implications for theory and research. *American Psychologist, 65*, 237–251.

Shadel, W. G., Edelen, M., & Tucker, J. S. (2011). A unified framework for smoking assessment: The PROMIS Smoking Initiative. *Nicotine & Tobacco Research, 13*(5), 399–400.

Smith, T. B., Rodríguez, M. D., & Bernal, G. (2011). Culture. *Journal of Clinical Psychology, 67*(2), 166–175.

Thorndike, A. N., Biener, L., & Rigotti, N. A. (2002). Effect on smoking cessation of switching nicotine replacement therapy to over-the-counter status. *American Journal of Public Health, 92*(3), 437–442.

Trinidad, D. R., Perez-Stable, E. J., Emery, S. L., White, M. M., Grana, R. A., & Messer, K. S. (2009). Intermittent and light daily smoking across racial/ethnic groups in the United States. *Nicotine & Tobacco Research, 11*(2), 203–210.

Trinidad, D. R., Perez-Stable, E. J., White, M. M., Emery, S. L., & Messer, K. (2011). A nationwide analysis of US racial/ethnic disparities in smoking behaviors, smoking cessation, and cessation-related factors. *American Journal of Public Health, 101*(4), 699–706.

Unger, J. B., Schwartz, S. J., Huh, J., Soto, D. W., & Baezconde-Garbanati, L. (2014). Acculturation and perceived discrimination: Predictors of substance use trajectories from adolescence to emerging adulthood among Latinos. *Addictive Behaviors, 39*(9), 1293–1296.

Ussher, M. H., Taylor, A. H., Faulkner, G. E. (2014). Exercise interventions for smoking cessation. *Cochrane Database Systematic Review, 29*(8), CD002295.

U.S. Department of Health and Human Services. (2014). The Health Consequences of Smoking: 50 Years of Progress. A Report of the Surgeon General. Atlanta, GA: U.S. Department of Health and Human Services, Centers for Disease Control and Prevention, Office on Smoking and Health.

Vidrine, J. I., Reitzel, L. R., Figueroa, P. Y., Velasquez, M. M., Mazas, C. A., Cinciripini, P. M., & Wetter, D. W. (2013). Motivation and Problem Solving (MAPS): Motivationally based skills training for treating substance use. *Cognitive and Behavioral Practice, 20*, 501–516.

Vidrine, J. I., Shete, S., Cao, Y., Greisinger, A., Harmonson, P., Sharp, B., … Wetter, D. W. (2013). Ask-advise-connect: A new approach to smoking treatment delivery in health care settings. *JAMA Internal Medicine, 173(6)*, 458–464.

Vidrine, J. I., Shete, S., Li, Y., Cao, Y., Alford, M. H., Galindo-Talton, M., … Wetter, D. W. (2013). The Ask-Advise-Connect approach for smokers in a safety net healthcare system: A group-randomized trial. *American Journal of Preventive Medicine, 45(6)*, 737–741.

Warren, G. W., Marshall, J. R., Cummings, K. M., Zevon, M. A., Reed, R., Hysert, P., … Reid, M. E. (2014). Automated tobacco assessment and cessation support for cancer patients. *Cancer, 120(4)*, 562–569.

Webb Hooper, M., & Kolar, S. K. (2015). Distress, race/ethnicity, and smoking cessation in treatment-seekers: Implications for disparity elimination. *Addiction, 110*, 1495.

Webb, M. S., Rodriguez-Esquivel, D., & Baker, E. A. (2010). Smoking cessation interventions among Latinos in the United States: A systematic review and mini meta-analysis. *American Journal of Health Promotion, 25*(2), 109–118.

West, R., Walia, A., Hyder, N., Shahab, L., & Michie, S. (2010). Behavior change techniques used by the English Stop Smoking Services and their associations with short-term quit outcomes. *Nicotine & Tobacco Research, 12*(7), 742–747.

Wetter, D. W., Mazas, C., Daza, P., Nguyen, L., Fouladi, R. T., Li, Y., & Cofta-Woerpel, L. (2007). Reaching and treating Spanish-speaking smokers through the National Cancer Institute's Cancer Information Service. A randomized controlled trial. *Cancer, 109(2 Suppl)*, 406–413.

Whitlock, E. P., Orleans, C. T., Pender, N., & Allan, J. (2002). Evaluating primary care behavioral counseling interventions: An evidence-based approach. *American Journal of Preventive Medicine, 22*(4), 267–284.

Wilkinson, A. V., Koehly, L. M., Vandewater, E. A., Yu, R. K., Fisher-Hoch, S. P., Prokhorov, A. V., … Shete, S. (2015). Demographic, psychosocial, and genetic risk associated with smokeless tobacco use among Mexican heritage youth. *BMC Medical Genetics, 16*, 43.

Wilkinson, A. V., Spitz, M. R., Strom, S. S., Prokhorov, A. V., Barcenas, C. H., Cao, Y., … Bondy, M. L. (2005). Effects of nativity, age at migration, and acculturation on smoking among adult Houston residents of Mexican descent. *American Journal of Public Health, 95(6)*, 1043–1049.

Williams, J. M., Steinberg, M. L., Griffiths, K. G., & Cooperman, N. (2013). Smokers with behavioral health comorbidity should be designated a tobacco use disparity group. *American Journal of Public Health, 103*(9), 1549–1555.

Woodruff, S. I., Talavera, G. A., & Elder, J. P. (2002). Evaluation of a culturally appropriate smoking cessation intervention for Latinos. *Tobacco Control, 11*(4), 361–367.

Zhu, S.-H., Pulvers, K., Zhuang, Y., & Baezconde-Garbanati, L. (2007). Most Latino smokers in California are low-frequency smokers. *Addiction, 102*(Suppl 2), 104–111.

Chapter 14
Chronic Disease Management and Integrated Care Among Hispanic Populations

Olga Cirlugea and Janice Ta

The most frequently chronic diseases encountered in integrated healthcare include diabetes, hypertension, heart disease, and cancer for both Hispanic and non-Hispanic populations (CDC, 2016a). These costly conditions are, in some cases, preventable (CDC, 2016a). Prevalence among Hispanics varies by disease. Some conditions (e.g., diabetes, heart disease) are more prevalent among Hispanics than their non-Hispanic counterparts while others (e.g., cancer, hypertension) occur at a lower prevalence among Hispanics (American Cancer Society, 2015a, 2015b; American Diabetes Association, 2014; American Heart Association, 2013). Regardless of prevalence, these chronic conditions have a significant impact on the quality of life of this population, with the first two leading causes of death among Hispanics being cancer and heart disease (CDC, 2016b). Additionally, research indicates that Hispanics with chronic care conditions are more likely to be diagnosed and begin treatment after the disease has progressed, less likely to engage with the treatment recommended, more likely to report more barriers to the self-management of their conditions, and to overall experience a poorer quality of life following diagnosis (e.g., American Cancer Society, 2015a, 2015b; CDC, 2013; Glasgow et al., 2006; Hall, Lee, Clark, & Perilla, 2016; Lloyd-Jones et al., 2010; McGruder, Malarcher, Antoine, Greenlund, & Croft, 2004; Nwasuruba, Osuagwu, Bae, Singh, & Egede, 2009; Wen, Shepherd, & Parchman, 2004).

Integrated behavioral health allows Behavioral Health Providers (BHPs) to work coordinate care with Primary Care Providers (PCPs) when patients present to them with behavioral problems (O'Donohue, Cummings, Cucciare, Runyan, & Cummings, 2005). For example, in the case of the diabetic patient who is not testing his or her blood sugars regularly and is also having difficulties eating a healthier

O. Cirlugea, M.A. (✉)
Department of Psychology, University of Nevada, Reno, NV 89557, USA
e-mail: olgacirlugea@gmail.com

J. Ta
Reno, NV 89519, USA

© Springer International Publishing Switzerland 2016

L.T. Benuto, W. O'Donohue (eds.), *Enhancing Behavioral Health in Latino Populations*, DOI 10.1007/978-3-319-42533-7_14

diet, a behavioral health provider can assess for barriers and co-occurring mental health problems and assist the medical team in forming a more comprehensive care plan. This makes integrated healthcare the ideal setting to begin to address barriers to and disparities in the care received by Hispanic patients. However, when discussing any research conducted with Hispanics or making any recommendations for working with this population, it is important to note that Hispanics in the United States are an incredibly heterogeneous group with regard to the location from which they migrated (whether Mexico, Puerto Rico, Cuba, or Central America), immigration status (e.g., undocumented, holding work visa, naturalized, etc.), acculturation status (immigrant, first generation, etc.) and other factors (Office of the Surgeon General, 2001). Additionally, there is relatively limited research on integrated care, and even more so when Hispanics are included. Randomly controlled trials, the gold standard of research, are few and far in between in this area with Hispanics and this, coupled with the diversity of the group, makes it very difficult to generalize any findings.

Thus, the aim of this chapter is to explore the most commonly diagnosed chronic conditions in Hispanics in integrated care, how these affect the Hispanic patient, and to illustrate how BHPs can work with the Primary Care Provider (PCPs) in order to improve the health of Hispanics living with chronic conditions while drawing from evidence-based guidelines, when available. BHPs can be introduced to Hispanic patients by PCPs through warm handoffs (essentially pulling the BHP into the consultation room at some point during the PCP visit) or referrals for co-located behavioral health for consultation. Once contact with behavioral health is made BHPs utilize a stepped-care model (O'Donohue & Draper, 2011) in order to address issues related to chronic conditions in the most efficient way, and thus employ a more patient-centered approach rather than a one-size-fits all intervention. This and the warm handoff are described below.

Warm Handoff

Warm handoff is the procedure by which primary care providers (PCPs) assist behavioral health providers (BHPs) in making contact with patients in real time (i.e. while at their PCP visit). This process promotes collaboration between behavioral health and primary care, and although research on warm handoffs in integrated care has only begun to be conducted, data from a quarterly report for an integrated care program at a local primary clinic in Reno, NV has revealed that both PCPs and patients have been satisfied with the BHPs and the services they provide. Warm handoffs have been used in integrated healthcare to increase the likelihood that a patient will follow through with a referral to behavioral health. Not only can a BHP reduce the stigma of mental health for the Hispanic patient by normalizing reactions to life events, such as stress, and by using nonstigmatizing language (e.g., behavioral health versus mental health), the BHP can also being an intervening with the patient during the warm handoff in order to begin symptom reduction as soon as possible and ensure that the patient will return for a follow-up visit. Ideally BHPs would be bilingual and thus better able to communicate with Hispanic patients in their preferred language. However, in the case of English-speaking BHPs, a translation line may be used.

When PCPs determine that a patient could benefit from behavioral health services, they first discuss this with the patient and after obtaining the patient's consent, provide the BHP with a quick description of the case and referral question. Primary care providers are generally interested in one of the following: (a) Are the patient's medical problems being exacerbated by a mental health concern (e.g., is the patient's hypertension being exacerbated by difficult life events for which the patient has limited coping skills; is the patient's heart disease worsened by alcohol/drug/nicotine use?); (b) Why is the patient not adhering to his or her medication/exercise/dietary regiment and how can adherence be increased? (c) What is the patient's level of need for mental/behavioral health services and would the patient benefit from several sessions with a BHP or is a referral to specialty care warranted? The BHP then introduces him or herself to the patient and explains his or her role. Depending on the referral question, the BHE will first conduct a brief assessment of the patient's symptoms or problems and begin to formulate a hypothesis about what may be maintaining these and develop a plan for how to intervene with the patient. The BHP goes on to communicate his or her findings to the PCP, and how he or she plans to address the problems identified. One way to address problems in integrated healthcare is through a stepped-care approach, described below.

The warm handoff process described above does not require any tailoring for the Hispanic patient beyond making sure that contact with the patient occurs in his or her preferred language and should this be Spanish, that either a bilingual BHP or translation line is used. Whether specific elements of the encounter (for example, addressing the nonadherence to dietary and exercise plan) need cultural adaptations will be discussed as they arise in the context of each chronic condition.

Stepped Care

Stepped care refers to providing patients with interventions ranging from the least intrusive to the most, based on the individual patient's level of need (O'Donohue & Draper, 2011). Not all patients require individual weekly psychotherapy. This is a costly and time intensive treatment modality that is not necessary for every problem encountered in integrated care. Instead, some patients may just need information for their problem, e.g., education about nutritious foods like whole grains, while others may need one or several MI sessions to increase motivation to change and overcome barriers. Some patients may have co-occurring anxiety or depression that can be quickly address with brief CBT in several 30-min sessions or via a self-help book, yet others may have a history of chronic depression that warrants a referral to specialty care. The idea is that many patients can benefit from lower levels of intervention and it isn't until they "fail" at that level (i.e., do not show treatment response) that more intensive treatment ought to be provided. BHPs working with Hispanic patients within a stepped care model must first ensure that language barriers are taken care of, either using bilingual BHPs or a translation line. Many of the stepped care interventions (e.g., bibliotherapy, psychoeducation) are available in Spanish (for example, Choosemyplate.gov, a website with diet and exercise advice, has handouts in both English and Spanish). Others, for example self-help websites, do not. While some of the interventions themselves may not need specific cultural adaptation for Hispanic clients, BHPs must be aware that certain resources are not available to a monolingual Hispanic patient. Stepped care interventions are as follows (adapted from O'Donohue & Draper, 2011):

Watchful Waiting. Watchful waiting may be employed for mild cases that do not include suicidal ideation/severe mental illness and where the patient is willing to wait for several weeks to see if symptoms improve on their own.

Psychoeducation. The BHP provides information via pamphlets and handouts to the patient about any diagnoses assigned, treatments for those diagnoses, lifestyle changes, etc., for example, the Choosemyplate.gov handouts for healthy eating or American Lung Association for quitting smoking. A challenge that may arise when working with Hispanic patients is finding Psychoeducation resources in Spanish. While some major organizations (e.g. National Institute of Health, Mayo Clinic) have printable handouts in both English and Spanish, others do not.

Bibliotherapy. Bibliotherapy refers to self-help books that BHPs may hand out to their patients. There are books that have been demonstrated to be effective in reducing psychological distress (e.g., David Burns' *Feeling Good*). This treatment modality is relatively cheap (or even free if the BHP has extra copies of a book) and the patient can go through the treatment on his or her own time. Some, although not all, self-help books have Spanish translations.

E-Health. E-Health utilizes the Internet to deliver interventions via websites that combine psychoeducation, treatment, and even feedback/help from a therapist. Like bibliotherapy, E-Health is relatively cheap, or free in certain cases. However, few websites have Spanish-speaking versions. Large healthcare systems such as the Mayo Clinic and National Institute for Health have both English- and Spanish-speaking pages, while others resources (such as the self-help website MoodGym for depression) do not. This is problematic when working with Hispanic patients whose English proficiency is limited.

Group Therapy. Cheaper than individual therapy, group therapy is more efficient as more patients can be seen at one time, for example in healthy living groups that combines a walking component with psychoeducation or a substance abuse group. Group therapy has often been showed to be just as effective as individual therapy.

Individual Outpatient. This treatment modality is the most widely used one in psychology and although useful, it is not always feasible or necessary. Additionally, when working with Hispanic patient, a BHP may find that resources are limited for psychotherapy services provided in Spanish.

Medication. Although medication is a more intensive step in the stepped-care model, it is generally the first line of intervention in a primary care clinic. Thus, it is likely that many Hispanic patients will come to their BHP appointment after having already been prescribed psychotropic medication such as antianxiety or antidepressant medication.

Inpatient Therapy. The most intensive treatment modality, inpatient therapy is recommended when patients demonstrate severe life threatening behaviors (e.g., self harm, suicidal ideation with a plan/intent, etc.).

In regards to working with Hispanic patients, this stepped-care model may actually increase the likelihood that patients will get the care they need, thus beginning to reduce the disparities in access to healthcare. Spanish-speaking psychologists are hard to come by, even in a city where about 25 % of the population identifies itself as Hispanic (United States Census Bureau, 2015). In the United States, only 1 % of licensed psychologists identify themselves as Hispanic, and there are only 29 Hispanic mental health professionals for every 100,000 Hispanics compared to 174 Caucasians per 100,000 (Center for Mental Health Services, 2001; Williams & Kohout, 1999). Further, many problems related to living with chronic conditions can be addressed in a faster and cheaper manner that doesn't require a specialty referral. Thus, having Hispanic patients come into contact with behavioral health via warm handoffs or a referral for consultation can improve the quality of life of this underserved population, provided that language barriers are addressed via bilingual BHP or the use of a translation line. A discussion of major chronic conditions with which Hispanic patients present in integrated care, as well as how the BHP can work with the PCP to address these, follows.

Diabetes Mellitus

Diabetes Mellitus is a collection of diseases that affect the way the body processes blood sugar, or glucose. Diabetes indicates that there is too much glucose in the blood as a result of too little insulin (whether due to the body not making enough or not being able to use it adequately). Type 1 diabetes is generally developed during childhood or adolescence (although not always) and is the result of the body no longer making enough insulin. Type 2 diabetes is diagnosed in 90–95 % of patients with diabetes (NIH, 2014) and is more common in individuals over 40 who are overweight although the condition can develop at any age. Although the cause of Type 2 diabetes haven't been clearly established, risk factors have been identified including a sedentary lifestyle, high blood pressure, high cholesterol, heart disease, race, a history of gestational diabetes and having a close relative who has been diagnosed with diabetes (Mayo Clinic, 2016a). Other types of diabetic include prediabetes (a condition in which blood glucose levels are higher than normal but not high enough to be considered diabetes) and gestational diabetes (diabetes developed during the pregnancy, usually around 24 weeks) (American Diabetes Association, 2016). In the United States 29.1 million individuals (9.3 %) had diabetes in 2012

(American Diabetes Association, 2014). However, race is a risk factor for diabetes, with Hispanics (and other minorities such as African Americans) being at higher risk of developing diabetes; thus 12.8 % of Hispanics are living with diabetes, compared to 7.6 % of non-Hispanic whites (American Diabetes Association, 2014).

Prior to an individual being diagnosed with diabetes, he or she may present to his or her primary care provider with prediabetes, which refers to when a patient has higher than normal glucose levels (i.e., an A1C of 5.7–6.4 %, fasting blood glucose of 100–125 mg/dl, or an OGTT 2 h blood glucose of 140–199 mg/dl) but not high enough to be considered diabetes (American Diabetes Association, 2016). Although many patients with prediabetes will go on to develop diabetes, there are several steps that an individual can take in order to avoid or delay having the prediabetes turn into diabetes, and primary care providers will generally advise prediabetic patients decrease their body weight by eating more healthy, decreasing overall food consumption, and increasing exercise. Additionally, yearly blood glucose level checks are recommended.

In some cases, patients will present to their doctor after they have already developed diabetes and are experiencing diabetic symptoms. Symptoms of both type 1 and type 2 diabetes include frequent urination, blurred vision, increased thirst and hunger, ketones in the urine, irritability, and frequent infections (e.g., skin or vaginal infections) although individuals with type 2 diabetes may not experience any symptoms initially. Thus, ADA guidelines recommend that anyone with a body mass index (BMI) of 25 or over with additional risk factors and/or over 45 years of age be screened for diabetes (American Diabetes Association, 2016). Because Hispanics are more likely to be overweight or obese and thus have a higher BMI (NHCSL, 2010), PCPs should pay particular attention to Hispanic patients in order to ensure that they are screened for diabetes.

Diabetes Screening

Several tests are widely used in the screening of diabetes and subsequent monitoring of management of the disorder. These included the A1C, fasting plasma glucose test, oral glucose tolerance test, and random plasma glucose test. All tests are performed in the primary care clinic and vary in their method of administration, cost and ease of administration, whether fasting is required, and so on.

A1C. The A1C test, also referred to as glycated hemoglobin, glycosylated hemoglobin, hemoglobin A1C, and HbA1c, measures average blood glucose (i.e., sugar) levels for the past 2–3 months, and an A1C greater than or equal to 6.5 % is indicative of diabetes (American Diabetes Association, 2016). Blood glucose levels refer specifically to what percentage of one's hemoglobin is coated with sugar. This test is used both for diabetes detection and monitoring of the treatment plan and varies in how often it is used based on the condition and management of the disease (e.g., once a year for prediabetics, twice a year for type 2 diabetics whose disease is under control, etc.) (Mayo Clinic, 2016b). One of the benefits of using this test is that the patient does not need to fast or drink anything prior to its administration.

Fasting Plasma Glucose Test. The fasting plasma glucose test checks fasting blood glucose levels, i.e. blood glucose levels after an individual has not have had anything to eat or drink (except water) for at least 8 h of test administration, and thus the test is generally administered first thing in the morning before breakfast (American Diabetes Association, 2016). A fasting blood glucose level greater than or equal to 126 mg/dl is indicative of diabetes. This test is the most commonly used one in the diagnosis of diabetes because of convince and cost over the next test described, the Oral Glucose Tolerance Test (NIH, 2014).

Oral Glucose Tolerance Test. The OGTT checks blood glucose levels before and 2 h after the patient drinks a syrupy glucose solution. This test measures the body's response to sugar and a 2-h blood glucose of greater than or equal to 200 mg/dl is representative of diabetes (American Diabetes Association, 2016). Just like with the fasting plasma test, patients have to fast for at least 8 h before the test administration. Because many factors may affect the accuracy of this test, including illness and certain medications, the test may be repeated at a later date in order to ensure reliability of the results (Mayo Clinic, 2016c, 2016d).

Random Plasma Glucose Test. Random Plasma Glucose Test (or casual plasma glucose test) is a simple blood sugar test that can be used at any time of the day. Fasting is not required, and diabetes is diagnosed at blood glucose of greater than or equal to 200 mg/dl (American Diabetes Association, 2016). This test is generally administered when patients experience diabetes symptoms.

Other Tests. In addition to the tests described above, primary care providers frequently perform other tests including dilated eye exams and foot tests in diabetics. Dilated eye exams check for diabetic retinopathy while foot tests evaluate for diabetic neuropathy, both diabetic complications that result in damage to nerves and blood vessels through prolonged exposure to high blood sugar. Additionally, PCPs recommend regular checking of blood glucose levels using a glucose-monitoring meter with test strips as part of the self-management of diabetes.

There is no evidence that the tests mentioned about would need any cultural adaptation to better fit the Hispanic patient given that all these tests measure some sort of physiological function that is similar across ethnicities. PCPs only need to be aware that language barriers may play a role in the Hispanic patient's understanding of what the tests are used for, what requirements exist (e.g., fasting), and what results mean in order to ensure that the patient has comprehended the purpose of the test and its implications.

Diabetes Management and the Hispanic Patient

Overall, research indicates that Hispanics with type 2 diabetes are less likely to adequately self-manage their disease when compared to non-Hispanic whites; specifically, 36.8 % of Hispanics versus 60 % of non-Hispanic whites have their A1C under control, and Hispanics are 2 times less likely to engage in the recommended exercises and to meet dietary guidelines, 36 % less likely than non-Hispanic whites to self-monitor blood glucose levels (e.g., Agency for Healthcare Research and Quality, 2011; AHRQ AfHRaQ, 2009; Glasgow et al., 2006; McGruder et al., 2004; Nwasuruba et al., 2009; Wen et al., 2004). Additionally, approximately three-fourths of Hispanics are either overweight or obese (NHCLS, 2010).

Studies of diabetes self-management have shown that this population has identified several factors including low income and education, low acculturation, language barriers, low social support, differing beliefs and values, and comorbidities with other conditions as barriers to adequate management of their diabetes (e.g., Ghaddar, Brown, Pagán, & Díaz, 2010; González, Vega, Rodríguez, Tarraf, & Sribney, 2009; Mainous, Diaz, & Geesey, 2008; McCloskey & Flenniken, 2010; Weiler & Crist, 2009). Hispanics are more likely to be living in poverty, to have poor access to healthcare, to not have health insurance and to not be able to afford medications than their non-Hispanic white counterparts (e.g., Bailey et al., 2012; Benavides-Vaello, Garcia, Brown, & Winchell, 2004; DeNavas-Walt, Proctor, & Smith, 2011; Lopez-Class & Jurkowski, 2010). Additionally, Hispanics are more likely to encounter language barriers such as misunderstanding of directions and miscommunication, (i.e., due to limited or no English proficiency), to have low literacy that contributes to low knowledge of diabetes management, and less likely to receive information on dietary needs and exercise (e.g., Agency for Healthcare Research and Quality, 2011; Chilton, Hu, & Wallace, 2006; González et al., 2009; Lopez-Quintero, Berry, & Neumark, 2009; Mainous, Diaz, Saxena, & Geesey, 2007; Rosal, Goins, Carbone, & Cortes, 2004). Further, family support plays an integral role in the diabetes management of Hispanic patients and a lack of such support/certain beliefs and values may interfere with effective self management (Hu, Amirehsani, Wallace, & Letvak, 2013). Cultural values that place the need of the family above that of the individual dictate that the Hispanic patient must to attend to the needs of his or her family first, and even more so for Hispanic females, who encounter greater challenges when trying to make lifestyle changes while also keeping the other family members happy (Clark, Vincent, Zimmer, & Sanchez, 2009; John, Resendiz, & De Vargas, 1997). Lastly, Hispanic foods such as rice and beans, tortillas, and soda tend to generally be higher in fat, carbohydrates, and total calories, and lower in nutrients and thus Hispanics with diabetes are less likely to meet recommended dietary guidelines (Glasgow et al., 2006; Wen et al., 2004). Further, societal pressures may exist for Hispanic patients to continue to consume those items (Caban, Walker, Sanchez, & Mera, 2008; Weiler & Crist, 2009).

In order to assist Hispanics to overcome barriers to diabetes self-management and increase their quality of life, a behavioral health referral can help increase Hispanic patients' management of their chronic condition in addition to referring prediabetic or diabetic patients to a registered dietitian and endocrinologist. The clinical training obtained by behavioral health providers lends itself to resolving many of the problems related to diabetes in integrated healthcare. Primary care providers may refer patients for nonadherence to medication treatment, nonadherence to diet and exercise regimen, comorbid mental disorder, or a combination of the three.

Nonadherence to Testing/Medication Regimen. Eighteen percent of Hispanic patients with diabetes have never tested their blood sugar and 32 % have not had an A1C test done in the past 12 months (Nwasuruba et al., 2009). Further, Hispanics are less likely to take insulin or oral medications such as Metformin (Thackeray, Merrill, & Neiger, 2004). The BHP can assist in first determining what is getting in the way of the Hispanic patient fully adhering to the medication treatment (e.g., (a) is it a lack of education or misunderstanding that has resulted in the patient not knowing how often he or she is supposed to test blood sugar levels and/or take the medication; (b) is it a matter of motivation that has resulted in the patient only monitoring levels sometimes or only taking medications when symptoms increase; (c) is it a matter of financial difficulties that has resulted in the patient not being able to afford testing materials/medications; or (d) is it something else entirely, such as a fear of needles), then work to increase adherence. BHPs can increase consumer literacy by providing psychoeducation, either verbally or via handouts, to Hispanic diabetic patients. The National Institute of Health (https://www.nlm.nih.gov/medlineplus/spanish/ency/article/001214.htm) and Mayo Clinic (http://www.mayoclinic.org/espanol/enfermedades-y-tratamientos/diabetes) both provide health literacy resources in Spanish for diabetes. BHPs can also use Motivational Interviewing (MI; Miller, 1983) to increase motivation and elicit behavior change in a nonjudgmental, patient-centered manner. During MI the behavioral health provider asks open-ended questions and utilizes other therapeutic techniques including asking permission, reflective listening, normalizing, affirmations, and eliciting/evoking change talk in order to resolve any ambivalence the patient may have. This style is very different from what patients may be used to in primary care (e.g., a more directive "This is what you need to do and why" approach) and has been shown to increase adherence to medication regiment in Hispanic diabetic patients (e.g., Dellasega, Añel-Tiangco, & Gabbay, 2012). Additionally, a brief cultural adaptation of MI (Osborn et al., 2010) was shown to be effective in decreasing A1C values in Puerto Ricans with Type 2 Diabetes.

Nonadherence to Diet and Exercise Regimen. Because Hispanics consume foods that are high in carbohydrates and fat and low in other nutrients, for example tortillas, rice and beans, meat, soda and juice, many living with diabetes do not meet recommended dietary guidelines (Glasgow et al., 2006; Wen et al., 2004). However, what specifically constitutes a healthy Hispanic diet has not been clearly defined. The *2015–2020 Dietary Guidelines for Americans* released by the Office of Disease Prevention and Health fail to take culture into consideration, instead taking a "one size fits all" approach to dietary guidelines (ODPHP, 2016). Some organizations such as the Dairy Council of California published guidelines tailored for Hispanics, including cooking with low fat dairy products (Heller, 2006). However, there is no evidence that these guidelines are supported by the literature and that suggestions made (e.g., emphasizing dairy products in a diet) would actually be healthy. The importance of food in the Hispanic culture cannot be understated, and the impact of a diabetes diagnosis on not just the patient, but also his or her own family, should not be minimized. Hispanic patients may encounter difficulties in not being able to enjoy the meals with family members or in having to eat different meals from the rest of the family as mealtime an important event in the Hispanic patients' daily lives.

Even though some could argue that the occupations generally taken by Hispanics (e.g., construction, leisure, and hospitality—i.e., housekeeping; Buerau of Labor Statistics, 2015) are more physically demanding, Hispanics are overall less likely than their Caucasian counterparts to get the exercise they need, with studies showing that as many as 67.6% of Hispanics do not get the recommended 150 min of weekly activity (Bautista, Reininger, Gay, Barroso, & McCormick, 2011). Thus, even if Hispanics who are employed are more active while at work, they overall do not get sufficient exercise and this is supported by evidence that Hispanics are more overweight than their Caucasian counterparts (CDC, 2009). Once again, behavioral health providers can assist in identifying the barriers to engaging in dietary and exercise regimen recommended by their primary care physicians, whether these are related to literacy (e.g., lack of understanding what appropriate foods are for a diabetic, what should be avoided, how much to exercise), motivation, lack of familial support, or some other factor. A randomized control trial conducted by Rosal and colleagues (2011) evaluated the effects of a group-based intervention consisting of 12 weekly and 8 monthly sessions on the knowledge, attitudes, and self-management behaviors of low income Hispanics with Type 2 diabetes and found that the intervention group had significantly HbA_1 levels and increased knowledge about diabetes. Interestingly, the authors tailored the intervention to the participants' culture by using educational soap operas, bingo games, addressing family preferences, and emphasizing making traditional foods healthier. Additionally, a prospective randomized study found that Hispanic patients newly diagnosed with Type 2 Diabetes receiving services from trained community health workers had better health status and improved dietary habits, physical activity, and medication adherence and lower emergency department utilizations than controls (Babamoto et al., 2009).

BHPs can also use MI to increase motivation to make diet and activity level changes and assist Hispanic patients in establishing concrete goals for their diabetes management (e.g., lower A1C levels from 9.4 to the 8 range) and breaking those down into smaller, more manageable steps (e.g., walk 30 min per day 5 days per week, reduce soda consumption from 3 to 1 per week, swap white rice for brown). BHPs may also enlist the help of family members in addressing the diabetes nonadherence. This could be an important step in overcoming some of the barriers to as enlisting family support and involvement in the patient's diabetes management provides the family with opportunities to learn about diabetes and its treatment (Hu et al., 2013). Additionally, getting the whole family on board with the lifestyle changes required to promote good diabetes self-management could be integral in eliciting the social support needed for the Hispanic patient to effectively make the necessary changes (e.g., if the whole family adopts a new, healthy diet and the Hispanic patient now feels included in meals).

Co-occurring Mental Disorders. BHPs can provide therapeutic interventions/make appropriate referrals for any mental disorders co-occurring with and exacerbating the diabetes. For example, patients who have a difficult time controlling their eating habits and who report eating to manage negative emotions may be taught alternative ways of coping with negative emotions (e.g., through distress tolerance skills), or to reduce stress (e.g., via mindfulness training). One quasi-experiment was found that evaluated the effects of collaborative depression care in Hispanic diabetic patients and have found that patients receiving collaborative depression (i.e., protocol-driven depression care by providers of a disease management program) care had overall lower depression scores, improved depression remission, reduced functional impairment, and fewer patients met criteria for moderate or severe depression, than those receiving usual care in which PCPs translated and employed evidence-based depression care (B. Wu et al., 2014). Additionally, a study is currently underway evaluating the effects of technology-facilitated (i.e., E-health) depression care management in a predominantly Hispanic sample receiving services at eight county-operated clinics in Los Angeles (S. Wu et al., 2014).

Heart Disease

Heart disease encompasses a variety of conditions that could negatively impact the person's coronary system. Types of heart disease include coronary artery disease, blood vessel diseases, or heart defects that appear when the individual is born (congenital heart defects) (Mayo Clinic, 2016e). Hispanics have a higher risks compared to non-Hispanic whites in regards to cardiovascular diseases (American Heart Association, 2016). Of Hispanic adults who are 20 years or older, 30.7 % of females and 33.4 % of males suffer from cardiovascular disease, while 6.7 % of Hispanic males 20 or older 5.3 % of Hispanic females suffer from coronary heart disease (American Heart Association, 2013). Causes for a heart disease could vary depending on the disease.

Various risks for heart disease have been identified. As an individual ages, the risk for heart disease increases from damaged/narrow arteries and potentially weakened/thickened heart muscle (Mayo Clinic, 2016f). Gender is also a risk factor, with men having at a higher risk for heart disease in general but women having an increase in risk after menopause (Mayo Clinic, 2016f). A genetic predisposition is also a risk, especially if a good portion of the person's family has had an onset of a heart disease early in life (before 55 for males, and before 65 for women) (Mayo Clinic, 2016f). Other risk factors include having a poor diet (e.g. extremely high cholesterol, sugar, salt, fat), lack of physical activity, hypertension (high blood pressure), high cholesterol levels, diabetes, stress, and even poor hygiene (Mayo Clinic, 2016f). Hispanics who are at a higher risk for cardiovascular diseases tend to have risk factors including high blood pressure, diabetes, and/or obesity (American Heart Association, 2016).

Diagnostic Screening

PCPs are generally first alerted to the possibility of heart disease when patients present with chest pain. A number of tests are used to screen for and diagnose heart disease in integrated care. These vary on method of administration, specific indicator utilized (e.g., blood flow, heart beats), etc. based on the condition of interest.

Cardiac Catheterization. The process of the cardiac catheterization is a sheath (short tube) being inserted in a patient's vein in order to guide a catheter (a tiny hollow tube) and view the regulations of the heart (Mayo Clinic, 2016g). This procedure measures the heart's pressure, and injected dye can be utilized to help view blood flow on an X-ray (Mayo Clinic, 2016g).

Cardiac Computerized Tomography (CT) Scan. A CT scan is a type of X-ray that yields a very detailed image of organs and tissues of the patient (Mayo Clinic, 2016g). This kind of scan provides a detailed image of the heart and chest to detect any abnormalities.

Cardiac Magnetic Resonance Imaging (MRI). MRI scans refer to cross-sectional scans using magnetic fields that provide detailed imagery of the patient's heart in order for the doctor to examine the condition of the heart (Mayo Clinic, 2016g).

Echocardiogram. This kind of diagnostic tests involves a ultrasound on the patient's chest and can provide images of the heart and its functioning (Mayo Clinic, 2016g).

Electrocardiogram (ECG). The electrocardiogram has the capability to read electrical signals of the heart. The doctor will be able to notice any irregular rhythms of the heart and/or its structure (Mayo Clinic, 2016g).

Holter Monitoring. Holter monitoring refers to a portable device that records a consistent ECG that ranging from 24 to 72 h (Mayo Clinic, 2016g). This sampling allows doctors to notice abnormal heart rhythms that may not appear on regular ECG exams (Mayo Clinic, 2016g).

Stress Test. A stress test can help doctors diagnose coronary heart disease (CHD) as well as detect the abnormality in blood pressure or heart rate, symptoms, and abnormality in the rhythm of the heart or electrical activity (Department of Health and Human Services, 2016). Patients undergoing stress tests engage in exercises such as walking/running on treadmills or possibly using a stationary bike to make the heart work harder during physical stress (Department of Health and Human Services, 2016). The physical stress on the heart helps doctors assign a more definite diagnosis.

There is no research to indicate that tests that used to screen for heart disease need cultural adaptation for Hispanic patients other than making sure that language barriers are addressed.

Heart Disease Management and the Hispanic Patient

Many of the common causes and risk factors for heart disease, including high blood pressure, diabetes, smoking, excessive use of alcohol or caffeine, drug abuse and stress, can be managed by BHPs in integrated healthcare. This may be particularly important for Hispanic patients, who are more likely to have some form of heart disease but less likely than their Caucasian counterparts to receive adequate treatment and to effectively self manage the condition (CDC, 2013). Thus, the BHP may be enlisted by the PCP to assist with one or more of the following:

Nonadherence to Medication Treatment. As noted in the section on diabetes self-management, some patients may be referred to behavioral health providers for not taking their medications as prescribed. BHPS can work to identify barriers to adhering to the medication treatment (e.g., poor health literacy, low motivation). The National Institute of Health (http://www.nhlbi.nih.gov/health/educational/hearttruth/espanol/index.htm) provides health literacy resources in Spanish for heart disease.

Smoking. Although Hispanics report smoking at lower rates than their Caucasian counterparts (11.2 % versus 18.2 %; CDC, 2015), when they present to primary care they are less likely to be screened for smoking, to receive advice about quitting smoking, and to use nicotine replacement therapy as a smoking cessation aid (Fiore et al., 2008; Houston, Scarinci, Person, & Greene, 2005; Jamal et al., 2012; Levinson, Pérez-Stable, Espinoza, Flores, & Byers, 2004). This is problematic because smoking can significantly negatively impact heart disease (i.e., by making blood vessels more vulnerable to atherosclerosis, or plaque buildup, which in turns increases the risks of heart attacks and stroke). Behavioral health providers can assist in screening Hispanic patients with heart disease who also smoke and providing smoking cessation counseling. Motivational interviewing has been successfully used as an intervention for smoking and although no studies have specifically evaluated MI with Hispanic smokers, Hispanics have been included in efficacy and effectiveness studies of MI (for a review, see Hettema & Hendricks, 2010).

Drug and Alcohol Use. Drugs from all classes (e.g., stimulants, amphetamines, barbituates, hallucinogens) have been linked to cardiovascular problems such as abnormal heart rate, heart attacks, collapsed veins, and bacterial infections of heart valves (National Institute on Drug Abuse, 2012). Hispanics are less likely than Caucasians to use drugs and alcohol, although research has shown that acculturation negatively impacts these rates, with Hispanics born in the United States being more likely to use drugs and alcohol than their immigrant counterparts (Escarce, Morales, & Rumbaut, 2006). Behavioral health providers can assist in the detection, treatment, and/or referral to specialty care of Hispanic patients with heart disease who also use substances and/or alcohol. Motivational interviewing has been shown to reduce alcohol consumption in heavy-drinker Hispanic males, and significant decrease in consumption was found for both a culturally adapted and nonadapted MI, although effects were stronger for the culturally adapted MI (Lee et al., 2013).

Diabetes. As previously mentioned, Hispanics have higher rates of diabetes (American Diabetes Association, 2014). Further, diabetes may increase an individual's risk of heart diseases. Please refer to the section on diabetes for more information on how behavioral health providers can assist in the management of diabetes.

Poor Diet and Physical Inactivity. A diet high in fat, salt, sugar, and cholesterol combined with low or no physical activity is associated with many forms of heart disease. Research has shown that Hispanic diets tend to be higher in fat and calories, and that Hispanics tend to engage in less activity than their Caucasian counterparts (Glasgow et al., 2006; Wen et al., 2004). Behavioral health providers can work with Hispanic patients to make positive lifestyle changes that include eating healthier foods and increasing activity levels. This may be achieved by providing psychoeducation about healthy eating and exercise, utilizing MI to increase motivation for change, etc.

Obesity. Related to some of the other risk factors discussed (e.g., poor diet and physical inactivity, diabetes), being overweight or obese also increases the risk of developing heart disease and Hispanics are more likely than non-Hispanic whites to be overweight (CDC, 2016b). For a discussion of managing obesity with Hispanic patients in integrated healthcare, please refer to Ch. X.

Stress. Primary care providers often refer patients with heart disease who also report having other stressors in their lives (e.g., marriage issues, financial difficulties, etc.). Stress that is poorly managed may damage the arteries and increase other risk factors for heart disease. Some research has found that chronic stress is associated with higher cardiovascular risk and prevalence in Hispanics (Gallo et al., 2014). Research has identified stressors unique to Hispanics including stress from immigration and acculturation, low socioeconomic status, and neighborhood stress (i.e., living in a neighborhood with poor-quality housing and unsafe conditions) (National Research Council, 2006; Ornelas & Perreira, 2011). Behavioral health providers can teach Hispanic patients various stress management techniques or utilize problem solving to help them navigate through stressful situations as well as help connect patients to resources. For example, behavioral health providers can provide rationale for, demonstrate, and practice muscle relaxation and deep breathing with the Hispanic patient in order to help him or her reduce stress. Behavioral health providers can also address stressors, for example by bringing in the significant other or referring patients to marital counseling for marital discord. Accurate diagnosing is integral in providing appropriate treatment for the stressors identified. For example, if the Hispanic patient reports she has been experiencing stress after being the victim of sexual assault, whether the symptoms experienced meet criteria for PTSD should be evaluated as prolonged exposure for PTSD (Foa, Hembree, & Rothbaum, 2007) rather than a stress management technique such as muscle relaxation, is the gold standard for the treatment of trauma symptoms.

Depression. Like stress, depression can increase the risk of heart disease significantly. Hispanics report a slightly lower 12-month prevalence rate of depression than their non-Hispanic white counterparts (5.4% versus 7.1%; NIMH, 2014).

However, they are less likely to seek out specialty care services, and less likely overall to receive treatment for their depression (Lewis-Fernández, Das, Alfonso, Weissman, & Olfson, 2005). Behavioral health providers can work to detect and treat/make appropriate referrals for depression. For a discussion of treating depression in Hispanic patients in integrated healthcare, please refer to Ch. Y.

Hypertension

Hypertension refers to a person's high blood pressure, which tends to be a common potential precursor to various health issues. A person's blood pressure considers the factors of how much blood is pumped by the heart and how much resistance in the arteries during blood flow (Mayo Clinic, 2016h). Hypertension will not always exhibit symptoms, but this condition can still affect a person's health by causing damage to the heart. Hispanic adolescents have a greater prevalence of high blood pressure and pre-high blood pressure compared to non-Hispanic whites, and these include both males and females (American Heart Association, 2013). Control of hypertension is also problematic as only of 39.3 % of Hispanics have been found to have their condition under control to 54.9 % of non-Hispanic whites (American Heart Association, 2013).

The condition may either be diagnosed as primary/essential hypertension or secondary hypertension. Primary hypertension refers to the trend of gradual development of high blood pressure that has no identifiable cause (Mayo Clinic, 2016i). Secondary hypertension identifies underlying conditions in the individual and tends to develop more drastically and suddenly (Mayo Clinic, 2016i). Some conditions that could influence the development of secondary hypertension include kidney problems, alcohol abuse, and certain medications (Mayo Clinic, 2016i).

Diagnostic Tests

Blood pressure is generally taken as a part of any primary care appointment. Guidelines for having blood pressure monitored includes having blood pressure taken every 2 years after 18, every year if the patient is ages 19–39 with a high risk of the condition, and more frequently if already diagnosed with it.

Sphygmomanometer. Sphygmomanometers are the devices with the arm cuffs that can be inflated with air. This device has the capability to measure the patient's blood pressure when looking at the pressure-measure gauge attached. Blood pressure is measured in millimeters of mercury (mm Hg) (Mayo Clinic, 2016j). Two measures when recording blood pressure is the individual's pressure in arteries in the moment of a heart beating (systolic pressure) and the diastolic pressure which is the pressure within the arteries between the heart beats (Mayo Clinic, 2016j).

Normal blood pressure. Normal blood pressure for someone less than 60 years old would be if the systolic pressure is less than 140 mmHg and/or the diastolic is less than 90 mmHg. For someone who is 60 years old or older, normal blood pressure should have the systolic pressure less than 150 mmHg, and/or the diastolic pressure less than 90 mmHg.

High blood pressure. High blood pressure for someone who is less than 60 years old would be if the systolic is greater than 150 mmHg and/or the diastolic pressure is greater than 90 mmHg. For someone who is 60 years old or older, high blood pressure is when the systolic is greater than 150 mmHg and/or the diastolic is greater than 90 mmHg.

There is no evidence that any cultural adaptations are needed when taking the blood pressure of Hispanic patients.

Hypertension Management and the Hispanic Patient

Hispanics have been found to have lower rates of hypertension compared to other minorities, but once detected, this group is least likely to have the disease adequately controlled (Lloyd-Jones et al., 2010). In fact, one study found that only about half of Hispanic migrant/seasonal farmworkers adhered to their medication treatment and factors such as lack of blood pressure knowledge, perceived stress, acculturation, health literacy, and health care access affected adherence to the hypertension treatment (Hall et al., 2016).

Hispanic patients with hypertension may be referred to behavioral health for treatment nonadherence, lifestyle changes including eating a healthier diet with less salt, exercising regularly, quitting smoking, and other substances, limiting alcohol use, and losing weight in the case of overweight patients or maintaining a healthy weight. Although research has been conducted on Hispanics and factors impacting hypertension diagnosis/treatment, no studies have evaluated the effects of psychological/behavioral interventions on hypertension in this population. Nevertheless, the integrated health care setting may be the ideal place to begin to address some of the healthcare disparities experienced by Hispanics with hypertension.

Treatment Nonadherence. Poor medical treatment adherence for hypertension has been found among Hispanics with hypertension. In fact, one study found that only about half of Hispanic migrant/seasonal farmworkers adhered to their medication treatment and factors such as lack of blood pressure knowledge, perceived stress, acculturation, health literacy, and health care access affected adherence to the hypertension treatment (Hall et al., 2016). BHPs can work to identify whatever barriers are present for the individual Hispanic patient (e.g., health literacy), and provide the patient with appropriate interventions (e.g., psychoeducation about the chronic illness). The National Institute of Health (http://www.nhlbi.nih.gov/health-spanish/health-topics/temas/hbp) provides health literacy resources in Spanish for hypertension. Currently, a practice-based randomized controlled trial is underway to improve medication adherence among Latinos with hypertension (Schoenthaler et al., 2015).

Lifestyle Changes. More Hispanics in the United States are overweight or obese compared to their Caucasian counterparts and this may be due to a higher carbohydrate/calorie diet combined with a more sedentary lifestyle and potential genetic factors (CDC, 2011). BHPs can provide education about making healthier choices when picking out ingredients, for example swapping out quesadillas, refried beans, and sour cream (all high in fats and sodium) for chicken fajitas with pico de gallo and borracho beans (American Heart Association, 2014). BHPs can also use MI to help the patient identify important things that will motivate them to change their behavior (e.g., increasing activity level). Further, BHPs can problem solve barriers to behavior change such as economic constraints. For example, they may discuss with the Hispanic patient about using the local food pantry (or a food pantry collaborating with the primary care clinic) and utilizing the Internet for exercises such as YouTube for free workout videos.

Alcohol and Drug Use. Once again, MI may be employed to help Hispanic patients recognize how alcohol and drug use is impacting their health and overcome any ambivalence they have about reducing or eliminating alcohol and substance use. BHPs may also decide to run alcohol and substance-use group at the primary care clinic, or refer patients out (e.g., to Alcoholics Anonymous) should such groups not be available in the integrated care setting.

Stress. Perceived stress and anxiety sensitivity have been shown to be related to hypertension self care in Hispanics (Alcántara et al., 2014; Hall et al., 2016). BHPs can work with Hispanic patients on stress management techniques such as meditation, guided relaxation, and deep breathing described in an earlier section. There is no evidence that these basic techniques require cultural tailoring beyond making them available in Spanish. First, the BHP may chose to just teach a technique such as deep breathing and thus no resources would be required. In the case that the BHP wants the Hispanic patient to practice a technique such as guided mediation, there are various resources available in Spanish. For example, the BHP may give the Hispanic patient a list of YouTube links to videos for guided meditation in Spanish or direct them to other websites that have audio and video resources, for example the Association for Contextual Behavioral Sciences (https://contextualscience.org/audioact).

Cancer

Cancer refers to a collection of diseases characterized by the development of abnormal cells that multiply, penetrate, and destroy normal body tissue (Mayo Clinic, 2016k). Cancer varies regarding where it's located on the body and how it spreads and can affect areas such as the breasts, bone marrow, lungs, and blood. The risk of developing cancer increases with age, with a 86 % chance in people 50 years of age or older in the United States (American Cancer Society, 2016a). According to the American Cancer Society (2016b), Hispanics tend to have lower rates for the most common cancers compared to non-Hispanics (American Cancer Society, 2016b) Cancers that are frequently diagnosed in Hispanics include stomach, liver, and gallbladder cancers, and these tend to be more common in developing countries, although first generation immigrants in the United States have higher rates of stomach and cervical cancers compared to non-Hispanics (American Cancer Society, 2016b). Cancers are caused by external factor(s) and/or internal factor(s). External factors include an unhealthy diet, infectious organisms, or tobacco. Internal factors of the causes of cancer include the person's immune conditions or a genetic mutation (American Cancer Society, 2016a). External and internal factors could influence the development of cancerous cells together or sequentially and the appearance of cancer in different areas of the individual could share similar or have different characteristics (American Cancer Society, 2016c).

One feature all cancers share is how they affect the individual's normal cells (i.e., abnormal cells take over and grow out of control). However, different cancers spread at different paces, have different reactions to treatment, etc. For example, there are some cancers that can be treated through procedures such as surgery, but there are some kinds of cancers that are much more responsive to treatments such as chemotherapy (American Cancer Society, 2016c).

Cancer also varies in the stage at which it is when first diagnosed/treated. These stages are labeled with roman numerals I through IV, with higher numbers representing a more advanced stage of the cancer. The stage of the cancer depends on its size as well as whether cancer has affected other body parts and/or lymph nodes (American Cancer Society, 2016c).

Diagnostic Tests

There are some tests that could be used when regarding the screening of cancer and the stage of it. The diagnostic tests for cancer may help indicate the detection of cancer and physiological changes of the body with consideration of the developing cancer. These include different types of scans, biopsies, and other laboratory examinations.

Biopsy. A biopsy utilizes sample cells or tissues from any part of the body. Biopsies may be conducted in various ways including removing the organ (by a surgeon), taking tumor samples with a needle, shaving layers of skin, or doing sentinel lymph node mapping to locate lymph node areas for removal (e.g. in the case of breast cancer, melanoma) (American Cancer Society, 2016d).

Computed Tomography (*CT*) *Scan*. A computed tomography scan refers to a scan similar to a standard X-ray test that has capability to create images of bones, soft tissues, and organs in a much more defined manner (American Cancer Society,

2016e). CT scans tend to be conducted in an outpatient setting, and may require the patient to take a contrast dye/liquid before having the test (American Cancer Society, 2016e). Downsides of using CT scans include cost and side effects/complications of using a contrast dye such as wheezing, nausea, and itching (American Cancer Society, 2016e).

Fiber-optic Endoscopic Evaluation. This procedure utilizes an endoscope, which has a long, thin tube attached to a miniature camera (MedlinePlus, 2016). The tube is moved through a body passageway in order to detect abnormalities, e.g., inside an organ (MedlinePlus, 2016).

Laboratory tests. These tests include urine and blood tests that help detect abnormalities that may be results of cancer developing in the body (Mayo Clinic, 2016l).

Magnetic Resonance Imaging (MRI). The MRI is a type of diagnostic test that scans an image of the specific cancer. MRI scans provide cross-sectional images to show soft tissue areas in a person's body and are often conducted in an outpatient setting (American Cancer Society, 2016f). Prepping for an MRI scan could require the patient to follow specific instructions such as taking contrast material before an upcoming MRI appointment (American Cancer Society, 2016f).

Ultrasound. Ultrasounds are used to find cancerous cells during biopsies, or to get a better picture of the patient's tissues than one generated by an X-ray. An ultrasound is often conducted in an outpatient setting, but is not as detailed as an MRI or CT scan (American Cancer Society, 2016g). This type of diagnosis test provides no exposure to radiation and can look at fluid-filled cysts apart from solid tumors (American Cancer Society, 2016g).

X-rays/Radiographs. Radiographs are scans that provide images of bones and certain organs/tissues. Images generated by general radiograph may not be particularly detailed but patients do have the option of getting an MRI or CT scan for increased detail (American Cancer Society, 2016h). More detailed X-rays include MRIs and CT scans, which are more commonly used as contrast studies to view the stage(s) of cancer in organs/tissues.

The tests mentioned above need no cultural adaptation. However, PCPs ought to be aware that Hispanics are less likely to follow through with cancer screenings and may need to be more proactive about addressing this with the Hispanic patient.

Cancer and the Hispanic Patient

Cancer is the leading cause of death among Hispanics and although this population is less likely to develop cancer than non-Hispanic whites, it is also more likely to be diagnosed with an advanced stage of cancer, wait longer for a conclusive diagnosis and to begin treatment, and to experience worse quality of life (American Cancer Society, 2015b). Among Hispanic females, breast cancer is the leading cause of cancer-related death while among Hispanic males, lung cancer is (American Cancer Society, 2015b). Behavioral health providers can be of help to Hispanic patients with cancer and address quality of life issues as there is growing evidence for the link between psychosocial factors and the disease. For example, distress and social support have been shown to be associated with changes in the cellular immune response at the tumor level (Lutgendorf et al., 2005). Research has also revealed links between stress, depression, isolation, and the trajectory of cancer (Lutgendorf, Sood, & Antoni, 2010).

BHPs can be utilized in integrated care (for example, during a warm handoff) to screen cancer patients for psychological distress. Cancer patients may be referred to the BHP for stress management, lack of social support, anxiety, depression, fear, pain, and lifestyle changes including smoking, diet, and exercise. BHPs may also help increase the medical literacy of Hispanic patients. The National Institute of Cancer (http://www.cancer.gov/espanol) and Mayo Clinic (http://www.mayoclinic.org/espanol/enfermedades-y-tratamientos) both provide health literacy resources in Spanish for cancer. Psychosocial interventions have been largely conducted with breast-cancer patients and have been shown to have positive effects on anxiety, depression, pain, and quality of life (e.g., Andersen et al., 2007; Antoni et al., 2006; Goodwin et al., 2001). Further, some studies have provided evidence for the effectiveness of psychological interventions in increasing survival, although generally the research is conflicting and none has looked specifically at Hispanic cancer patients. For example, Andersen and colleagues (2008) conducted a study in which Nonhispanic patients with stage 2 and 3 breast cancer were assigned to two conditions, standard care and group-based cognitive behavioral intervention including relaxation and coping skills training post surgery. The authors found that participants who had received the intervention showed a significant decrease in overall and breast cancer-specific mortality rates and decreased risk of breast cancer recurrence at 11 years follow-up. Although research with Hispanics in this area is limited, there is little reason to believe that these interventions would not be effective and ought not to be used with this population, with a few recommendations for attendance to culture-specific values.

One of these values, *fatalismo*, refers to the belief that our life is predetermined and thus there isn't much we can do to change events. This has been studied in relation to beliefs about cancer and research indicates that Latinos, who endorse fatalismo more than their non-Hispanic white counterparts, are more likely to believe that cancer is not preventable and death after diagnosis is inevitable (Perez-Stable & Sabogal, 1992). Some studies point to fatalismo playing a role in Hispanics underutilizing cancer screenings (for a review see Espinosa de los Monteros & Gallo, 2011) although the research is conflicting and some (e.g., Abraído-Lanza et al., 2007) have cautioned against using this construct to explain Hispanic engagement in prevention and treatment for cancer. Additionally, fatalismo has been associated with worse quality of life among breast cancer survivors (Ashing-Giwa, Padilla, Bohórquez, Tejero, & Garcia, 2006; Graves et al., 2012). BHPs could potentially ask patients of any beliefs that may get in the way of patients utilizing resources for cancer and work with the PCP to challenge any misperceptions. Some cultural values have been shown to have very positive effects on cancer patients. For example, religiosity/spirituality has been associated with greater quality of life for Hispanics (Wildes, Miller, de Majors, & Ramirez, 2009). BHPs should not be afraid to ask the Hispanic patient with cancer about his or her spiritual/religious beliefs and promote them in this population (Hunter-Hernández, Costas-Muñíz, & Gany, 2015).

Stress. BHPs can teach Hispanic patients with cancer stress management techniques such as meditation, guided relaxation, and CBT techniques for modifying worry thoughts. BHPs first provide the rationale for the technique, then demonstrate it, and practice it with the patients. Technology can be of great help in teaching stress management techniques as many websites (for example, YouTube) contain audio/videos of guided mediation, relaxation, deep breathing, etc. Only one study has evaluated stress management intervention with Hispanics although Hispanics have been included in other research (e.g., Stagl et al., 2015). Specifically, Penedo and colleagues (2007) found that a 10-week group-based cognitive-behavioral stress management intervention increased physical well-being, emotional well-being, sexual functioning, and total well-being in Hispanic males with prostate cancer.

Social Support. Social support has been shown to be directly linked to health outcomes in cancer patients (Cohen, 2004). Further, some studies have demonstrated that social support moderates the effects of stress (e.g., Oh & Ell, 2015). The Hispanic cultural values of familismo may work to provide the individual with cancer with the support of family members. However, it may also be problematic as the individual does not want to be a burden for the family and may be reluctant to reach out to others for social support. Therefore, a focus of the BHP working with the Hispanic patient with cancer ought to be on activating social support.

Anxiety and Depression. Psychological disorders such as anxiety and depression are relatively common in cancer patients. For example, Zabora and colleagues (2001) evaluated approximately 4500 adult patients with cancer and found that of patients with the 14 most common types of cancer, 29–43 % of them reported significant psychological distress. Specific to Hispanics, research indicates that Hispanic females with cancer are more likely than their Caucasian counterparts to also suffer from depression and anxiety (for a review see Yanez, Thompson, & Stanton, 2011). Further, anxiety and depression have both been shown to negatively impact cancer screening rates in Hispanics (Pabon-Nau, 2010). One randomly controlled trial addressing depression with 'collaborative care' in Hispanic patients with cancer was identified (Ell et al., 2008). Results indicated that the patients receiving collaborative care (a 12-month intervention including the use of problem-solving therapy, antidepressants, symptom monitoring, and relapse prevention overseen by a depression care manager) had significantly reduced depressive symptoms and pain levels and improvement in quality of life when compared to usual care. At 1-year follow-up, many of the outcomes were sustained (Ell et al., 2011). However, no measures related to cancer were evaluated. Depending on the severity of the disorder, the BHP may choose to intervene at any one of the levels in the stepped care model. Managing anxiety and depression in integrated healthcare with Hispanics are discussed elsewhere in this volume and will not be covered here.

Fear. Fear of cancer-related problems, whether of its recurrence, of the treatment itself, or of death, may be addressed by a BHP. Fear has been identified as a barrier to cancer screenings in Hispanics, including fear of the pain of the screening procedure and of detecting any cancerous tissue (e.g., Jing, Moehring, Stuhr, & Krug, 2013; Livaudais et al., 2010). Acceptance of one's (potentially) terminal disease is a challenging undertaking, and the BHP can work with the Hispanic patient to address any misconceptions or medical literacy issues and normalize the fear in order to move the patient towards that acceptance and away from hopelessness and helplessness. Additionally, any one of the other techniques described in this section can work to reduce the fear (e.g., engaging in mindfulness exercises).

Lifestyle. A healthy lifestyle, including one in which the patient eats a healthy diet high in fruit and vegetables, is physically active, and abstains from smoking, has been shown to be positively associated with greater quality of life in cancer survivors (Koutoukidis, Tish Knobf, & Lanceley, 2015). BHPs can work with the Hispanic patient to increase knowledge and motivation about a living a healthy lifestyle and promote behavior change.

Pain. Pain is reported in one third to one half of patients undergoing active treatment for cancer, with pain developing from the cancer, its treatment, or comorbid diseases; additionally, pain may continue to persist even after the cancer has been successfully treated (Adler & Page, 2008). Culture specific factors that affect the management and expression of pain specific to Hispanics include family, religion, and stoicism and these may lead to an underreporting of the pain (Juarez, Ferrell, & Borneman, 1998). Additionally, Hispanics have been found to rely more on folk beliefs and nondrug interventions (Juarez et al., 1998). More problematic is that the pain with which Hispanics present in primary care appears to be undertreated and Hispanics overall report less pain relief (Cleeland, Gonin, Baez, Loehrer, & Pandya, 1997; Delgado, Lin, & Coffey, 1995; Eley et al., 1994). Thus, BHPs can work with the Hispanic patient to address his or her pain via mindfulness, acceptance, and other techniques, for example by normalizing the cancer-related pain and promoting acceptance of pain as a part of the disease process.

Conclusion

When Hispanic patients present to their Primary Care Providers with chronic conditions including diabetes, heart disease, hypertension, and cancer, successfully treating the chronic conditions may not be so straightforward. Barriers to adequate screening and treatment have been identified including language barriers, low income and education, low acculturation, and differing beliefs and values (e.g., Ghaddar et al., 2010; González et al., 2009; Mainous et al., 2008; McCloskey & Flenniken, 2010; and Weiler & Crist, 2009). Additionally, risk factors and comorbid conditions may exacerbate chronic conditions and make their management more challenging for the Hispanic patient. Integrated care is a system in which Behavioral

Health Providers can work with PCPs in order to improve the health of Hispanics living with chronic conditions by addressing barriers, improving treatment adherence, and promoting positive lifestyle changes. Although research with Hispanics in integrated care has been limited, and the heterogeneity of this population makes it difficult to generalize results, there is little evidence to suggest that interventions utilized in integrated care ought not to work for the Hispanics patient (for example, a mindfulness training for stress reduction) as long as cultural factors are taken into consideration and language barriers are addressed.

References

Abraído-Lanza, A. E., Viladrich, A., Flórez, K. R., Céspedes, A., Aguirre, A. N., & De La Cruz, A. A. (2007). Commentary: Fatalismo reconsidered: A cautionary note for health-related research and practice with Latino populations. *Ethnicity & Disease, 17*(1), 153–158.

Adler, N. E., & Page, A. K. (2008). *Cancer care for the whole patient: Meeting psychosocial health needs*. Washington, DC: National Academies Press.

Agency for Healthcare Research and Quality. (2011). National *healthcare disparities report*. Retrieved from http://www.ahrq.gov/qual/nhdr10/nhdr10.pdf.

AHRQ AfHRaQ Minority Health. (2009). *Recent findings*. Retrieved from http://www.ahrq.gov/research/minorfind.pdf.

Alcántara, C., Edmondson, D., Moise, N., Oyola, D., Hiti, D., & Kronish, I. M. (2014). Anxiety sensitivity and medication nonadherence in patients with uncontrolled hypertension. *Journal of Psychosomatic Research, 77*(4), 283–286. doi:10.1016/j.jpsychores.2014.07.009.

American Cancer Society. (2015a). *Cancer facts and figures 2015*. Retrieved from http://www.cancer.org/acs/groups/content/@epidemiologysurveilance/documents/document/acspc-036845.pdf.

American Cancer Society. (2015b). *Cancer facts and figures for Hispanics/Latinos 2015–2017*. Retrieved from http://www.cancer.org/acs/groups/content/@epidemiologysurveilance/documents/document/acspc-034778.pdf.

American Cancer Society. (2016a). *Cancer facts and figures 2016*. Retrieved from http://www.cancer.org/acs/groups/content/@research/documents/document/acspc-047079.pdf.

American Cancer Society. (2016b). *Cancer facts and figures for Hispanics/Latinos*. Retrieved from http://www.cancer.org/acs/groups/content/@research/documents/document/acspc-046405.pdf.

American Cancer Society. (2016c). *What is cancer? A guideline for patients and families*. Retrieved from http://www.cancer.org/cancer/cancerbasics/what-is-cancer.

American Cancer Society. (2016d). *Types of biopsies used to look for cancer*. Retrieved from http://www.cancer.org/treatment/understandingyourdiagnosis/examsandtestdescriptions/testingbiopsyandcytologyspecimensforcancer/testing-biopsy-and-cytology-specimens-for-cancer-biopsy-types.

American Cancer Society. (2016e). *CT scan for cancer*. Retrieved from http://www.cancer.org/treatment/understandingyourdiagnosis/examsandtestdescriptions/ct-scan-for-cancer.

American Cancer Society. (2016f). *MRI for cancer*. Retrieved from http://www.cancer.org/treatment/understandingyourdiagnosis/examsandtestdescriptions/mri-for-cancer.

American Cancer Society. (2016g). *Ultrasound for cancer*. Retrieved from http://www.cancer.org/treatment/understandingyourdiagnosis/examsandtestdescriptions/ultrasound-for-cancer.

American Cancer Society. (2016h). *X-rays and other radiographic tests for cancers*. Retrieved from http://www.cancer.org/treatment/understandingyourdiagnosis/examsandtestdescriptions/x-rays-and-other-radiographic-tests.

American Diabetes Association. (2014). *Diabetes among Hispanics: All are not equal*. Retrieved from http://www.diabetes.org/newsroom/press-releases/2014/diabetes-among-hispanics-all-are-not-equal.html?referrer=https://www.google.com/.

American Diabetes Association. (2016). *Diagnosing diabetes and learning about prediabetes*. Retrieved from http://www.diabetes.org/diabetes-basics/diagnosis/?referrer=https://www.google.com/.

American Heart Association. (2013). *Hispanics/Latinos & CVD – 2013 statistical fact sheet*. Retrieved from https://www.heart.org/idc/groups/heart-public/@wcm/@sop/@smd/documents/downloadable/ucm_319572.pdf.

American Heart Association. (2014). *Tips for eating Mexican food*. Retrieved from http://www.heart.org/HEARTORG/HealthyLiving/HealthyEating/DiningOut/Tips-for-Eating-Mexican-Food_UCM_308411_Article.jsp#.VuRwOJMrI_U.

American Heart Association. (2016). *Hispanics and heart disease, stroke*. Retrieved from http://www.heart.org/HEARTORG/Conditions/More/MyHeartandStrokeNews/Hispanics-and-Heart-Disease-Stroke_UCM_444864_Article.jsp#.VukcguIrLRY.

Andersen, B. L., Farrar, W. B., Golden-Kreutz, D., Emery, C. F., Glaser, R., Crespin, T., & Carson, W. I. (2007). Distress reduction from a psychological intervention contributes to improved health for cancer patients. *Brain, Behavior, and Immunity, 21(7)*, 953–961. doi:10.1016/j.bbi.2007.03.005.

Andersen, B. L., Yang, H., Farrar, W. B., GoldenKreutz, D. M., Emery, C. F., Thornton, L. M., … Carson, W. E. (2008). Psychologic intervention improves survival for breast cancer patients: A randomized clinical trial. *Cancer*, *113(12)*, 3450–3458.

Antoni, M. H., Lechner, S. C., Kazi, A., Wimberly, S. R., Sifre, T., Urcuyo, K. R., … Carver, C. S. (2006). How stress management improves quality of life after treatment for breast cancer. *Journal of Consulting and Clinical Psychology*, *74(6)*, 1143–1152.

Ashing-Giwa, K. T., Padilla, G. V., Bohórquez, D. E., Tejero, J. S., & Garcia, M. (2006). Understanding the breast cancer experience of Latina women. *Journal of Psychosocial Oncology, 24*, 19–52. Retrieved from http://dx.doi.org/10.1300/J077v24n03_02.

Babamoto, K., Sey, K., Camilleri, A., Karlan, V., Catalasan, J., & Morisky, D. (2009). Improving diabetes care and health measures among Hispanics using community health workers: Results from a randomized controlled trial. *Health Education & Behavior, 36*(1), 113–126. doi:10.1177/1090198108325911.

Bailey, G. R., Barner, J. C., Weems, J. K., Leckbee, G., Solis, R., Montemayor, D., & Pope, N. D. (2012). Assessing barriers to medication adherence in underserved patients with diabetes in Texas. *The Diabetes Educator, 38*(2), 271–279. doi:10.1177/0145721711436134.

Bautista, L., Reininger, B., Gay, J. L., Barroso, C. S., & McCormick, J. B. (2011). Perceived barriers to exercise in Hispanic adults by level of activity. *Journal of Physical Activity & Health, 8*(7), 916–925.

Benavides-Vaello, S., Garcia, A. A., Brown, S. A., & Winchell, M. (2004). Using focus groups to plan and evaluate diabetes self-management interventions for Mexican Americans. *The Diabetes Educator, 30*(2), 238–256. doi:10.1177/014572170403000217.

Buerau of Labor Statistics. (2015). *Hispanics and Latinos in industries and occupations*. Retrieved from http://www.bls.gov/opub/ted/2015/hispanics-and-latinos-in-industries-and-occupations.htm.

Caban, A., Walker, E. A., Sanchez, S., & Mera, M. S. (2008). "It feels like home when you eat rice and beans": Perspectives of urban Latinos living with diabetes. *Diabetes Spectrum, 21*(2), 120–127.

CDC. (2009). *Differences in prevalence of obesity among Black, White, and Hispanic adults – United States, 2006-2008*. Retrieved from http://www.cdc.gov/mmwr/preview/mmwrhtml/mm5827a2.htm.

CDC. (2013). *Cardiovascular disease is the leading cause of death among US Hispanics*. Retrieved from http://www.cdc.gov/features/MillionHeartsHispanic/.

CDC. (2015). Fast facts: Smoking & tobacco use. Retrieved from http://www.cdc.gov/tobacco/data_statistics/fact_sheets/fast_facts/.

CDC. (2016a). *Chronic disease overview*. Retrieved from http://www.cdc.gov/chronicdisease/overview.

CDC. (2016b). *Health of Hispanic or Latino population*. Retrieved from http://www.cdc.gov/nchs/fastats/hispanic-health.htm.

Center for Mental Health Services. (2001). *Cultural competence standards in managed care mental health services: Four underserved/underrepresented racial/ethnic groups*. Retrieved from http://www.mentalhealth.org/publications/allpubs/SMA00-3457/.

Centers for Disease Control and Prevention. (2011). *Obesity: Halting the epidemic by making health easier: At a glance*. Retrieved from http://www.cdc.gov/chronicdisease/resources/publications/aag/obesity.htm.

Chilton, L., Hu, J., & Wallace, D. C. (2006). Health-promoting lifestyle and diabetes knowledge in Hispanic American adults. *Home Health Care Management & Practice, 18*(5), 378–385. doi:10.1177/1084822306288059.

Clark, L., Vincent, D., Zimmer, L., & Sanchez, J. (2009). Cultural values and political economic contexts of diabetes among low-income Mexican Americans. *Journal of Transcultural Nursing, 20*(4), 382–394.

Cleeland, C. S., Gonin, R., Baez, L., Loehrer, P., & Pandya, K. J. (1997). Pain and treatment of pain in minority patients with cancer: The Eastern Cooperative Oncology Group Minority Outpatient Pain Study. *Annals of Internal Medicine, 127*(9), 813–816.

Cohen, S. (2004). Social relationships and health. *American Psychologist, 59*(8), 676–684. doi:10.1037/0003-066X.59.8.676.

Delgado, D. J., Lin, W. Y., & Coffey, M. (1995). The role of Hispanic race/ethnicity and poverty in breast cancer survival. *Puerto Rico Health Sciences Journal, 14*(2), 103–116.

Dellasega, C., Añel-Tiangco, R., & Gabbay, R. (2012). How patients with type 2 diabetes mellitus respond to motivational interviewing. *Diabetes Research & Clinical Practice, 95*(1), 37–41.

DeNavas-Walt, C., Proctor, B. D., & Smith, J. C. (2011). *Income, poverty, and health insurance coverage in the United States*. Washington, DC: U.S. Government Printing Office.

Department of Health and Human Services. (2016). *What is stress testing*?. Retrieved from https://www.nhlbi.nih.gov/health/health-topics/topics/stress.

Eley, J. W., Hill, H. A., Chen, V. W., Austin, D. F., Wesley, M. N., Muss, H. B., … Hunter, C. P. (1994). Racial differences in survival from breast cancer: Results of the National Cancer Institute Black/White Cancer Survival Study. *JAMA, 272(12)*, 947–954.

Ell, K., Xie, B., Kapetanovic, S., Quinn, D., Lee, P., Wells, A., & Chou, C. (2011). One-year follow-up of collaborative depression care for low-income, predominantly Hispanic patients with cancer. *Psychiatric Services, 62(2)*, 162–170. doi:10.1176/appi.ps.62.2.162.

Ell, K., Xie, B., Quon, B., Quinn, D., Dwight-Johnson, M., & Lee, P. (2008). Randomized controlled trial of collaborative care management of depression among low-income patients with cancer. *Journal of Clinical Oncology, 26*(27), 4488–4496.

Escarce, J. J., Morales, L. S., & Rumbaut, R. G. (2006). The health status and health behaviors of Hispanics. In M. Tienda, F. Mitchell, M. Tienda, & F. Mitchell (Eds.), *Hispanics and the future of America* (pp. 362–409). Washington, DC: National Academies Press.

Espinosa de los Monteros, K., & Gallo, L. (2011). The relevance of fatalism in the study of Latinas' cancer screening behavior: A systematic review of the literature. *International Journal of Behavioral Medicine, 18*(4), 310–318. doi:10.1007/s12529-010-9119-4.

Fiore, M. C., Jaén, C. R., Baker, T. B., Bailey, W. C., Benowitz, N. L., Curry, S. J., … Henderson, P. N. (2008). *Treating tobacco use and dependence: 2008 Update—Clinical practice guideline*. Retrieved from http://www.ahrq.gov/sites/default/files/wysiwyg/professionals/clinicians-providers/guidelines-recommendations/tobacco/clinicians/update/treating_tobacco_use08.pdf.

Foa, E. B., Hembree, E. A., & Rothbaum, B. O. (2007). *Prolonged exposure therapy for PTSD: Emotional processing of traumatic experiences: Therapist guide*. New York, NY: Oxford University Press.

Gallo, L. C., Roesch, S. C., Fortmann, A. L., Carnethon, M. R., Penedo, F. J., Perreira, K., … Isasi, C. R. (2014). Associations of chronic stress burden, perceived stress, and traumatic stress with cardiovascular disease prevalence and risk factors in the Hispanic Community Health Study/ Study of Latinos sociocultural ancillary study. *Psychosomatic Medicine, 76(6)*, 468–475. doi:10.1097/PSY.0000000000000069.

Ghaddar, S., Brown, C. J., Pagán, J. A., & Díaz, V. (2010). Acculturation and healthy lifestyle habits among Hispanics in United States-Mexico border communities. *Revista Panamericana de Salud Pública, 28*(3), 190–197.

Glasgow, R., Strycker, L., King, D., Toobert, D., Rahm, A., Jex, M., & Nutting, P. (2006). Robustness of a computer-assisted diabetes self-management intervention across patient characteristics, healthcare settings, and intervention staff. *American Journal of Managed Care, 12(3)*, 137–145.

González, H. M., Vega, W. A., Rodríguez, M. A., Tarraf, W., & Sribney, W. M. (2009). Diabetes awareness and knowledge among Latinos: Does a usual source of healthcare matter? *Journal of General Internal Medicine, 24*(3), 528–533.

Goodwin, P. J., Leszcz, M., Ennis, M., Koopmans, J., Vincent, L., Guther, H., … Navarro, M. (2001). Effect of group psychosocial support on survival in metastatic breast cancer. *New England Journal of Medicine, 345(24)*, 1719–1726.

Graves, K. D., Jensen, R. E., Cañar, J., Perret-Gentil, M., Leventhal, K.-G., Gonzalez, F., … Mandelblatt, J. (2012). Through the lens of culture: Quality of life among Latina breast cancer survivors. *Breast Cancer Research and Treatment, 136*, 603–613. Retrieved from http://dx.doi.org/10.1007/s10549-012-2291-2.

Hall, E., Lee, S., Clark, P. C., & Perilla, J. (2016). Social ecology of adherence to hypertension treatment in Latino migrant and seasonal farmworkers. *Journal of Transcultural Nursing, 27*(1), 33–41. doi:10.1177/1043659614524788.

Heller. (2006). *New Hispanic nutrition guidelines promote healthy eating*. Retrieved from http://www.foodnavigator-usa.com/Suppliers2/New-Hispanic-nutrition-guidelines-promote-healthy-eating.

Hettema, J. E., & Hendricks, P. S. (2010). Motivational interviewing for smoking cessation: A meta-analytic review. *Journal of Consulting and Clinical Psychology, 78*(6), 868–884. doi:10.1037/a0021498.

Houston, T. K., Scarinci, I. C., Person, S. D., & Greene, P. G. (2005). Patient smoking cessation advice by health care providers: The role of ethnicity, socioeconomic status, and health. *American Journal of Public Health, 95*(6), 1056–1061.

Hu, J., Amirehsani, K., Wallace, D. C., & Letvak, S. (2013). Perceptions of barriers in managing diabetes: Perspectives of Hispanic immigrant patients and family members. *The Diabetes Educator, 39*(4), 494–503. doi:10.1177/0145721713486200.

Hunter-Hernández, M., Costas-Muñíz, R., & Gany, F. (2015). Missed opportunity: Spirituality as a bridge to resilience in Latinos with cancer. *Journal of Religion & Health, 54*(6), 2367. doi:10.1007/s10943-015-0020-y.

Jamal, A., Dube, S. R., Malarcher, A. M., Shaw, L., Engstrom, M. C., & Centers for Disease Control and Prevention (CDC). (2012). Tobacco use screening and counseling during physician office visits among adults—National ambulatory medical care survey and national health interview survey, United States, 2005–2009. *Morbidity and Mortality Weekly Report, 61*(Suppl), 38–45.

Jing, W., Moehring, J., Stuhr, S., & Krug, M. (2013). Barriers to colorectal cancer screening in Hispanics in the United States: An integrative review. *Applied Nursing Research, 26*(4), 218–224. doi:10.1016/j.apnr.2013.08.005.

John, R., Resendiz, R., & De Vargas, L. W. (1997). Beyond familism?: Familism as explicit motive for eldercare among Mexican American caregivers. *Journal of Cross-Cultural Gerontology, 12*(2), 145–162.

Juarez, G., Ferrell, B., & Borneman, T. (1998). Influence of culture on cancer pain management in Hispanic patients. *Cancer Practice, 6*(5), 262–269.

Koutoukidis, D. A., Tish Knobf, M., & Lanceley, A. (2015). Obesity, diet, physical activity, and health-related quality of life in endometrial cancer survivors. *Nutrition Reviews, 73*(6), 399–408.

Lee, C. S., López, S. R., Colby, S. M., Rohsenow, D., Hernández, L., Borrelli, B., & Caetano, R. (2013). Culturally adapted motivational interviewing for Latino heavy drinkers: Results from a randomized clinical trial. *Journal of Ethnicity in Substance Abuse*, *12*(*4*), 356–373. doi:10.1080/15332640.2013.836730.

Levinson, A. H., Pérez-Stable, E. J., Espinoza, P., Flores, E. T., & Byers, T. E. (2004). Latinos report less use of pharmaceutical aids when trying to quit smoking. *American Journal of Preventive Medicine, 26*(2), 105–111.

Lewis-Fernández, R., Das, A. K., Alfonso, C., Weissman, M. M., & Olfson, M. (2005). Depression in US Hispanics: Diagnostic and management considerations in family practice. *The Journal of the American Board of Family Practice, 18*(4), 282–296.

Livaudais, J., Coronado, G., Espinoza, N., Islas, I., Ibarra, G., & Thompson, B. (2010). Educating Hispanic women about breast cancer prevention: Evaluation of a home-based promotora-led intervention. *Journal of Women's Health, 19*(11), 2049–2056. doi:10.1089/jwh.2009.1733.

Lloyd-Jones, D., Adams, R., Brown, T., Carnethon, M., Dai, S., De Simone, G., … Lisabeth, L. (2010). Heart disease and stroke statistics -- 2010 Update: A report from the American Heart Association. *Circulation*, *121*(*7*), e46–215. doi:10.1161/CIRCULATIONAHA.109.192667.

Lopez-Class, M., & Jurkowski, J. (2010). The limits of self-management: Community and health care system barriers among Latinos with diabetes. *Journal of Human Behavior in the Social Environment, 20*(6), 808–826.

Lopez-Quintero, C., Berry, E. M., & Neumark, Y. (2009). Limited English proficiency is a barrier to receipt of advice about physical activity and diet among Hispanics with chronic diseases in the United States. *Journal of the American Dietetic Association, 109*(10), 1769–1774.

Lutgendorf, S., Sood, A., Anderson, B., McGinn, S., Maiseri, H., Dao, M., … Lubaroff, D. (2005). Social support, psychological distress, and natural killer cell activity in ovarian cancer. *Journal of Clinical Oncology*, *23*(*28*), 7105–7113.

Lutgendorf, S., Sood, A., & Antoni, M. (2010). Host factors and cancer progression: Biobehavioral signaling pathways and interventions. *Journal of Clinical Oncology, 28*(26), 4094–4099. doi:10.1200/JCO.2009.26.9357.

Mainous, A. G., Diaz, V. A., Saxena, S., & Geesey, M. E. (2007). Heterogeneity in management of diabetes mellitus among Latino ethnic subgroups in the United States. *The Journal of the American Board of Family Medicine, 20*(6), 598–605.

Mainous, A. G., Diaz, V. A., & Geesey, M. E. (2008). Acculturation and healthy lifestyle among Latinos with diabetes. *The Annals of Family Medicine, 6*(2), 131–137.

Mayo Clinic. (2016a). *Diabetes risk factors*. Retrieved from http://www.mayoclinic.org/diseases-conditions/diabetes/basics/risk-factors/con-20033091.

Mayo Clinic. (2016b). *A1C test*. Retrieved from http://www.mayoclinic.org/tests-procedures/a1c-test/home/ovc-20167930.

Mayo Clinic. (2016c). *Glucose tolerance test*. Retrieved from http://www.mayoclinic.org/diseases-conditions/diabetes/basics/definition/prc-20014814.

Mayo Clinic. (2016d). *Oral glucose tolerance test*. Retrieved from http://www.mayoclinic.org/tests-procedures/glucose-tolerance-test/basics/results/prc-20014814.

Mayo Clinic. (2016e). *Heart Disease*. Retrieved from http://www.mayoclinic.org/diseases-conditions/heart-disease/basics/definition/con-20034056.

Mayo Clinic. (2016f). *Heart disease risk factors*. Retrieved from http://www.mayoclinic.org/diseases-conditions/heart-disease/basics/risk-factors/con-20034056.

Mayo Clinic. (2016g). *Heat disease tests and diagnosis*. Retrieved from http://www.mayoclinic.org/diseases-conditions/heart-disease/basics/tests-diagnosis/con-20034056.

Mayo Clinic. (2016h). *High blood pressure (hypertension)*. Retrieved from http://www.mayoclinic.org/diseases-conditions/high-blood-pressure/basics/definition/con-20019580.

Mayo Clinic. (2016i). *High blood pressure (hypertension) causes*. Retrieved from http://www.mayoclinic.org/diseases-conditions/high-blood-pressure/basics/causes/con-20019580.

Mayo Clinic. (2016j). *High blood pressure (hypertension) tests and diagnosis*. Retrieved from http://www.mayoclinic.org/diseases-conditions/high-blood-pressure/basics/tests-diagnosis/con-20019580.

Mayo Clinic. (2016k). *Cancer definition*. Retrieved from http://www.mayoclinic.org/diseases-conditions/cancer/basics/definition/con-20032378.

Mayo Clinic. (2016l). *Cancer tests and diagnosis*. Retrieved from http://www.mayoclinic.org/diseases-conditions/cancer/basics/tests-diagnosis/con-20032378.

McCloskey, J., & Flenniken, D. (2010). Overcoming cultural barriers to diabetes control: A qualitative study of southwestern new Mexico Hispanics. *Journal of Cultural Diversity, 17*(3), 110.

McGruder, H. F., Malarcher, A. M., Antoine, T. L., Greenlund, K. J., & Croft, J. B. (2004). Racial and ethnic disparities in cardiovascular risk factors among stroke survivors United States 1999 to 2001. *Stroke, 35*(7), 1557–1561.

MedlinePlus. (2016). *Endoscopy*. Retrieved from https://www.nlm.nih.gov/medlineplus/endoscopy.html.

Miller, W. R. (1983). Motivational interviewing with problem drinkers. *Behavioural Psychotherapy, 11*(02), 147–172.

National Hispanic Caucus of State Legislators (NHCSL). (2010). *Hispanic obesity: An American crisis*. Retrieved from http://www.nhcsl.org/issues/healthcare/Hispanic-Obesity-An-American-Crisis.pdf.

National Institute on Drug Abuse. (2012). *Medical consequences of drug abuse*. Retrieved from https://www.drugabuse.gov/publications/medical-consequences-drug-abuse/cardiovascular-effects.

NIH. (2014). *Diagnosis of diabetes and prediabetes*. Retrieved from http://www.niddk.nih.gov/health-information/health-topics/Diabetes/diagnosis-diabetes-prediabetes/Pages/index.aspx.

NIMH. (2014). *Major depression among adults*. Retrieved from http://www.nimh.nih.gov/health/statistics/prevalence/major-depression-among-adults.shtml.

Nwasuruba, C., Osuagwu, C., Bae, S., Singh, K. P., & Egede, L. E. (2009). Racial differences in diabetes self-management and quality of care in Texas. *Journal of Diabetes and its Complications, 23*(2), 112–118. doi:10.1016/j.jdiacomp.2007.11.005.

O'Donohue, W. T., Cummings, N. A., Cucciare, M. A., Runyan, C. N., & Cummings, J. L. (Eds.). (2005). *Integrated behavioral health care: A guide to effective intervention*. Amherst, NY: Humanity Books (Prometheus).

O'Donohue, W. T., & Draper, C. (2011). *Stepped care and e-health: Practical applications to behavioral disorders*. New York, NY: Springer Science+Business Media. doi:10.1007/978-1-4419-6510-3.

ODPHP. (2016). *2015–2020 Dietary Guidelines for Americans*. Retrieved from http://health.gov/dietaryguidelines/2015.

Office of the Surgeon General. (2001). Mental health: Culture, race, and ethnicity. In *Supplement to mental health: A report of the Surgeon General*. Washington, DC: GPO.

Oh, H., & Ell, K. (2015). Social support, a mediator in collaborative depression care for cancer patients. *Research on Social Work Practice, 25*(2), 229–239.

Ornelas, I. J., & Perreira, K. M. (2011). The role of migration in the development of depressive symptoms among Latino immigrant parents in the USA. *Social Science & Medicine, 73*, 1169–1177. doi:10.1016/j.socscimed.2011.07.002.

Osborn, C., Amico, K., Cruz, N., O'Connell, A., Perez-Escamilla, R., Kalichman, S., … Fisher, J. (2010). A brief culturally tailored intervention for Puerto Ricans with type 2 diabetes. *Health Education & Behavior, 37(6)*, 849–862. doi:10.1177/1090198110366004.

Pabon-Nau. (2010). *Effects of anxiety or depression on cancer screening among Hispanic immigrants*. Retrieved from https://www2.massgeneral.org/disparitiessolutions/z_files/Lina%20Pabon%20Nau_CHIS.pdf.

Penedo, F. J., Traeger, L., Dahn, J., Molton, I., Gonzalez, J. S., Schneiderman, N., & Antoni, M. H. (2007). Cognitive behavioral stress management intervention improves quality of life in Spanish monolingual Hispanic men treated for localized prostate cancer: Results of a randomized controlled trial. *International Journal of Behavioral Medicine, 14(3)*, 164–172.

Perez-Stable, E. J., & Sabogal, F. (1992). Misconceptions about cancer among Latinos and Anglos. *JAMA, 268*(22), 3219.

Rosal, M. C., Goins, K. V., Carbone, E. T., & Cortes, D. E. (2004). Views and preferences of low-literate Hispanics regarding diabetes education: Results of formative research. *Health Education & Behavior, 31*(3), 388–405.

Rosal, M., Ockene, I., Restrepo, A., White, M., Borg, A., Olendzki, B., … Reed, G. (2011). Randomized trial of a literacy-sensitive, culturally tailored diabetes self-management intervention for low-income Latinos: Latinos en control. *Diabetes Care, 34(4)*, 838–844. doi:10.2337/dc10-1981.

Schoenthaler, A., De La Calle, F., Barrios-Barrios, M., Garcia, A., Pitaro, M., Lum, A., & Rosal, M. (2015). A practice-based randomized controlled trial to improve medication adherence among Latinos with hypertension: Study protocol for a randomized controlled trial. *Trials, 16(1)*, 1. doi:10.1186/s13063-015-0815-x.

Stagl, J. M., Bouchard, L. C., Lechner, S. C., Blomberg, B. B., Gudenkauf, L. M., Jutagir, D. R., … Antoni, M. H. (2015). Long-term psychological benefits of cognitive-behavioral stress management for women with breast cancer: 11-Year follow-up of a randomized controlled trial. *Cancer, 121(11)*, 1873–1881. doi:10.1002/cncr.29076.

Thackeray, R., Merrill, R., & Neiger, B. (2004). Disparities in diabetes management practice between racial and ethnic groups in the United States. *The Diabetes Educator, 30*(4), 665–675.

Tienda, M., Mitchell, F., & National Research Council (Eds.). (2006). *Hispanics and the future of America*. Washington, DC: The National Academies Press.

United States Census Bureau. (2015). *Quick facts Reno, Nevada*. Retrieved from http://www.census.gov/quickfacts/table/PST045215/3260600.

Weiler, D. M., & Crist, J. D. (2009). Diabetes self-management in a Latino social environment. *The Diabetes Educator, 35*(2), 285–292.

Wen, L. K., Shepherd, M. D., & Parchman, M. L. (2004). Family support, diet, and exercise among older Mexican Americans with type 2 diabetes. *The Diabetes Educator, 30*(6), 980–993.

Wildes, K., Miller, A., de Majors, S., & Ramirez, A. (2009). The religiosity/spirituality of Latina breast cancer survivors and influence on health-related quality of life. *Psycho-Oncology, 18*(8), 831–840. doi:10.1002/pon.1475.

Williams, S., & Kohout, J. L. (1999). *A survey of licensed practitioners of psychology: Activities, roles, and services*. Washington, DC: American Psychological Association.

Wu, S., Ell, K., Gross-Schulman, S. G., Sklaroff, L. M., Katon, W. J., Nezu, A. M., … Guterman, J. J. (2014). Technology-facilitated depression care management among predominantly Latino diabetes patients within a public safety net care system: Comparative effectiveness trial design. *Contemporary Clinical Trials, 37(2)*, 342–354. doi:10.1016/j.cct.2013.11.002.

Wu, B., Jin, H., Vidyanti, I., Lee, P., Ell, K., & Wu, S. (2014). Collaborative depression care among Latino patients in diabetes disease management, Los Angels 2011–2013. *Preventing Chronic Disease, 11*, E148. doi:10.5888/pcd11.140081.

Yanez, B., Thompson, E. H., & Stanton, A. L. (2011). Quality of life among Latina breast cancer patients: A systematic review of the literature. *Journal of Cancer Survivorship, 5*(2), 191–207.

Zaboraa, J., Brintzenhofeszoc, K., Curbow, B., Hooker, C., & Piantadosi, S. (2001). The prevalence of psychological distress by cancer site. *Psycho-Oncology, 10*(1), 19–28.

Chapter 15
Seriously Mentally Ill and Integrated Care Among Hispanic Populations

Brian D. Leany

Introduction

Public Law 102-321 put forth by the Substance Abuse and Mental Health Services Administration funds programs and research for Serious Mental Illness (SMI), which they define as any DSM diagnosis (other than a substance-use disorder) with a duration of more than 12 months and functional impairment in at least two domains. SAMSHA also clarified that impairment should be measured by a Global Assessment of Functioning (GAF) score of less than 60. Clinically, we most often see this in Schizophrenia, Bipolar I Disorder, and Delusional or other Psychotic Disorders (excluding those resulting from acute substance intoxication).

As a psychologist who has worked in state and community-based health care settings as well as private practice and managed care I've had the opportunity to observe a variety of systems function (or attempt to function) in treating serious mental illness (SMI). Though state- and community-based settings, do provide individuals with SMI access to a spectrum of health care providers both within the organization as well as outside contracted providers, it is more often the case in these settings that the individual, as a result of a serious degradation in functioning (occasionally as the result of a legal entanglement) is ultimately hospitalized. Hospitalization results in significantly increased costs, both in real dollars for treating the individual, as well as costs from that individual no longer functioning in their traditional psychosocial environment (e.g. family, work, school). A primary challenge with serious mental illness is the limited continuum of care across the transition between in and outpatient care, which frequently occurs with SMI (Clarke et al., 2000). Not all hospitals provide an integrated approach to treating SMI, which is ultimately detrimental to the patient and the hospital. When comparing an

B.D. Leany, Ph.D. (✉)
Lake's Crossing Center, Nevada State Forensic Hospital,
Sparks, NV 89431, USA
e-mail: leanyb@gmail.com

© Springer International Publishing Switzerland 2016

L.T. Benuto, W. O'Donohue (eds.), *Enhancing Behavioral Health in Latino Populations*, DOI 10.1007/978-3-319-42533-7_15

integrated approach to mental health treatment with a general medical approach within the same hospital, researchers found that the patients demonstrated not only greater satisfaction with the care received, but also greater participation in prevention programs. Additionally, those individuals who participated in the integrated treatment were less likely to be seen in the Emergency Room and were also demonstrated better overall improvement in symptom presentation both mentally and physically, while those in the general medical treatment model reported a physical and mental decline (Druss, Rohrbaugh, Levinson, & Rosenheck, 2001). This suggests that there is likely a lot of variability among hospitals in the care provided, which can create a disparity of outcomes between those who provide integrated care and those who do not.

For SMI, Mueser and colleagues (2003) describe the implementation and components of evidence-based practice within integrated care. These components, in an integrated setting include: collaborative psychopharmacology; assertive community treatment (ACT); family psychoeducation; supported employment; illness management and recovery and for those with comorbid substance-use disorders, integrated dual disorders treatment. While most of these interventions, on their face, are intuitively understood, ACT is a process described as an integrated approach that utilizes "assertive" community outreach to engage community providers and resources to address the comorbid issues of homelessness, unemployment, and legal entanglements that are common in SMI. For a more comprehensive understanding of ACT, one should visit their informational site (https://www.centerforebp.case.edu/resources/tools/act-getting-started-guide).

From a primary care perspective, the authors indicate a strong body of literature identifying the overriding benefits of medication in reducing symptoms associated with severe mental illness (e.g. psychosis), and the secondary ability to address underlying affective symptoms as well as greater amenability to behavioral interventions and follow-up care. However, given the side-effects and problems with compliance that arise in SMI, the integrated specialty care and selective use of neuroleptics (Whitaker, 2004), underscore the need to emphasize the latter components of Mueser, Torrey, Lynde, Singer, and Drake's (2003) recommendations (e.g. that of family psychoeducation, supported employment).

The most recent data from the National Institute of Mental Health indicate that over 4 % of the adults were diagnosed in that year with a serious mental illness (SAMHSA, 2013), constituting over nine million adults in the US who are diagnosed with a serious mental illness. Of those diagnosed with serious mental illness, Hispanics constitute a large percentage, second only to those who identify as American Indian or Native Alaskan. Additionally, McGovern and colleagues (2006) found that between 16 and 21 % of those with comorbid substance-use disorders also were diagnosed with SMI.

The Affordable Care Act and mental health parity in the U.S. has led to an expansion of coverage that should theoretically increase access to mental health treatment, and that treatment should also be largely covered by a combination of public and private insurance providers (Mechanic, 2012). This is particularly salient to the treatment of serious mental illness, which was previously costly with limited reimbursement, limiting profitability, and thus relegated the responsibility of providing services to public/state hospitals. Though budgets have been expanded to cover mental health treatment (for example California's Proposition 63 Mental Health Services Act, while in Nevada, state agencies have adopted the role of coordinating care among newly available private beds), and researchers (Patel et al., 2013) while investigating challenges in integrating mental health care called for specific emphasis on serious mental illness. However, though these changes increase coverage and in some ways improve technology that would facilitate integrated care, they do not require integrated care, which is particularly problematic when treating serious mental illness. Specific to integrated care, it is estimated that between 20 and 25 % of patients in a primary care setting have a mental illness (Spitzer, Kroenke, & Williams, 1999), with only 2/3 of those being referred for mental health treatment seeing the referral through (Grembowski et al., 2002).

The challenge with serious mental illness is daunting, due in large part to its chronic nature and high costs (estimated to be over 192 Billion annually; Insel, 2008), as well as the nature of the condition itself (e.g. psychosis and avolitional behaviors that contribute to overall poor health and quality of life). However, mental illness is not alone in being a chronic disease. Diabetes provides us with a good example of how to manage chronic, and potentially life-threatening illness with a stepped-care approach. Researchers (Von Korff, Glasgow, & Sharpe, 2002) proposed just such a process for effectively managing chronic illness that can be applied across domains.

Von Korff and colleagues (2002) suggested that the common elements to care for chronic conditions (in their case, diabetes) include not only reaction to the presenting systems, but also indicated a need to be preemptive in planning follow-up visits utilizing a protocol to implement the stepped-care. Similarly, the World Health Organization recognizing the variability in health care systems and, in particular the limited number of mental health providers, proposed a systematic approach to treating mental health diagnoses, including serious mental illness, via a stepped-care approach formally presenting this information at the 2008 Geneva Convention (WHO, 2010). Eventually, this was formalized and expanded with specific recommendations, that included recommendations at all levels of the stepped-care system (psychoeducation, community involvement, patient follow-up and monitoring, involvement of specialists, etc.) specific to the most chronic mental health issues including: substance use, psychosis, depression, and bipolar disorder as well as broader issues of Alzheimer's and developmental and childhood behavioral disorders (WHO, 2010). However, the challenge of SMI as compared to those that serve as the foundation for this model, include the severity of symptoms and a higher degree of noncompliance both as a direct (Wang, Demler, & Kessler, 2002) and indirect result of those symptoms (e.g. the loss of support benefits due to a commitment, homelessness or incarceration; Ries & Comtois, 1997).

Population Characteristics

The most recent U.S. Census data for Hispanic populations indicated over 55 million people identified as Hispanic, with California, Texas, and Florida (in rank order) having the highest numbers of Hispanics (Krogstad & Lopez, 2015). This is described as representing a slowing in the previous growth rate of 4.8 % annually (reported in the decade between 200 and 2010) to a more modest 2.1 % growth rate. However, it still represents an increase to 17.5 % of the population, meaning nearly one in five individuals identifies as Hispanic. Finally, the authors indicated that the median age for this population has increased from 27 in 2010 to 29 in 2014, which still represents a younger demographic group, when compared to non-Hispanic Blacks (34); non-Hispanic Whites (43) and Asians (36).

Prevalence Rates of Serious Mental Illness in Hispanics

As discussed in the outset of this chapter, the most recent data indicates the prevalence rate of 3.5 % for SMI in U.S. Hispanic populations, which is slightly lower than the 4.1 % prevalence rate of the overall U.S. population. This suggests a prevalence rate of SMI for Hispanics that approximate the overall population.

Barriers to Treatment in Serious Mental Illness

Across treatment domains (e.g. mental health, substance use) a primary barrier to care has been the ability to pay for the services (Mojtabai, Chen, Kaufmann, & Crum, 2014), but it is proposed that the Affordable Care Act will address this issue of affordability. However, as will be discussed below, this assumption is problematic for some Hispanics. The second most commonly reported barrier, specifically relevant to SMI, was the fear of being committed, followed by a lack of information about where to get services, and finally the perception that an individual should be able to resolve their own mental health problems. The authors also described a lack of a perceived need as a potential additional barrier, specifically in the context of those individuals with comorbid disorders of substance use and mental illness.

When we look at actual treatment rates for those with SMI we see that only 40–55 % receive "minimally adequate treatment" [this term was defined by best practices based in the empirical literature and corresponding to the diagnosis] (Wang et al., 2002). That same research also shows that among those that did not receive minimally adequate treatment over 95 % of them had a "nonaffective" psychosis (e.g. Schizophrenia). Further, the best outcomes were those that were treated by specialty mental health care and the worst outcomes were those that were treated in a general medical setting or that utilized both general and specialized care (not through a program of integrated care). Finally, specific to Hispanics, the evidence is mixed with some research (Wang et al., 2002) showing that there was a greater likelihood that Hispanics were likely to benefit from care, once accessed, as well as be more likely (as compared to non-Hispanic Whites and Black/African Americans) to be treatment compliant, which the authors attributed to a greater cultural perception of the severity of psychosis and serious mental illness. However, others found lower treatment compliance (based on a percentage of the sample rather than a comparison among ethnic and racial groups), in particular for studies that included only Hispanics (Lanouette, Folsom, Sciolla, & Jeste, 2009), which they attributed to barriers of language, affordability of the treatment regimen and related problems related to socioeconomic issues (e.g. transportation, the ability to access specific services or systems based on legal status).

Culture-Specific Barriers

From a practical standpoint, the primary barrier to treatment for Hispanics, in particular those with limited or no proficiency in English, is language. In a review of the literature Timmins (2002) found that language was a primary barrier to access to care for Hispanics, largely due to the limited number of Spanish speaking providers, as well as a lack of appropriately qualified interpreters. Specific to mental health, it has been shown that the language barrier directly leads to an overdiagnosis of SMI (Flores, 2006). Once access was achieved, a lack of a provider or interpreter for the individual's language corresponded with poorer ratings for quality of care as well as worse health outcomes. Similarly, Hispanic patients are vulnerable to the same barriers to access and treatment that exist for individuals of low socioeconomic status in general (Benuto & Leany, 2011), including issues of transportation and a general inability to navigate the healthcare system (Timmins, 2002). Though it might seem intuitive to hire interpreters for the provision of services (and research has shown that an ad-hoc interpreter is better than no interpreter; Brisset, Leanza, & Laforest, 2013), professional guilds are likely to regulate the qualifications and use of translators (e.g. the APA code of ethics related to translators) and there are potentially life altering consequences due to misinterpretation by an unqualified or poorly qualified interpreter (e.g. an inappropriate referral to child protective services for undocumented immigrants or a referral and subsequent prescription of psychotropic medication; Flores, 2006). Thus, we may wish to consider as a field a program of training or perhaps a paraprofessional field for bilingual mental health translators.

Given the aforementioned challenge of the cost of care, one needs to consider the eligibility of the Hispanic client for coverage under the Affordable Care Act. In fact, it was predicted that although differences in insured and un-insured rates among race and ethnicity would be reduced by the Affordable Care Act, Hispanics would remain underinsured (Clemans-Cope, Kenney, Buettgens, Carroll, & Blavin, 2012). This projected residual difference is posited due to the Act's application limited to "Lawfully residing immigrants". The authors also indicated a need for programs to accommodate income and language barriers as well as develop programs for retention.

Though varying to some degree across Hispanic cultures and socioeconomic status among those cultures, values related to family, interpersonal relations, and religion are most prominent. When we consider the barrier of individual's ability to address mental health cultural beliefs that one should be able to overcome any issues on their own, or a fatalistic view that the symptoms were God's will, may overlap or superimpose itself on a lack of a perceived need for services (Caplan et al., 2013; Vargas et al., 2015), and can often be seen in phrases such as "that's just how they are" or "They're just lazy (capricious, etc.)", and thus the primary care provider's awareness of this barrier is critical in this initial contact (Ishikawa et al., 2014).

Stepped-Care Approach General

Though integrated care is indicative of a systematic approach, the application has flexibility in application that is reflective of available resources. For example, Thornicroft and Tansella (2004) describe approaches that divide this systematic approach by resources. The resources are categorized into low, medium, and high (in terms of resources available), recommending lower resource areas emphasize primary care that utilizes specialists as a fallback while high resource areas would utilize outpatient teams and clinics with a high degree of specialization. Logically, medium resource areas would utilize a blend of clinics and outpatient teams dependent on available resources (e.g. if a high number of specialists were available, one could create a specialty outpatient clinic).

The notion of integrated care, and specifically integrating mental health care into primary care settings has many benefits (Patel et al., 2013) that also address barriers to health care access for minorities in general (Benuto & Leany, 2011). Primarily, integrated care is intended to improve both physical and mental health by reducing the barriers and strengthening the overall system, through a process of patient-centered care that utilizes screening in the primary or prominent care system to identify auxiliary challenges to the person as a whole (Patel et al., 2013). Researchers have shown that when integrating care, even in systems that integrate public and private services, there is a substantial cost reduction, in particular when that integrated system incorporates a system of checks for quality assurance (Unutzer et al., 2012). Further, a primary component of the ACA is a reduction in rapid readmissions (which is defined as those that occur within 30 days of the initial admission), which can result in reduced payments from insurers such as Medicare (Katon & Unützer, 2013). In a review of how stigma impacts mental health treatment Corrigan, and colleagues (2014) found that integrated care in and of itself is an evidence-based practice that has been found to help reduce stigma, and that the ability to further reduce the impact could be augmented by developing better understandings of culture-specific conceptualizations of stigma, in an effort to help provide better tailored psychoeducation for overcoming that stigma.

Both the chronic-illness approach (Von Korff et al., 2002) and the WHO mhGAP (2010, 2015) approach, lend themselves well to the current emphasis on providing culturally sensitive, person-centered treatment. This is because many of the identified components of this approach incorporate individualized treatment based on patient perspectives, which are applicable across cultures (for example identifying personal barriers to treatment implementation, but also taking into consideration individual and familial beliefs). However, this approach does not suggest avoiding best practices because of a patient's (or family's) beliefs, but rather, indicates that the team should agree upon a standard of evidence that incorporates support from a specialist for the domain of interest.

Aligning Stepped Care to Overcoming Identified Barriers

To implement effective stepped care in mental health requires systematic changes in the structure of the current healthcare system that spans from or current healthcare culture through models for provision of services, adapting current limitations in technology, payment, and ideology (Pincus et al., 2015). Researchers have suggested (through an evaluation of a cross-section of integrated models; Pincus et al., 2015) that current payment systems and structure (e.g. the private practice model of mental health services) creates challenges to implementing stepped care on a broader level that can be addressed through training (e.g. emphasizing the imperative nature and benefits of a more integrated system), but also need to be addressed through better collaboration and coordination among providers and payers of service (for example reorganizing the structure of payment to reinforce effective implementation of more cost-effective treatment).

When we consider that the primary barrier to mental health treatment is cost (Mojtabai et al., 2014), it makes sense to improve the method and systems of payment across may reduce this barrier. For example, it would be challenging to provide support services for an individual with SMI or their family, if the services are not coordinated/covered under their existing insurance. Additionally, the leveraging of technology to reduce costs and increase the number of providers, particularly in areas with low to medium resources may help overcome traditional barriers, and facilitate the integrated treatment model. For example, research (Mohr, Burns, Schueller, Clarke, & Klinkman, 2013) has shown the efficacy of telehealth for psychotherapy that, though not directly assessed for SMI, could provide the supportive home or tertiary care. Similarly, Ben-Zeev, and colleagues (2013) have shown an increasing utilization of mobile phone technology, with a high interest in utilizing the phone specifically for mental health treatment. Given the high degree of homelessness and number of emergent situations that individuals with SMI are likely to encounter, the ability to utilize this technology may serve both as a method of reducing cost, but also a method of improving the continuity of care across services (e.g. by improving the ability to coordinate supportive services and follow-up on compliance with those services). The latter issue also suggests that a primary role of behavioral health professionals (e.g. social workers and caseworkers, would be related to connecting these individuals to the supportive home or tertiary care previously discussed).

WHO mhGAP (2010, 2015)

The WHO mhGAP (2010, 2015) provides a simple to use decision-making chart (available at http://www.drugsandalcohol.ie/13984/1/WHO_mhGAP_intervention_guide.pdf) that uses color-coded decision trees and easy to identify alerts. This system can be used across disciplines, and lends itself well to overcoming many of the barriers to treatment (identified earlier), and thus can serve as the primary screening tool for primary care physicians. Though this guide is specific to nonspecialized care settings (e.g. those outside of mental health facilities) it can be beneficial to provide this resource to all providers within the integrated system for continuity of care and clarity of referral purposes.

The benefit of this guide is that it is color coded by possible disorder, and is organized into three sections classified as "assess, decide, and manage". The assessment and decision points are very brief and often include iconic indicators (e.g. "!" for potential problem issues or a pill bottle for medication decisions). A major benefit promoted by WHO is that the chart provides recommendations about "what to do, but not how to do it", with the specific intention being that the "how" of intervention is to be determined by the specialists to which the primary or secondary care provider refers the patient to.

Additionally, the mhGAP guide emphasizes six "General Principles of Care" that align with the overall notion of integrated care (e.g. that described by Pincus et al., 2015; Thornicroft & Tansella, 2004), including: communication (to include caregivers and family); assessment; treatment and monitoring; mobilizing social support; protection of human rights and overall well-being. Again, these principles provide opportunities to address culture-specific barriers, in particular at the points of communication and mobilizing social support.

mhGap is designed to be used within a system of care, thus it is assumed that the initial barrier of cost has initially been addressed once the system has been accessed. However, the aforementioned emphasis on what and not how to provide services helps to reduce costs, by allowing the administrator(s) to determine cost-effective models of specialized service. Further, because this process is one that emphasizes the protection of human it is designed to reduce unnecessary involuntary hospitalizations. The principle of communication along with processes that mobilize social supports help to reduce the stigma associated with mental health treatment, and again provides an opportunity to generate culturally appropriate interventions. Again, the actual implementation, of those culturally appropriate interventions would occur after the warm handoff, but serves primarily to reduce stigma as well as assuage concerns about hospitalization.

Kessler K6 Nonspecific Distress Scale (K6; Kessler et al., 2002)

The K6 is derived from the K10 as a screening instrument for SMI (Kessler et al., 2002). This scale, as the name implies, consists of six, self-report items scored with a value of 1–4 for each. A score greater than or equal to 13 indicates the likely presence of SMI, with some research indicating that a score between 5 and 13 indicating subthreshold clinical treatment needs (Kessler et al., 2010). Thus, this measure has been identified as a reliable and valid screen for SMI in less than 2 min. Though it does not provide the robust recommendations related to system flow and possible interventions, it is like of the most utility in a Primary Care setting. When compared to other screening instruments (e.g. the WHO-DAS or the CIDI-SF and even the K10) it has the greatest sensitivity, takes the least amount of time to administer and is the least cumbersome to administer (Kessler et al., 2003). Thus, this measure appears to be the most pragmatic screener in a primary care setting.

Primary Care in Behavioral Health Settings

Given the aforementioned issues of co-occurring chronic health conditions and SMI, it is likely that a PCP would be co-located in a Behavioral Health Setting. The intent being to facilitate access to ongoing care and increased treatment compliance for chronic health issues such as diabetes and obesity. SAMSHA and HRSA have developed specific funding to study the integration of primary care in behavioral health settings (PCBHI Grants), but early research has been variable in terms of identifying clear determinants or predictors of success in treatment, with researchers most often citing difficulties related to licensing, patient recruitment as well as patient and staff retention as confounds in the evaluation of the programs (Gerity, n.d.; Scharf et al., 2013). Nevertheless, those studies describe perceptions about benefits that include the ability to collaborate and share patient healthcare information that are continuing to be studied, especially in light of their report that many states are now legislating required integration of PCP care in behavioral healthcare settings.

Recommendations

As discussed, a primary issue for treating Hispanic patients with SMI, is the need to incorporate Spanish, medical interpreters (specifically interpreters with sufficient mental health training) and bilingual practitioners (as well as paraprofessionals) into the primary care setting. It may well be time to create a program of training of Associate or Bachelor's level paraprofessionals who are bilingual, in order to fill the gap of non-Spanish speaking providers.

Once we can overcome the logistical issues of language, there is an overarching need to improve understanding of the process of stepped care in mental health in general, and specific to this chapter, a need to improve the understanding across practitioners who service individuals with serious mental illness. A primary resource guide to help improve understanding and expectations is the mhGAP intervention guide for mental, neurological, and substance-use disorders in nonspecialized health settings (WHO, 2015).

Though the guide provides the foundation and explicit protocols for implementing stepped care, many of the identified barriers to implementation are issues related to real costs and availability of providers, which has consistently been identified as the most prominent barrier to mental health treatment in general. As discussed, the implementation of stepped care has the potential to reduce costs across a variety of systems, primarily through early identification and intervention for historically chronic and thus expensive mental health problems. If we recall the recommendations of Thornicroft and Tansella (2004) the goal is to provide the services within the system that exists, and this is true for mhGAP guidelines, which were designed to raise global standards of care for SMI. However, in terms of sheer efficiency, the K6 appears to serve as an excellent screener for identifying SMI, and taking the next step in handing off the patient to a behavioral healthcare specialist.

Particularly relevant to the issue of SMI, the next largest barrier to cost (involuntary commitment; Mojtabai et al., 2014) is a real and salient issue. Thus, practitioners, and more importantly health care administrators, need to create and or evaluate their integrated care system to ensure it not only supports a program that reduces the probability of hospitalization, but also a system that promotes education and a message for how intermediate services can reduce or prevent the likelihood of hospitalizing an individual with SMI. This is a role that can be largely accomplished by non-primary care practitioners, and paraprofessionals.

We need to train and utilize new types of healthcare works to fill the intermediary steps that are shown to be part of an effective process of reducing costs and maintaining mental health. In developed systems, such as the U.S., the challenge is not just the cost, but the coordination among professional licensing boards to define what these positions are, and are not. Specific to Hispanic patients, these newly trained workers would benefit by introducing more individuals who are fluent in Spanish at critical points in the stepped-care process (e.g. psychoeducation, social skills training, and monitoring). Given the critical role of monitoring, it is important that the individual have a clinical base of knowledge to assess compliance with treatment recommendations (e.g. at least a rudimentary ability to assess mental status, for example to assess and report back to other members of the treatment community about compliance, noncompliance or potential points of intervention such as stressors or failed interventions).

In addition to trained professionals and paraprofessionals, the role of nonprofessionals plays a critical role, in particular for psychosocial interventions, specifically those recommended (Dua et al., 2011) for vocational and economic inclusion as well as those designed to improve community attitudes. For the Hispanic population, this would include community outreach that includes both monolingual

Spanish speakers as well as bilingual community members. Given the research (Clarke et al., 2000) on re-hospitalization and other negative outcomes (e.g. homelessness and arrest) which is directly correlated to the time to implementation of comprehensive support services, the primary importance of these nonprofessionals is ensuring the continuity of care by persisting in implementing the external support systems as the patients transition from inpatient settings back to the community.

References

Ben-Zeev, D., Davis, K. E., Kaiser, S., Krzsos, I., & Drake, R. E. (2013). Mobile technologies among people with serious mental illness: Opportunities for future services. *Administration and Policy in Mental Health and Mental Health Services Research, 40*(4), 340–343.

Benuto, L., & Leany, B. D. (2011). Reforms for ethnic minorities and women. Understanding the behavioral healthcare crisis: The promise of integrated care and diagnostic reform, 367–394.

Brisset, C., Leanza, Y., & Laforest, K. (2013). Working with interpreters in health care: a systematic review and meta-ethnography of qualitative studies. *Patient Education and Counseling, 91*(2), 131–140.

Caplan, S., Escobar, J., Paris, M., Alvidrez, J., Dixon, J. K., Desai, M. M., … Whittemore, R. (2013). Cultural influences on causal beliefs about depression among Latino immigrants. *Journal of Transcultural Nursing, 24(1)*, 68–77.

Clarke, G. N., Herinckx, H. A., Kinney, R. F., Paulson, R. I., Cutler, D. L., Lewis, K., & Oxman, E. (2000). Psychiatric hospitalizations, arrests, emergency room visits, and homelessness of clients with serious and persistent mental illness: Findings from a randomized trial of two ACT programs vs. usual care. *Mental Health Services Research, 2(3)*, 155–164.

Clemans-Cope, L., Kenney, G. M., Buettgens, M., Carroll, C., & Blavin, F. (2012). The Affordable Care Act's coverage expansions will reduce differences in uninsurance rates by race and ethnicity. *Health Affairs (Millwood), 31*, 920.

Corrigan, P. W., Druss, B. G., & Perlick, D. A. (2014). The impact of mental illness stigma on seeking and participating in mental health care. *Psychological Science in the Public Interest, 15*(2), 37–70.

Druss, B. G., Rohrbaugh, R. M., Levinson, C. M., & Rosenheck, R. A. (2001). Integrated medical care for patients with serious psychiatric illness: A randomized trial. *Archives of General Psychiatry, 58*(9), 861–868.

Dua, T., Barbui, C., Clark, N., Fleischmann, A., Poznyak, V., van Ommeren, M., … Saxena, S. (2011). Evidence-based guidelines for mental, neurological, and substance use disorders in low-and middle-income countries: summary of WHO recommendations. *PLoS Medicine, 8(11)*, e1001122.

Flores, G. (2006). Language barriers to health care in the United States. *New England Journal of Medicine, 355*(3), 229–231.

Gerrity, M. (n.d.) *Integrating primary care into behavioral health settings: What works*. Retrieved from http://www.integration.samhsa.gov/integrated-care-models/Integrating-Primary-Care-Report.pdf.

Grembowski, D. E., Martin, D., Patrick, D. L., Diehr, P., Katon, W., Williams, B., … Goldberg, H. I. (2002). Managed care, access to mental health specialists, and outcomes among primary care patients with depressive symptoms. *Journal of General Internal Medicine, 17*, 258–69.

Insel, T. R. (2008). Assessing the ECONOMIC COSTS OF SERIOUS MENTAL ILLNESS. *The American Journal of Psychiatry, 165*(6), 663–665. See more at: https://www.nami.org/Learn-More/Mental-Health-By-the-Numbers#sthash.OqF9reiH.dpuf.

Ishikawa, R. Z., Cardemil, E. V., Alegría, M., Schuman, C. C., Joseph, R. C., & Bauer, A. M. (2014). Uptake of depression treatment recommendations among Latino primary care patients. *Psychological Services, 11*(4), 421.
Katon, W. J., & Unützer, J. (2013). Health reform and the Affordable Care Act: the importance of mental health treatment to achieving the triple aim. *Journal of Psychosomatic Research, 74*(6), 533.
Kessler, R. C., Andrews, G., Colpe, L. J., Hiripi, E., Mroczek, D. K., Normand, S. L., … Zaslavsky, A. M. (2002). Short screening scales to monitor population prevalences and trends in non-specific psychological distress. *Psychological medicine, 32(6)*, 959–976.
Kessler, R. C., Barker, P. R., Colpe, L. J., Epstein, J. F., Gfroerer, J. C., Hiripi, E., … Zaslavsky, A. M. (2003). Screening for serious mental illness in the general population. *Archives of General Psychiatry, 60(2)*, 184–189.
Kessler, R. C., Green, J. G., Gruber, M. J., Sampson, N. A., Bromet, E., Cuitan, M., … Lara, C. (2010). Screening for serious mental illness in the general population with the K6 screening scale: Results from the WHO World Mental Health (WMH) survey initiative. *International Journal of Methods in Psychiatric Research, 19(1)*, 4.
Krogstad, J. M., & Lopez, H. M. (2015). *Hispanic population reaches record 55 million, but growth has cooled.* The Pew Research Center. Retrieved from http://www.pewresearch.org/fact-tank/2015/06/25/u-s-hispanic-population-growth-surge-cools/.
Lanouette, N. M., Folsom, D. P., Sciolla, A., & Jeste, D. V. (2009). Psychotropic medication non-adherence among United States Latinos: A comprehensive literature review. *Psychiatric Services, 60*, 157.
McGovern, M. P., Xie, H., Segal, S. R., Siembab, L., & Drake, R. E. (2006). Addiction treatment services and co-occurring disorders: Prevalence estimates, treatment practices, and barriers. *Journal of Substance Abuse Treatment, 31*(3), 267–275.
Mechanic, D. (2012). Seizing opportunities under the Affordable Care Act for transforming the mental and behavioral health system. *Health Affairs, 31*(2), 376–382.
Mohr, D. C., Burns, M. N., Schueller, S. M., Clarke, G., & Klinkman, M. (2013). Behavioral intervention technologies: Evidence review and recommendations for future research in mental health. *General Hospital Psychiatry, 35*(4), 332–338.
Mojtabai, R., Chen, L. Y., Kaufmann, C. N., & Crum, R. M. (2014). Comparing barriers to mental health treatment and substance use disorder treatment among individuals with comorbid major depression and substance use disorders. *Journal of Substance Abuse Treatment, 46*(2), 268–273.
Mueser, K. T., Torrey, W. C., Lynde, D., Singer, P., & Drake, R. E. (2003). Implementing evidence-based practices for people with severe mental illness. *Behavior Modification, 27*(3), 387–411.
Patel, V., Belkin, G. S., Chockalingam, A., Cooper, J., Saxena, S., & Unützer, J. (2013). Grand challenges: integrating mental health services into priority health care platforms. PLoS Med, 10(5), e1001448.
Pincus, H. A., Jun, M., Franx, G., van der Feltz-Cornelis, C., Ito, H., & Mossialos, E. (2015). How can we link general medical and behavioral health care? International models for practice and policy. *Psychiatric Services, 66*, 775.
Ries, R. K., & Comtois, K. A. (1997). Illness severity and treatment services for dually diagnosed severely mentally ill outpatients. *Schizophrenia Bulletin, 23*(2), 239.
Scharf, D. M., Eberhart, N. K., Schmidt, N., Vaughan, C. A., Dutta, T., Pincus, H. A., & Burnam, M. A. (2013). Integrating primary care into community behavioral health settings: Programs and early implementation experiences. *Psychiatric Services, 64*, 660.
Spitzer, R. L., Kroenke, K., & Williams, J. B. (1999). Validation and utility of a self-report version of PRIME-MD: The PHQ primary care study. Primary care evaluation of mental disorders. Patient health questionnaire. *JAMA, 282*, 1737–1744.
Substance Abuse and Mental Health Services Administration. (2013). *Results from the 2012 National survey on drug use and health: Mental health findings, NSDUH series H-47, HHS publication no. (SMA) 13-4805*. Rockville, MD: Author.

Thornicroft, G., & Tansella, M. (2004). Components of a modern mental health service: A pragmatic balance of community and hospital care Overview of systematic evidence. *The British Journal of Psychiatry, 185*(4), 283–290.

Timmins, C. L. (2002). The impact of language barriers on the health care of Latinos in the United States: a review of the literature and guidelines for practice. *Journal of Midwifery & Women's Health, 47*(2), 80–96.

Unutzer, J., Chan, Y. F., Hafer, E., Knaster, J., Shields, A., Powers, D., & Veith, R. C. (2012). Quality improvement with pay-for-performance incentives in integrated behavioral health care. *American Journal of Public Health, 102*, e41–e45.

Vargas, S. M., Cabassa, L. J., Nicasio, A., De La Cruz, A. A., Jackson, E., Rosario, M., … Lewis-Fernández, R. (2015). Toward a cultural adaptation of pharmacotherapy: Latino views of depression and antidepressant therapy. *Transcultural Psychiatry, 52*(2), 244–273.

Von Korff, M., Glasgow, R. E., & Sharpe, M. (2002). ABC of psychological medicine: Organising care for chronic illness. *BMJ [British Medical Journal], 325*(7355), 92.

Wang, P. S., Demler, O., & Kessler, R. C. (2002). Adequacy of treatment for serious mental illness in the United States. *American Journal of Public Health, 92*(1), 92–98.

Whitaker, R. (2004). The case against antipsychotic drugs: a 50-year record of doing more harm than good. *Medical Hypotheses, 62*(1), 5–13.

World Health Organization. (2010). *Mental Health Gap Action Programme: MhGAP intervention guide for mental, neurological and substance use disorders in non-specialized health settings: Version 1.0*. Geneva: World Health Organization.

World Health Organization. (2015). MhGAP intervention guide for mental, neurological and substance use disorders in non-specialized health settings. *The Lancet, 376*, 1274.

Chapter 16
Marital Problems and Relationship Difficulties and Integrated Care Among Hispanic Populations

Kristin M. Lindahl and Sara Wigderson

Health disparities are vast for Hispanic families in the United States and access to behavioral health care may be particularly underutilized (U.S. Dept. of Health and Human Services, 2001). For example, several studies suggest that Hispanics, as compared to non-Hispanic Whites, are less likely to receive appropriate care for disorders related to depression or anxiety (Alegría, Jackson, Kessler, & Takeuchi, 2008; Young, Klap, Sherbourne, & Wells, 2001). Data are lacking, however, for other domains of mental health such as marital distress. Marital distress, despite its known links with poorer mental and physical health (Kiecolt-Glaser & Newton, 2001; Papp, Goeke-Morey, & Cummings, 2004), has received scant attention in the health disparities field of study.

Though limited in scope and quantity, research to date suggests that Hispanic couples experience marital distress at a similar rate to other couples, at least as compared to non-Hispanic white couples (Bulanda & Brown, 2007). In addition, as has been found with other couples, marital distress is both longitudinally and cross-sectionally related to depressive symptoms for Hispanic couples (Hollist, Miller, Falceto, & Fernandez, 2007; Treviño, Wooten, & Scott, 2007). Given that Hispanics now comprise the largest minority group in the United States and the proportion of married couples that are Hispanic doubled between 1980 and 2000 (Amato, Johnson, Booth, & Rogers, 2003), a research base on marital quality for Hispanics is long overdue. Some studies suggest that marital functioning for Hispanic couples more closely resembles non-Hispanic whites than Blacks (Bulanda & Brown, 2007), but very little is known about what factors might be uniquely important to Hispanic couples.

One movement that is actively gaining traction to try and reduce health care disparities is the integrated care model whereby medical and behavioral health

K.M. Lindahl, Ph.D. (✉) • S. Wigderson
Department of Psychology, University of Miami, Coral Gables,
FL 33124-0751, USA
e-mail: kristin.lindahl@gmail.com

© Springer International Publishing Switzerland 2016
L.T. Benuto, W. O'Donohue (eds.), *Enhancing Behavioral Health in Latino Populations*, DOI 10.1007/978-3-319-42533-7_16

professionals work side-by-side and in concert with one another. Numerous empirically supported programs and interventions exist to reduce and alleviate marital or couple distress, but given the separate silos medical and behavioral health professionals have historically worked in, it is likely the exception far more than the rule that distressed couples find their way to marital therapy or a marital educational group via their primary care physician. The goals of this chapter are to provide a brief review of marital distress and its impact on individual functioning, an overview of integrated behavioral health care and a stepped care model for addressing marital distress, including attention to cultural considerations and how they can be applied to interventions for marital distress to better serve Hispanic couples, and a review of the types of empirically supported marital interventions that are available.

Relationship Health

Social relationships affect mental health, health behavior, and physical health (Umberson & Montez, 2010) and perhaps no social relationship affects adult well-being as much as the marital relationship. Many couples will encounter difficulty at some point in their relationship and if these problems are not ameliorated, a whole host of potential negative consequences can occur for both the couple, and if there are children, their family. It is estimated that about one-third of couples experience distress or discord at any one point in time (Whisman, Beach, & Snyder, 2008). Marital satisfaction drops considerably over the first 10 years of marriage (Bradbury, Fincham, & Beach, 2000) and chronic relationship distress can sufficiently erode the positive elements of a relationship such that couples ultimately divorce. Divorce is common in the United States and it is estimated that nearly 50 % of marriages end within the first 20 years (Copen, Daniels, Vespa, & Mosher, 2012). Marital distress also is associated with an increased risk for a variety of psychiatric concerns including anxiety, mood, bipolar, and substance-abuse disorders (Whisman, 2007) as well as compromised endocrine and immune functioning (Kiecolt-Glaser & Newton, 2001).

The limited literature to date suggests that, overall, Hispanic couples are at similar risk for marital difficulties as non-Hispanic Whites. Confounding effects of ethnicity and economic stress, however, may place some Hispanic couples at higher risk. Negy and Snyder (2000) found inter-ethnic and non-Hispanic White couples to be similar in their levels of marital satisfaction; however, monoethnic Mexican-American couples experienced less satisfaction compared to inter-ethnic couples. Several studies suggest that external stressors impact marital satisfaction indirectly for non-Hispanic White couples and a couple of recent studies suggest that this is the case for Hispanic couples as well. In a study of 120 first-generation Mexican immigrant couples, Helms et al. (2014) found economic pressure and cultural adaptation stress to be linked with depressive symptoms, which in turn was associated with negativity in marital interaction and low marital satisfaction. Similarly,

Falconier, Nussbeck, and Bodenmann (2013) found how couples cope can mitigate the link between immigration stress and marital satisfaction for Hispanic couples, especially for wives.

Although research is starting to grow with Hispanic couples, relatively few studies have focused on issues that may be specifically relevant to Hispanic couples. One of the issues that has been the subject of several studies, however, is that of acculturation or acculturative stress. Acculturation can be operationalized in different ways, but it commonly refers to the degree to which an individual endorses beliefs, attitudes, and behaviors of their culture of origin, the dominant culture in their new environment, or both (Negy & Snyder, 1997). A couple of studies suggest a link between acculturation and marital distress for Mexican Americans (Negy & Snyder, 2000; Vega, Kolody, & Valle, 1988), and Negy, Hammons, Reig-Ferrer, and Carper (2010) found acculturative stress to be associated with marital distress in a sample of Hispanic immigrant women. Acculturation differences between husbands and wives also have been linked to lower marital quality in Mexican-origin couples, with the relationship between acculturation (adoption of American cultural practices) and enculturation (maintenance or retention of culture of origin) implicated in understanding the complex role of acculturation and how it relates to relationship functioning (Cruz et al., 2014). Cruz and colleagues found cultural similarities between couples to generally be associated with positive marital quality, though interactive effects between acculturation and enculturation show the importance of assessing cultural orientation in a multi-dimensional manner. In addition, generation status, which is often considered a marker for acculturation, also has been linked to marital distress for Hispanic couples (e.g., Casas & Ortiz, 1985). Although findings are varied, studies tend to find greater marital distress for couples with higher levels of acculturation toward the dominant culture, especially when wives are more dominant-culture oriented than husbands. An assessment of acculturation would seem to be a potentially important component when conducting a culturally sensitive marital intervention.

Integrated Care and Hispanic Families

Hispanic families are the largest ethnic minority in the United States. Estimates project that by 2050, Hispanic families will make up nearly 30 % of the U.S. population (Ennis, Rios-Vargas, & Albert, 2011; Gutierrez, Barden, & Tobey, 2014; Passel & Cohn, 2008). In recent decades, the United States has made significant efforts to improve the quality of health care and access to health care and reduce disparities, but ongoing economic, social, and racial/ethnic disparities continue to exist. In fact, with regard to Hispanics specifically, according to the 2012 report of the Roundtable on the Promotion of Health Equity and the Elimination of Health Disparities, health disparities between Hispanics and other populations have minimally improved over the last decade. Underutilization of mental health care in particular is an area of growing concern (Gutierrez et al., 2014). Even when differences in the prevalence of mental health difficulties are controlled for, Hispanics are less likely to access mental health services than non-Hispanic Whites (Cabassa, Zayas, & Hansen, 2006).

Numerous economic factors are cited as contributing to the disparity in health care access including financial limitations and geographical concerns (Gutierrez et al., 2014). The socioeconomic status of Hispanic couples in the United States is difficult to summarize globally as they occupy all rungs of the socioeconomic ladder. Given the diverse cultural, political, and economic circumstances in their heritages that lead them or their forebearers to immigrate to this country, even the terms "Hispanic" and "Latino" are so broad and encompassing that many of the differences within this large group are lost. Nonetheless, on average and a collective group, Hispanics are more likely to experience economic distress than non-Hispanic whites and overall, they have lower levels of educational achievement than non-Hispanic whites (Casper & Bianchi, 2002; Fronczek, 2005). Hispanics also have substantially higher uninsured rates than non-Hispanic whites (CDC, 2011). All of these socioeconomic factors may inhibit access to care. In addition, economic instability is stressful for couples and may negatively affect the quality and stability of marriages (Conger, Conger, & Martin, 2010). Thus, economic struggles may not only be associated with marital stress but also may present a barrier to accessing interventions that might provide some relief.

Sociocultural factors also are cited as potential barriers to Hispanics receiving comparable mental health services as their non-Hispanic White counterparts. English language proficiency, for example, is a notable predictor of health care usage (Fiscella, Franks, Doescher, & Saver, 2002). A lack of Spanish-speaking providers likely limits mental health care utilization for many individuals. Some Hispanic individuals also may also fear questions about citizenship or risk of deportation (Shattell, Hamilton, Starr, Jenkins, & Hinderliter, 2008). Concerns about the cultural sensitivity of interventions is another concern for Hispanics seeking mental health services and culturally relevant services that are grounded in empirical science are in insufficient supply to keep up with demand (Flores, Olson, & Tomany-Korman, 2005). Even once services are accessed, less than optimal outcomes may result for Hispanics due to premature termination (Kouyoumdjian, Zamboanga, & Hansenmn, 2003). Some of the reasons for leaving therapy early are likely culturally related, including possible unintentional biases on the part of service providers (Bridges et al., 2014) and Vasquez (2007) found that ethnic minority clients may not establish as strong a therapeutic alliance with the service provider as majority culture White clients, especially when the care provider is White. For all of the above reasons, Hispanics have less access to and receive fewer mental health services than do non-Hispanic whites even though studies suggest that rates of mental health concerns are comparable across the two groups (U.S. Dept. of Health and Human Services, 2001).

One potential means to overcoming utilization disparities is through integrated health care. Integrated health care is an approach to health care that is characterized by a high degree of collaboration and communication among health professionals. In the broadest use of the term, "integrated behavioral health care" (IBHC) describes health care settings where behavioral health and medical providers work together. Integrated care can occur along a continuum of collaboration, however, from minimally to fully integrated. As articulated by Blount (1998), in the fully integrated model, there is close collaboration between behavioral health and medical professionals and they share the same sites, vision, and systems. All providers are "on the same team" and have developed an in-depth understanding of each other's roles and areas of expertise. In this scenario, facilities are shared and collaborative routines are regular and smooth. All providers chart in the same patient medical record and may even see clients together when this is appropriate. Informal consultation between health and mental health care workers occurs regularly.

Initial presentation in an integrated care clinic. Integrating mental health care into primary care services may be one way to reduce barriers to accessing services for Hispanic couples (Bridges et al., 2014). Some studies suggest that Hispanics are more likely to seek mental health care services from their primary care setting as compared to any other resources, including specialty mental health care (Bridges et al., 2014; Vega, Kolody, Aguilar-Gaxiola, & Catalano, 1999). Although primary care physicians often have limited training in the assessment, diagnosis, and treatment of mental health problems (Mitchell, Vaze, & Rao, 2009), this issue can be more easily overcome in an IBHC setting as compared to a traditional care setting.

There are several ways in which an individual with significant marital distress may initially present at an integrated care clinic with a concern other than marital problems. Mental health concerns often co-occur with medical conditions or can mimic medical conditions. For example, an individual might present with symptoms related to anxiety/depression, either with or without a co-occurring with a medical condition, or mood symptoms may be attributed to a medical condition (e.g., heart problem) that does not exist. Maritally distressed individuals also are overrepresented in those seeking help for psychological difficulties, regardless of whether or not marital distress is reported as one of their primary concerns (Lin, Goering, Offord, Campbell, & Boyle, 1996). Thus, for a variety of reasons, individuals may seek services from their primary care physician for needs that go beyond physical conditions and ailments, and may well include mental health issues.

Numerous studies indicate a bidirectional relationship between marital or couple functioning and mental health. In contrast to happily married persons, maritally distressed individuals are three time more likely to have a mood disorder (e.g., Whisman, 2001, 2007). Although depression may be the most common type of psychological disorder to be reciprocally related to marital distress, individuals in distressed or conflictual relationships are also more vulnerable to anxiety disorders and substance-use problems (Proulx, Helms, & Buehler, 2007; Whisman, 2007). Links between marital quality and risk for a psychological disorder have been replicated across numerous racial and ethnic groups, including several groups of Hispanic heritage (McShall & Johnson, 2015).

Couple distress also is associated with poor physical health (Umberson, Williams, Powers, Liu, & Needham, 2006). Marital conflict, in particular, has been shown to have direct adverse effects on cardiovascular, endocrine, immune, neurosensory, and other physiological systems that, in turn, can contribute to physical health problems (Kiecolt-Glaser & Newton, 2001). Whisman and Uebelacker (2012) found poor marital adjustment and divorce to be associated with risk for metabolic syndrome in women, and marital loss is associated with increased risk for cardiovascular disease (Zhang & Hayward, 2006).

Screening measures for marital distress. Given known links between emotional distress and marital difficulties, as part of the screening process to determine etiology of a presenting problem, one logical step for physicians is to utilize screening measures to detect for possible marital distress. Simple and short screening measures exist for marital distress and if these were given routinely by primary care physicians, with individuals with higher scores to be scheduled for a follow-up consult with a mental health specialist, many more couples may be referred to appropriate support and intervention.

Fortunately, several empirically supported screening measures for marital distress exist. One of the shortest questionnaires, containing just four items, is the Couple Satisfaction Index (CSI; Funk & Rogge, 2007). To develop the CSI, 176 potential items were culled from eight well-validated self-report measures of marital satisfaction. Using principal components analysis and item response theory, 32 items were selected for the CSI and then shorter versions of this measure were created by identifying the items that provided the largest amount information for the assessment of relationship satisfaction. The CSI items assess global satisfaction with the relationship and are rated on Likert-scales ranging from 0 to 6 or 0 to 5, with total scores ranging from 0 to 21. The cut-off score for marital distress is 13.5. The 4-item version of the CSI has demonstrated good convergent and construct validity and higher precision measurement of marital satisfaction than longer measures such as the Marital Adjustment Test (MAT; Locke & Wallace, 1959) and the Dyadic Adjustment Scale (DAS; Spanier, 1976).

Another recently developed questionnaire to assess for marital distress that is brief is the Marital Satisfaction Inventory-Brief form (MSI-B; Balderrama-Durbin, Snyder, & Balsis, 2015). The MSI-B is a shorter version of the Marital Satisfaction Inventory-Revised (Whisman et al., 2008). The MSI-B contains 10 items and total scores range from 0 to 10, with higher scores indicating greater distress. The MSI-B shows excellent discriminant validity in being able to distinguish community from clinical samples and scores ≥ 4 are classified as significantly distressed. Although the original MSI-R has been successfully translated and validated for use in Spanish (Negy & Snyder, 2000), and thus translation of the ten items of the MSI-B are available in Spanish, the MSI-B itself has yet to be formally assessed for reliability and validity in Spanish. Nonetheless, the impressive empirical care that has gone into translating the MSI-R items is a significant advantage of the MSI-B for cross-cultural samples.

Sabourin, Valois, and Lussier (2005) created the DAS(4) by using nonparametric IRT (Hambleton, Swaminathan, & Rogers, 1991) on the 32 items of the DAS to select the four items that consistently provided the most information at the distress threshold. Scores <13 are classified as distressed. The DAS-4 is as effective in predicting couple dissolution as the DAS-32 and is less affected by socially desirable responding. The DAS-4 also shows good stability over time.

The Quality of Marriage Index (QMI; Norton, 1983) is a 6-item measure of global relationship satisfaction. Five items are rated on Likert-scales which range from 1 to 7 (e.g., "We have a good relationship") and one item, regarding overall level of happiness in the marriage is rated on a scale that ranges from 1 to 10. Total scores range is from 6 to 45, with higher scores indicating greater satisfaction with the marriage. The QMI is well validated and has been shown to have good reliability (e.g., Funk & Rogge, 2007).

A stepped-care approach. Once marital distress is identified as a potentially contributing factor to an individual's distress, a behavioral health professional can intervene and in coordination with integrated care, a stepped-care model within ICBH can be applied. A stepped-care approach within an integrated care setting could include the following three sequentially organized steps.

As a first step, especially if marital distress is mild, information on relationship success could be provided to the individual in the form of handouts, bibliotherapy references, or e-health options. One of the more popular books written for couples to educate and assist them in improving their relationship quality is, The Seven Principles for Making Marriage Work, written by John M. Gottman, Ph.D., and Nan Silver. This book is also available in Spanish, Los Siete Pricipios para Hacer que el Matrimonio Funcione. On line, several websites are available to educate and assist couples about relationship health, including www.healthymarriageinfo.org, which also has most of its materials available in Spanish.

In addition to providing individuals with sources of information and education about marriage, another Step 1 intervention might be for behavioral health professionals to help clients engage in prevention programs. Several marriage and relationship education programs have been designed as preventative options for couples and for individuals with low or mild distress, these might be a good option. In a recent and inclusive meta-analysis of relationship education programs, Hawkins and colleagues (Hawkins, Blanchard, Baldwin, & Fawcett, 2008) found that relationship education programs result in increases in communication skills and relationship quality (small to medium effect sizes). Similarly, Stanley, Amato, Johnson, and Markman (2006) found that premarital education was associated with a lower divorce rate and was effective at enhancing satisfaction and commitment and lowering levels of conflict for couples of various races and income levels. In this study, Latinos participated in marital education programs at a rate similar to that of non-Hispanic Whites (and more so than Black couples) and also benefited similarly. This study is important as it among the few that have targeted a diverse and/or disadvantaged sample.

One of the more popular evidence-based programs aimed at preventing marital distress is the Prevention and Relationship Education Program (PREP; Markman, Renick, Floyd, Stanley, & Clements, 1993), which teaches couples communication and conflict resolution skills that are associated with marital success. The program utilizes features of behavioral and cognitive therapy, while placing particular emphasis on the problem-solving skills component. At a 5-year follow-up, PREP demonstrated effectiveness with couples in the program having higher levels of positive communication skills, lower levels of negative communication, and lower levels of marital violence compared to controls (Markman et al., 1993). A recent RCT of PREP used by couples through religious organizations, however, suggested that there were no overall differences in the divorce rate for couples using PREP versus naturally occurring services (i.e. premarital education provided by religious organizations; Markman, Rhoades, Stanley, & Peterson, 2013). PREP is one of the few programs that has begun to be empirically tested with underserved ethnic minority groups. Daire et al. (2012) conducted focus groups with Hispanic individuals who had completed 20 h of marital relationship education using a PREP-based curriculum. Participants reported learning and acquiring new communication skills and they also reported an increase in peace and calm at home.

There is some evidence that it may not be necessary to have intensive preventative education programs in order to achieve some measure of success. Rogge and colleagues (Rogge, Cobb, Lawrence, Johnson, & Bradbury, 2013) compared two time intensive relationship education programs, PREP and CARE, the latter being designed specifically for the trial, with a one session relationship awareness (RA) program. The RA program did not focus on building relationship skills but instead focused on increasing partners' awareness of the relationship through looking at current behaviors and deciding if these behaviors were constructive or destructive. There were no differences in relationship dissolution or satisfaction between couples receiving the time intensive skills training (PREP and CARE) and those in the RA session, suggesting that more intensive preventative education programs may be unnecessary, at least for some couples. The long-term effectiveness the RA session is not clear, however.

If Step 1 options are insufficient, Step 2 options that could be considered by the behavioral health professional might include brief or web-based interventions. One evidence-based brief intervention option for distressed couples is the Marriage-Checkup (MC; Cordova et al., 2014). The MC was designed to fill the gap between preventative relationship education and tertiary treatment by serving as a brief intervention for couples who are at risk for marital deterioration, but who are not otherwise seeking treatment for their marriage. The MC is a two-session assessment and feedback intervention which is designed for early problem detection and early intervention. In an RCT of the MC, Cordova et al. (2014) found that when compared to a control condition, the MC results in improvements in relationship satisfaction, intimacy, and acceptance. The effect sizes for MC were similar to other marital education programs and gains in intimacy and acceptance were maintained at the 2-year follow-up, when comparisons were made with the control group. The authors suggest that similarly to a yearly doctor visit, the MC should be provided annually to couples.

Web-based marital interventions have started to become popular in recent years and they address both preventative goals as well as provide interventions for distressed couples. Marital programs accessed via the internet address many obstacles couples commonly cite as interfering with treatment-seeking, such as financial limitations, geographical concerns, and the shame an individual or couple may feel by attending therapy (Hoge et al., 2004). Several web-based interventions have been developed to target relationship distress and these programs are often adaptations of previously proven in-person relationship education programs and couple therapies. ePREP, an online version of the PREP relationship program, was found to be effective at improving mental health and relationship relevant outcomes at a 10-month follow up as compared to a control condition (Braithwaite & Fincham, 2009). Another online relationship education program is "Power of Two Online". After completing the 2-month online program, participants reported improved marital satisfaction and conflict management compared to participants in a control condition (Kalinka, Fincham, & Hirsch, 2012). OurRelationship.com is a new web-based couple intervention program aimed at reducing couple distress (Doss, Benson, Georgia, & Christensen, 2013). An adaptation of IBCT, couples are taken through a three-step program aimed at increasing their awareness of a "core issue" in the couple's relationship, promoting acceptance of their partner's feelings and opinions around this issue, and learning skills that can help them talk about and work through their core issue. Web-based programs would seem to have a lot to offer Hispanic couples as the delivery of culturally responsive content could be individualized for couples. Increasing awareness of lower cost interventions such as on-line programs may be an important step for increasing access to marital interventions and this could easily be implemented in an integrated care setting, especially if primary care physicians were educated about these options.

For more severely distressed couples, or for couples for him Step 1 and Step 2 options were not effective or were not sufficient, several empirically supported, in-person treatment options exist. In a meta-analytic review of marital interventions for distressed couples, Shadish and Baldwin (2003) found a large effect size for marriage therapy. Specifically, the effect size for marriage therapy was $d=0.84$, suggesting that couples receiving marital therapy have more favorable outcomes than more than 80 % of couples who do not receive treatment. A more recent study found couple therapy to positively impact 70 % of couples receiving treatment (Lebow, Chambers, Christensen, & Johnson, 2012). Although these findings are very promising, it is important to note that most intervention studies for couples are based on samples where the majority of couples are White and middle class (and generally well educated). Limited data exist on how effective these interventions are with more diverse samples, but one of the purposes of this chapter is to consider how to apply these interventions to Hispanic couples.

There are a variety of evidence-based treatments that couples can choose from, with behavioral marital/couple therapy (BMT or BCT) being one of the most commonly studied approaches. BCT typically consists of some combination of communication training, problem-solving training, contingency contracting, behavior exchange, cognitive restructuring, and emotional expressiveness training. BCT has been evaluated in multiple randomized controlled trials, and Shadish and Baldwin (2005) conducted a meta-analysis to evaluate the overall effectiveness of BCT. The authors found an average effect size of $d=0.59$, which suggests that couples receiving BCT were better off than 72 % of couples who did not receive treatment.

However, the authors concluded that BCT did not necessarily result in better outcomes when compared to other forms of couple therapy. The outcomes generally assessed in studies of BCT include a variety of factors such as relationship satisfaction, improvement in desired areas of change for partners, and being indistinguishable from normative nondistressed couples (Halford, Sanders, & Behrens, 1993; Jacobson & Follette, 1985). More specifically, BCT can produce positive changes in the amount of direct expression, acceptance, and positive nonverbal behavior while decreasing the amount of critique, refusal, and negative nonverbal behavior (Hahlweg, Revenstorf, & Schindler, 1984).

Another couple intervention that has been evaluated in multiple trials is emotionally focused couple therapy (EFCT). This therapy focuses on relationships from an attachment perspective and emphasizes the formation of emotional responses that prime bonding events to then create new patterned, constructive cycles of caring within couples (Johnson, Hunsley, Greenberg, & Schindler, 1999). The therapy consists of nine steps as outlined in a meta-analytic review of EFCT conducted by Johnson et al. (1999). EFCT significantly reduces relationship distress (as measured by dyadic adjustment) compared to both wait-list controls and pretreatment scores. Additionally, in most of the studies in the Johnson et al. (1999) meta-analysis, over half of the couples enrolled in EFCT no longer met criteria for being maritally distressed post-therapy. When examining the four randomized clinical trials (RCTs) of EFCT in this meta-analysis, a very large effect size of $d=1.31$ was attained, suggesting that a treated couple performed better than 90 % of untreated couples. However, this effect size should be interpreted with caution given that it is based on only four RCTs.

There are three other commonly used couple therapies that have received significant empirical support. Integrative behavioral couple therapy (IBCT) is the most recently studied couples therapy and is built upon traditional BCT techniques, with an additional focus on emotional acceptance (Christensen et al., 2004). IBCT integrates traditional BCT's behavior change approach with an increased focus on empathy, intimacy, and emotional acceptance. This is achieved through detachment, in which relationship problems are understood as impartially as possible by the couple, and empathic joining, in which couples are taught to express emotions and feelings, leading to both individuals accepting the other's perspective and ultimately feeling closer to each other.

In a randomized clinical trial of 134 distressed couples, IBCT performed similarly to BCT, with 71 % of IBCT couples and 59 % of BCT couples demonstrating reliable improvement on relationship satisfaction (Christensen et al., 2004). IBCT and BCT also were found to have continued benefits over time and, at a 5-year follow up, 50 % of IBCT and 46 % of BCT couples maintained their gains with continued clinically significant improvement (i.e., reliable improvement or recovery; Christensen, Atkins, Baucom, & Yi, 2010).

The goal of insight-oriented couple therapy (IOCT) is to have couples resolve underlying conflictual emotional through addressing developmental issues, collusive interactions, irrational role assignments, and maladaptive relationship patterns (Snyder & Wills, 1989). IOCT was compared to BCT in a randomized clinical trial of 79 distressed couples. Both treatments performed similarly well with both demonstrating statistically and clinically significant improvement in marital satisfaction (Snyder & Wills, 1989). At a 4 year follow-up, a significantly higher proportion of BCT couples had experienced divorce compared to IOMT couples (38 % for BCT, 3 % for IOMT; Snyder, Wills, & Grady-Fletcher, 1991). These data are supported by only one study, however, and should be interpreted with this caution in mind.

Finally, in a randomized clinical trial of 42 couples, Goldman and Greenberg (1992) compared integrated systemic marital/couple therapy (ISMT/ISCT) with EFCT. The primary aim of ISCT is to reverse fight cycles by changing the meanings attributed to these negative cycles. The authors describe seven steps in the therapy, including restructuring and reframing the problem, encouraging the couple to take proceed slowly, and prescribing a relapse. In the trial, ISCT and EFCT were equally effective in lessening relationship distress. However, at a 4-month follow-up, ISCT couples showed a greater maintenance of gains than EFCT couples. These findings should be interpreted with caution, however, given that they are based on only one trial and the small sample size was relatively small.

The Step 3 therapies discussed thus far are well-established, evidence-supported options for treating couple/marital distress. There are no data to suggest, however, that any one approach is superior in its effectiveness than any other. In addition, it should be noted that a minority of couples (25–30 %) show no improvements from any of these therapies. Additionally, some treated couples fail to maintain their gains over time and up to 45 % will show significant deterioration when assessed 2 years or longer post-termination (Snyder & Halford, 2012). There are a few issues that still need to be addressed in future research and developing a better understanding of who the interventions best for and how to improve their effectiveness more broadly are two needed areas of research. One of the more obvious areas that needs be addressed is studying marital distress and its treatment in diverse cultures and ethnic groups. The therapies reviewed thus far have been examined in samples that are predominantly middle-class, heterosexual, and non-Hispanic White, and research to establish treatment validity among people of different socioeconomic statuses, sexualities, and ethnicities is very much needed.

Cultural Considerations for Evidence-Based Interventions

In order for marital interventions to be effective with Hispanic couples, some modifications are likely to be needed to make them fully applicable to diverse populations. Most marital intervention research to date has been done with white, middle-class, generally well-educated couples (Dion, 2005; Ooms & Wilson, 2004). Although there is some evidence that marital interventions can be effective among diverse populations (Daire et al., 2012; Hawkins & Fackrell, 2010; Owen, Quirk, Bergen, Inch, & France, 2012), cultural diversity factors are rarely directly incorporated into marital programs or interventions (Perez, Brown, Whiting, & Harris, 2013).

Acculturation and the migratory experience are two factors that may contribute to marital distress in Hispanic couples and are rarely directly addressed in marital interventions. In addition, many aspects of marital interaction and marital functioning likely differ according to cultural and ethnic factors, including communication skills, conflict management strategies, problem-solving approaches, and child rearing, and existing intervention approaches could widen their cultural appeal if they could accommodate some of these factors. Hispanics represent many different cultural traditions related to marriage, and while it is impractical to think that any intervention will accommodate each specific branch of Hispanic heritage, unless marital therapists can understand these differences and adapt interventions and materials in relevant ways, they are likely to struggle and to fail to meet the needs of Hispanic couples (Hawkins, Carroll, Doherty, & Willoughby, 2004).

Three of the specific factors have been proposed to be included in marital intervention programs to make them more culturally inclusive of issues important to Hispanic couples are respeto, familismo, and machismo/marianismo (Gutierrez et al., 2014; Perez et al., 2013). Respeto is a Hispanic family value that affects relationship health and it refers to the traditional perception of hierarchal authority in a family (Garza & Watts, 2010; Gutierrez et al., 2014). Gutierrez et al. (2014) advise marital educators and therapists to be well versed in this construct so that cultural norms are not unknowingly violated. In a qualitative study of Latino men and women who had participated in a marriage and relationship education program, Perez and colleagues (2013) found that their focus groups found attention to issues of familismo and machismo/marianismo to be valuable. Familismo has been described as the Latino culture's identification and loyalty to the nuclear and extended family (Lugo Steidel & Contreras, 2003). This construct emphasizes interdependence and connectedness among family members through their obligation to protect, honor, respect, and support the family and it prioritizes the family responsibilities over the individuals' needs (Falconier et al., 2013). The couples in the Perez et al. (2013) study indicated a keen awareness of how struggles in their marriage affected their children and extended family members, especially conflict that took place in front of their children. The couples in this study also reported it helpful for the marital program to address gender-typed differences in the roles men and women were expected to play in a marriage. No research to date has yet examined how acculturation issues are related to respeto, familismo, machismo/marianismo, or how interactions between these variations affect marital quality, but these are important directions for future studies.

Existing marital interventions and scientifically tested programs were developed in a particular linguistic and cultural context and it is a fair question to ask to what extent they are relevant for other ethnocultural groups that do not share the same language or cultural values (Bernal, Jiménez-Chafey, & Domenech Rodríguez, 2009). As Bernal and colleagues (2009) articulately point out, an over emphasis on the systematization of interventions, potentially resulting in a "one size fits all" type of approach, may undermine the very goal of the scientific approach (competent delivery of services). Clearly, a balance between the selection of appropriate and scientifically sound interventions and culturally competent practice is needed. Some cultural factors may be easier to address and incorporate than others. For example, issues regarding how marital conflict can impact children and larger family system relationships and how expectations regarding gender roles can impact couple communication and couple behavior are already incorporated into many marital interventions and it therefore seems that with further culturally responsive adjustments, existing programs could better meet the needs of Hispanic families without compromising integrity or fidelity of the interventions themselves.

Making modifications to well-established empirically supported interventions to accommodate the needs of minority groups without compromising fidelity of interventions is not a simple process, though models have been proposed as to the optimal ways of accomplishing this goal. The Ecological Validity Model (EVM; Bernal, Bonilla, & Bellido, 1995; Bernal et al., 2009) provides a systematic framework for adapting the content and methods of existing interventions to make them more culturally sensitive to specific minority groups. This model was originally specifically written with Latino populations in mind, and it addresses eight dimensions of interventions: language, persons, metaphors, content, concepts, goals, methods, and context. For example, using this model, Rosselló and Bernal (1999; Rosselló, Bernal, & Rivera-Medina, 2008) modified content from EBT therapies to incorporate cultural values of familismo and respeto in treating depressed adolescents. The model was later expanded to a more general cultural adaptation process model that consists of three general phases and ten specific target areas. As outlined by Domenech Rodríguez and Wieling (2004), the first phase is a collaborative effort between the change agent (researcher) and a community leader with the goal being to find a balance between community needs and scientific integrity. In the second phase, evaluation measures are selected and adaptations are made in line with adaptations made to the intervention. The third phase consists of integrating information learned and data collected in phase two into a newly packaged intervention.

In addition to the need for culturally informed and culturally competent marital interventions, there also is a need for culturally competent trainers to teach them. It will be important that those doing the training in culturally informed marital interventions have an understanding and appreciation for different values, customs, and ways of communicating. In particular, there is a significant need for more Spanish speaking interventionists so that Hispanic couples are able to speak in their language of choice. The importance of this issue cannot be overstated. It is not sufficient for existing intervention programs and materials to be merely translated into Spanish, they need to be appropriately adapted and interventions need to be led by people who are capable of conducting interventions in Spanish as needed. This is critical because many thoughts or ways of conveying emotion do not translate easily or well into English (Perez et al., 2013). In many cases, it is probably preferable to have the interventionist also be a person of Hispanic heritage to optimize cultural sensitivity. Although not yet studied in the context of marital therapy or marital education programs, there is some suggestion in the literature that more favorable therapeutic outcomes are obtained when there is an ethnic and linguistic match between the client and the therapist (Sue, Fujino, Hu, Takeuchi, & Zane, 1991; Vasquez, 2007).

In conclusion, given the high rate of marital distress and its associations with mental and physical health concerns, continuing to better understand these interconnections and how to intervene, is vitally important, especially for underserved and understudied minority groups such as Hispanic couples. Helping medical professionals be better tuned into marital stress and how it presents has the potential to promote better utilization of interventions that can reduce marital distress and perhaps even promote greater physical well-being for these couples.

References

Alegría, M., Jackson, J. S., Kessler, R., & Takeuchi, D. (2008). *Collaborative Psychiatric Epidemiology Surveys (CPES), 2001-2003* [United States] [Computer file]. ICPSR20240-v5. Ann Arbor, MI: Institute for Social Research, Survey Research Center [producer], 2007. Ann Arbor, MI: Inter-University Consortium for Political and Social Research [distributor], 2008-06-19. doi: 10.3886/ICPSR20240.

Amato, P. R., Johnson, D. R., Booth, A., & Rogers, S. J. (2003). Continuity and change in marital quality in marital quality between 1980 and 2000. *Journal of Marriage and the Family, 65*, 1–22.

Balderrama-Durbin, C., Snyder, D. K., & Balsis, S. (2015). Tailoring assessment of relationship distress using the marital satisfaction inventory—Brief form. *Couple and Family Psychology. Research and Practice, 4*, 127. doi:10.1037/cfp0000042.

Bernal, G., Bonilla, J., & Bellido, C. (1995). Ecological validity and cultural sensitivity for outcome research: Issues for cultural adaptation and development of psychosocial treatments with Hispanics. *Journal of Abnormal Child Psychology, 23*, 67–82.

Bernal, G., Jiménez-Chafey, M. I., & Domenech Rodríguez, M. M. (2009). Cultural adaptation of treatments: A resource for considering culture in evidence-based practice. *Professional Psychology: Research and Practice, 40*(4), 361–368. doi:10.1037/a0016401.

Blount, A. (1998). *Integrated primary care: The future of medical and mental health collaboration*. New York, NY: Norton.

Bradbury, T. N., Fincham, F. D., & Beach, S. R. H. (2000). Research on the nature and determinants of marital satisfaction: A decade in review. *Journal of Marriage and the Family, 62*(4), 964–980.

Braithwaite, S. R., & Fincham, F. D. (2009). A randomized clinical trial of a computer based preventive intervention: Replication and extension of ePREP. *Journal of Family Psychology, 23*(1), 32–38. doi:10.1037/a0014061.

Bridges, A. J., Andrews, A. R., Villalobos, B. T., Pastrana, F. A., Cavell, T. A., & Gomez, D. (2014). Does integrated behavioral health care reduce mental health disparities for Latinos? Initial findings. *Journal of Latina/o Psychology, 2*(1), 37–53.

Bulanda, J. R., & Brown, S. L. (2007). Race-ethnic differences in marital quality and divorce. *Social Science Research, 36*(3), 945–967. doi:10.1016/j.ssresearch.2006.04.001.

Cabassa, L. J., Zayas, L. H., & Hansen, M. C. (2006). Latino adults' access to mental health care: A review of epidemiological studies. *Administration and Policy in Mental Health and Mental Health Services Research, 33*, 316–330. doi:10.1007/s10488-006-0040-8.

Casas, J., & Ortiz, S. (1985). Exploring the applicability of the Dyadic Adjustment Scale for assessing level of marital adjustment with Mexican Americans. *Journal of Marriage and the Family, 47*, 1023–1027.

Casper, L. M., & Bianchi, S. M. (2002). *Continuity and change in the American family*. Thousand Oaks, CA: Sage Publications.

CDC. (2011). *Health disparities and inequalities report – United States 2011*. Retrieved from http://www.cdc.gov/minorityhealth/reports/CHDIR11FactSheet.pdf.

Christensen, A., Atkins, D. C., Baucom, B., & Yi, J. (2010). Marital status and satisfaction five years following a randomized clinical trial comparing traditional versus integrative behavioral couple therapy. *Journal of Consulting and Clinical Psychology, 78*(2), 225–235.

Christensen, A., Atkins, D. C., Berns, S., Wheeler, J., Baucom, D. H., & Simpson, L. E. (2004). Traditional versus integrative behavioral couple therapy for significantly and chronically distressed married couples. *Journal of Consulting and Clinical Psychology, 72*(2), 176–191.

Conger, R. D., Conger, K. J., & Martin, M. J. (2010). Socioeconomic status, family processes, and individual development. *Journal of Marriage and the Family, 72*, 685–704.

Copen, C. E., Daniels, K., Vespa, J., & Mosher, W. D. (2012). First marriages in the United States: Data from the 2006–2010 National Survey of Family Growth. *National Health Statistics Reports, 49.* Retrieved from http://www.cdc.gov/nchs/data/nhsr/nhsr049.pdf.

Cordova, J. V., Fleming, C. J. E., Morrill, M. I., Hawrilenko, M., Sollenberger, J. W., Harp, A. G., ... Wachs, K. (2014). The marriage checkup: A randomized controlled trial of annual relationship health checkups. *Journal of Consulting and Clinical Psychology, 82(4)*, 592–604.

Cruz, R. A., Gonzalez, N. A., Corona, M., King, K. M., Cauce, A. M., Robins, R. W., ... Conger, R. D. (2014). Cultural dynamics and marital relationship quality in Mexican-origin families. *Journal of Family Psychology, 28*, 844–854.

Daire, A. P., Harris, S. M., Carlson, R. G., Munyon, M. D., Rappleyea, D. L., Beverly, M. G., & Hiett, J. (2012). Fruits of improved communication: The experiences of Hispanic couples in a relationship education program. *Journal of Couple & Relationship Therapy, 11*(2), 112–129. doi:10.1080/15332691.2012.666498.

Dion, R. M. (2005). Healthy marriage programs: Learning what works. *The Future of Children, 15*, 139–156.

Domenech Rodríguez, M., & Wieling, E. (2004). Developing culturally appropriate, evidence based treatments for interventions with ethnic minority populations. In M. Rastogi & E. Wieling (Eds.), *Voices of color: First-person accounts of ethnic minority therapists* (pp. 313–333). Thousand Oaks, CA: Sage.

Doss, B. D., Benson, L. A., Georgia, E. J., & Christensen, A. (2013). Translation of integrative behavioral couple therapy to a web-based intervention. *Family Process, 52*, 139–153. doi:10.1037/t02125-000.

Ennis, S. R., Rios-Vargas, M., & Albert, N. G. (2011). *The Hispanic population: 2010* (Report No. c1010br-04). Retrieved from http://www.census.gov/prod/cen2020/briefs/c2010br-04.pdf.

Falconier, M. K., Nussbeck, F., & Bodenmann, G. (2013). Immigration stress and relationship satisfaction in Latino couples: The role of dyadic coping. *Journal of Social and Clinical Psychology, 32*(8), 813–843.

Fiscella, K., Franks, P., Doescher, M., & Saver, B. (2002). Disparities in health care by race, ethnicity, and language among the insured: Findings from a national sample. *Medical Care, 40*, 52–59.

Flores, G., Olson, L., & Tomany-Korman, S. C. (2005). Racial and ethnic disparities in early childhood health and health care. *Pediatrics, 115*, e183–e193. doi:10.1542/peds.2004-1474.

Fronczek, P. (2005). *Income, earnings, and poverty from the 2004 American community survey.* Washington, DC: United States Census Bureau.

Funk, J. L., & Rogge, R. D. (2007). Testing the ruler with item response theory: Increasing precision of measurement for relationship satisfaction with the Couples Satisfaction Index. *Journal of Family Psychology, 21*(4), 572–583. doi:10.1037/0893-3200.21.4.572.

Garza, Y., & Watts, R. E. (2010). Filial therapy and Hispanic values: Common ground for culturally sensitive helping. *Journal of Counseling & Development, 88*(1), 108–113. doi:10.1002/j.1556-6678.2010.tb00157.x.

Goldman, A., & Greenberg, L. (1992). Comparison of integrated systemic and emotionally focused approaches to couples therapy. *Journal of Consulting and Clinical Psychology, 60*(6), 962–969.

Gottman, J. M., & Silver, N. (1999). *The seven principles for making marriage work.* New York, NY: Crown Publishers.

Gutierrez, D., Barden, S. M., & Tobey, M. H. (2014). Mejorando Matrimonios: Relationship education as a vehicle to overcome barriers for Hispanic couples. *The Family Journal: Counseling and Therapy for Couples and Families, 22*(2), 148–155.

Hahlweg, K., Revenstorf, D., & Schindler, L. (1984). Effects of behavioral marital therapy on couples' communication and problem-solving skills. *Journal of Consulting and Clinical Psychology, 52*(4), 553–566.

Halford, W. K., Sanders, M. R., & Behrens, B. C. (1993). A comparison of the generalization of behavioral marital therapy and enhanced behavioral marital therapy. *Journal of Consulting and Clinical Psychology, 61*(1), 51–60.

Hambleton, R. K., Swaminathan, H., & Rogers, H. J. (1991). *Fundamentals of item response theory*. Thousand Oaks, CA: Sage Publications.

Hawkins, A. J., Blanchard, V. L., Baldwin, S. A., & Fawcett, E. B. (2008). Does marriage and relationship education work? A meta-analytic study. *Journal of Consulting and Clinical Psychology, 76*(5), 723–734.

Hawkins, A. J., Carroll, J. S., Doherty, W. J., & Willoughby, B. (2004). A comprehensive framework for marriage education. *Family Relations, 53*, 547–558.

Hawkins, A. J., & Fackrell, T. A. (2010). Does relationship and marriage education for lower-income couples work? A meta-analysis study. *Journal of Couple and Relationship Therapy, 9*, 181–191.

Helms, H. M., Supple, A. J., Su, J., Rodriguez, Y., Cavanaugh, A. M., & Hengstebeck, N. D. (2014). Economic pressure, cultural adaptation stress, and marital quality among Mexican-origin couples. *Journal of Family Psychology, 28*, 77–87.

Hoge, C. W., Castro, C. A., Messer, S. C., McGurk, D., Cotting, D. I., & Koffman, R. L. (2004). Combat duty in Iraq and Afghanistan, mental health problems and barriers to care. *New England Journal of Medicine, 351*(1), 13–22.

Hollist, C. S., Miller, R. B., Falceto, O. G., & Fernandez, C. L. C. (2007). Marital satisfaction and depression: A replication of the marital discord model in a Latino sample. *Family Process, 46*, 485–498.

Jacobson, N. S., & Follette, W. C. (1985). Clinical significance of improvement resulting from two behavioral marital therapy components. *Behavior Therapy, 16*(3), 249–262.

Johnson, S. M., Hunsley, J., Greenberg, L., & Schindler, D. (1999). Emotionally focused couples therapy: Status and challenges. *Clinical Psychology: Science and Practice, 6*(1), 67–79.

Kalinka, C. J., Fincham, F. D., & Hirsch, A. H. (2012). A randomized clinical trial of online–biblio relationship education for expectant couples. *Journal of Family Psychology, 26*(1), 159–164. doi:10.1037/a0026398.

Kiecolt-Glaser, J. K., & Newton, T. L. (2001). Marriage and health: His and hers. *Psychological Bulletin, 127*(4), 472–503.

Kouyoumdjian, H., Zamboanga, B. L., & Hansenmn, D. J. (2003). Barriers to community mental health services for Latinos: Treatment considerations. *Clinical Psychology: Science and Practice, 10*, 394–422.

Lebow, J. L., Chambers, A. L., Christensen, A., & Johnson, S. M. (2012). Research on the treatment of couple distress. *Journal of Marital and Family Therapy, 38*(1), 145–168. doi:10.1111/j.1752-0606.2011.00249.x.

Lin, E., Goering, P., Offord, D. R., Campbell, D., & Boyle, M. H. (1996). The use of mental health services in Ontario: Epidemiologic findings. *Canadian Journal of Psychiatry, 41*, 572–577.

Locke, H. J., & Wallace, K. M. (1959). Short marital adjustment and prediction tests: Their reliability and validity. *Marriage and Family Living, 21*, 251–255.

Lugo Steidel, A. G., & Contreras, J. M. (2003). A new familism scale for use with Latino populations. *Hispanic Journal of Behavioral Sciences, 25*, 312–330. doi:10.1177/0739986303256912.

Markman, H. J., Renick, M. J., Floyd, F. J., Stanley, S. M., & Clements, M. (1993). Preventing marital distress through communication and conflict management training: A 4- and 5-year follow-up. *Journal of Consulting and Clinical Psychology, 61*(1), 70–77.

Markman, H. J., Rhoades, G. K., Stanley, S. M., & Peterson, K. M. (2013). A randomized clinical trial of the effectiveness of premarital intervention: Moderators of divorce outcomes. *Journal of Family Psychology, 27*(1), 165–172.

McShall, J. R., & Johnson, M. D. (2015). The association between relationship distress and psychopathology is consistent across racial and ethnic groups. *Journal of Abnormal Psychology, 124*, 226–231.

Mitchell, A. J., Vaze, A., & Rao, S. (2009). Clinical diagnosis of depression in primary care: A meta-analysis. *Lancet, 374*, 609–619. doi:10.1016/S0140-6736(09)60879-5.

Negy, C., Hammons, M. E., Reig-Ferrer, A., & Carper, T. M. (2010). The importance of addressing acculturative stress in marital therapy with Hispanic immigrant women. *International Journal of Clinical and Health Psychology, 10*(1), 5–21.

Negy, C., & Snyder, D. K. (1997). Ethnicity and acculturation: Assessing Mexican American couples' relationships using the Marital Satisfaction Inventory—Revised. *Psychological Assessment, 9*(4), 414–421. doi:10.1037/1040-3590.9.4.414.

Negy, C., & Snyder, D. K. (2000). Relationship satisfaction of Mexican American and non-Hispanic White American interethnic couples: Issues of acculturation and clinical intervention. *Journal of Marital and Family Therapy, 26*, 293–304.

Norton, R. (1983). Measuring marital quality: A critical look at the dependent variable. *Journal of Marriage and the Family, 45*(1), 141–151. doi:10.2307/351302.

Ooms, T., & Wilson, P. (2004). The challenges of offering relationship and marriage education to low-income populations. *Family Relations, 53*, 440–447.

Owen, J., Quirk, K., Bergen, C., Inch, L. J., & France, T. (2012). The effectiveness of PREP with lower-income racial/ethnic minority couples. *Journal of Marital and Family Therapy, 38*(1), 296–307.

Papp, L. M., Goeke-Morey, M. C., & Cummings, E. M. (2004). Mothers' and fathers' psychological symptoms and marital functioning: Examination of direct and interactive links with child adjustment. *Journal of Child and Family Studies, 13*, 469–482. doi:10.1023/B:JCFS.0000044728.34058.c.

Passel, J. S., & Cohn, D. V. (2008). *U.S. Population projections: 2005–2050*. Washington. DC: Pew research Center. Retrieved from http://www.pewhispanic.org/files/reports/85.pdf.

Perez, C., Brown, M. D., Whiting, J. B., & Harris, S. M. (2013). Experiences of Latino couples in relationship education: A critical analysis. *The Family Journal, 21*(4), 377–385. doi:10.1177/1066480713488525.

Proulx, C. M., Helms, H. M., & Buehler, C. (2007). Marital quality and personal well-being: A metaanalysis. *Journal of Marriage and Family, 69*, 576–593.

Rogge, R. D., Cobb, R. J., Lawrence, E., Johnson, M. D., & Bradbury, T. N. (2013). Is skills training necessary for the primary prevention of marital distress and dissolution? A 3-year experimental study of three interventions. *Journal of Consulting and Clinical Psychology, 81*(6), 949–961.

Rosselló, J., & Bernal, G. (1999). The efficacy of cognitive-behavioral and interpersonal treatments for depression in Puerto Rican adolescents. *Journal of Consulting and Clinical Psychology, 67*(5), 734–745. doi:10.1037/0022-006X.67.5.734.

Rosselló, J., Bernal, G., & Rivera-Medina, C. (2008). Individual and group CBT and IPT for Puerto Rican adolescents with depressive symptoms. *Cultural Diversity and Ethnic Minority Psychology, 14*(3), 234–245. doi:10.1037/1099-9809.14.3.234.

Sabourin, S., Valois, P., & Lussier, Y. (2005). Development and validation of a brief version of the dyadic adjustment scale with a nonparametric item analysis model. *Psychological Assessment, 17*(1), 15–27. doi:10.1037/1040-3590.17.1.15.

Shadish, W. R., & Baldwin, S. A. (2003). Meta-analysis of MFT interventions. *Journal of Marital and Family Therapy, 29*(4), 547–570.

Shadish, W. R., & Baldwin, S. A. (2005). Effects of behavioral marital therapy: A meta-analysis of randomized controlled trials. *Journal of Consulting and Clinical Psychology, 73*(1), 6–14.

Shattell, M. M., Hamilton, D., Starr, S. S., Jenkins, C. J., & Hinderliter, N. A. (2008). Mental health needs of a Latino population: A community-based participatory research project. *Issues in Mental Health Nursing, 29*, 351–370. doi:10.1080/01612840801904316.

Snyder, D. K., & Halford, W. K. (2012). Evidence-based couple therapy: Current status and future directions. *Journal of Family Therapy, 34*(3), 229–249.

Snyder, D. K., & Wills, R. M. (1989). Behavioral versus insight-oriented marital therapy: Effects on individual and interspousal functioning. *Journal of Consulting and Clinical Psychology, 57*(1), 39–46.

Snyder, D. K., Wills, R. M., & Grady-Fletcher, A. (1991). Long-term effectiveness of behavioral versus insight-oriented marital therapy: A 4-year follow-up study. *Journal of Consulting and Clinical Psychology, 59*(1), 138–141.

Spanier, G. B. (1976). Measuring dyadic adjustment: New scales for assessing the quality of marriage and similar dyads. *Journal of Marriage and the Family, 38*, 15–28.

Stanley, S. M., Amato, P. R., Johnson, C. A., & Markman, H. J. (2006). Premarital education, marital quality, and marital stability: Findings from a large, random household survey. *Journal of Family Psychology, 20*(1), 117–126. doi:10.1037/0893-3200.20.1.117.

Sue, S., Fujino, D. C., Hu, L. T., Takeuchi, D. T., & Zane, N. W. (1991). Community mental health services for ethnic minority groups: A test of the cultural responsiveness hypothesis. *Journal of Consulting and Clinical Psychology, 59*, 533–540. doi:10.1037/0022-006X.59.4.533.

Treviño, Y. A., Wooten, H. R., & Scott, R. E. (2007). A correlational study between depression and marital adjustment in Hispanic couples. *The Family Journal, 15*(1), 46–52. doi:10.1177/1066480706294033.

U.S. Dept. of Health and Human Services. (2001). *Mental health: Culture, race, and ethnicity. A supplement to mental health: A report of the surgeon general*. Rockville, MD: Author.

Umberson, D., & Montez, J. K. (2010). Social relationships and health: A flashpoint for health policy. *Journal of Health and Social Behavior, 51*(1, Suppl), S54–S66. doi:10.1177/0022146510383501.

Umberson, D., Williams, K., Powers, D. A., Liu, H., & Needham, B. (2006). You make me sick: Marital quality and health over the life course. *Journal of Health and Social Behavior, 47*, 1–16. doi:10.1177/002214650604700101.

Vasquez, M. J. (2007). Cultural difference and the therapeutic alliance: An evidence-based analysis. *American Psychologist, 62*, 878–885. doi:10.1037/0003-066X.62.8.878.

Vega, W. A., Kolody, B., Aguilar-Gaxiola, S., & Catalano, R. (1999). Gaps in service utilization by Mexican Americans with mental health problems. *American Journal of Psychiatry, 156*, 928–934.

Vega, W. A., Kolody, B., & Valle, R. (1988). Marital strain, coping, and depression among Mexican-American women. *Journal of Marriage and the Family, 50*(2), 391–403. doi:10.2307/352005.

Whisman, M. A. (2001). Marital adjustment and outcome following treatments for depression. *Journal of Consulting and Clinical Psychology, 69*(1), 125–129. doi:10.1037/0022-006X.69.1.125.

Whisman, M. A. (2007). Marital distress and DSM-IV psychiatric disorders in a population-based national survey. *Journal of Abnormal Psychology, 116*(3), 638–643. doi:10.1037/0021-843X.116.3.638.

Whisman, M. A., Beach, S. R. H., & Snyder, D. K. (2008). Is marital discord taxonic and can taxonic status be assessed reliably? Results from a national, representative sample of married couples. *Journal of Consulting and Clinical Psychology, 76*(5), 745–755.

Whisman, M. A., & Uebelacker, L. A. (2012). A longitudinal investigation of marital adjustment as a risk factor for metabolic syndrome. *Health Psychology, 31*, 80–86. doi:10.1037/a0025671.

Young, A. S., Klap, R., Sherbourne, C. D., & Wells, K. B. (2001). The quality of care for depressive and anxiety disorders in the United States. *Archives of Psychiatry, 58*, 55–61. doi:10.1001/archpsyc.58.1.55.

Zhang, Z., & Hayward, M. D. (2006). Gender, the marital life course, and cardiovascular disease in late midlife. *Journal of Marriage and Family, 68*, 639–657.

Index

© Springer International Publishing Switzerland 2016
L.T. Benuto, W. O’Donohue (eds.), *Enhancing Behavioral Health in Latino Populations*, DOI 10.1007/978-3-319-42533-7

FSC
www.fsc.org
MIX
Papier | Fördert
gute Waldnutzung
FSC® C083411

Kolibri 360 GmbH
Ferdinand-Jühlke-Straße 7
99095 Erfurt, Deutschland
produktsicherheit@kolibri360.de